POISON DETECTION
IN
HUMAN ORGANS

Publication Number 988

AMERICAN LECTURE SERIES®

A Monograph in

The **BANNERSTONE DIVISION** *of*
AMERICAN LECTURES IN LIVING CHEMISTRY

Edited by

I. NEWTON KUGELMASS, M.D., Ph.D., Sc.D.
Consultant to the Departments of Health and Hospitals
New York, New York

Poison Detection
in
Human Organs

Third Edition

By

ALAN CURRY
M.A., Ph.D., F.R.I.C., F.R.C.Path.
Director of the
Home Office Central Research Establishment
Aldermaston, Reading, U.K.
Scholar of Trinity College, Cambridge

With an Introduction by
Keith Simpson
C.B.E., M.D., F.R.C. Path., M.D., (Ghent), F.R.C.P.
Emeritus Professor of Forensic Medicine
University of London

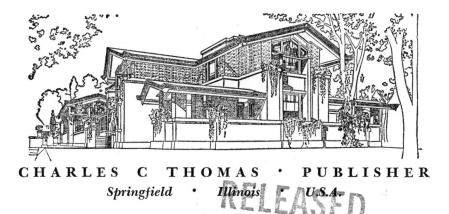

CHARLES C THOMAS · PUBLISHER
Springfield · Illinois · U.S.A.

Published and Distributed Throughout the World by
CHARLES C THOMAS • PUBLISHER
BANNERSTONE HOUSE
301-327 East Lawrence Avenue, Springfield, Illinois, U.S.A.

© *1963, 1969 and 1976 by* CHARLES C THOMAS • PUBLISHER
ISBN 0-398-03433-8
Library of Congress Catalog Card Number: 75 4742

First Edition, 1963
Second Edition, 1969
Third Edition, 1976

With THOMAS BOOKS *careful attention is given to all details of manufacturing and design. It is the Publisher's desire to present books that are satisfactory as to their physical qualities and artistic possibilities and appropriate for their particular use.* THOMAS BOOKS *will be true to those laws of quality that assure a good name and good will.*

Printed in the United States of America
N-1

Library of Congress Cataloging in Publication Data

Curry, Alan S
    Poison detection in human organs.

    (American lecture series; publication no. 988)
    Includes bibliographies and index.
    1. Poisons—Analysis. 2. Forensic toxicology. I. Title [DNLM. 1. Forensic
medicine. 2. Poisons. W750 C977p]
RA1221.C8 1975   615.9'07   75-4742
ISBN 0-398-03433-8

FOREWORD

O UR LIVING CHEMISTRY SERIES was conceived by editor and publisher to advance the newer knowledge of chemical medicine in the cause of clinical practice. The interdependence of chemistry and medicine is so great that physicians are turning to chemistry, and chemists to medicine in order to understand the underlying basis of life processes in health and disease. Once chemical truths, proofs and convictions become sound foundations for clinical phenomena, key hybrid investigators clarify the bewildering panorama of biochemical progress for application in everyday practice, stimulation of experimental research, and extension of postgraduate instruction. Each of our monographs thus unravels the chemical mechanisms and clinical management of many diseases that have remained relatively static in the minds of medical men for three thousand years. Our new series is charged with the *nisus élan* of chemical wisdom, supreme in choice of international authors, optimal in standards of chemical scholarship, provocative in imagination for experimental research, comprehensive in discussions of scientific medicine, and authoritative in chemical perspective of human disorders.

Dr. Curry presents a new, systematic approach to the chemical detection of unsuspected poisoning with maximum efficiency and minimum duplication of analytical procedure. Analyses of samples from the living or dead are considered within the framework of the organs on which they are performed to ensure that each poison is sought in the particular tissue in which it is most likely to concentrate. Rapid chemical detection of poisoning with accurate interpretation of results is paramount for crucial saving of life or establishing the cause of death. It can be done by simple color tests or by more modern techniques involving chromatography, ultraviolet spectrophotometry and infrared spectroscopy with complete satisfaction to both chemist and clinician faced with jars of organs and the knowledge of thousands of poisons.

v

The action of poison upon the animal organism was first observed in the ancient practice of divination which was well expressed by Ovid (10 B.C.) who considered the arrows of Hercules charged with the venoms of the Lerneian serpent. Poisons have always played a dominant role in literature, history, romance and crime. Each age had its own poisons, the silent and subtle weapons readily administered without violence or suspicion. Maccabees, x, 13, refers to poison as a suicidal agent. The Greeks were partial to hemlock juice, a galaxy of poisons. The Egyptians discovered the poisonous effects of animals, plants and minerals. Hippocrates described poisoning from fungi, herbs, plants and foods. The Medes appointed official food tasters to combat intentional food poisoning. The Romans (82 B.C.) enacted the first law against criminal poisoning. Nero's physician, Adromachus, developed the universal antidote of seventy-three components to combat poisoning. Avicenna (1010), a Persian, remained the authority on the diagnosis and treatment of poisoning until Orfila (1814), a Spaniard, founded modern toxicology as professor of legal medicine at the Sorbonne. It liberated the occult in toxicology from the ancient thralldom, replacing its threadbare garments with a raiment suited to a rapidly expanding science.

The tremendous rise in potentially poisonous substances in the homes, factories and fields is an index of degradation, a disgrace to mankind. It is only partially reflected in the vital statistics of civilized countries involving individual, occupational or mass poisoning in peace or war. The annual number exceeds 15,000 fatal, and 1 million nonfatal, poisons in the United States alone, and is ever on the increase. Acute poisoning cannot wait for the identification of the toxic agent or the use of specific antidote. Successful treatment depends on prompt action to prevent further exposure to the poison; to keep the airways clear; to control respiratory depression, shock, convulsions and infection; and to inactivate the toxic material.

Investigation of poisoning requires ingenious clinical detective work and painstaking chemical analyses by a team of trained technicians in close cooperation with the family and police. The mental process is identical with that by which Cuvier restored the extinct animals of Montmartre from fragments of their bones. Clues may be obtained from the common components of household drugs, medicines, cosmetics, insecticides, cleaning fluids and fuels; from exhaustive analyses of urines and stools; and from systematic chemical examination of specific organs. Clinical diagnosis alone may elude the medical examiner even though the toxic actions of most drugs are characteristic. There is scarcely a poisoning syndrome which does not stimulate some disease, e.g. acute poisoning by central nervous system stimulants may be mistaken for epilepsy or tetanus; poisoning by central nervous system depressants, uremic coma or brain tumor; chronic poisoning by manganese may be mistaken for parkinsonism; poisoning by carbon tetrachloride, hepatitis; and poisoning by bromides, neuropsychiatric disorders.

The analytical biochemistry of toxicology compels the determination of the poisonous substances found in the body and its excreta. Methods vary to enable the reader to choose the procedures that best fit his laboratory facilities, personal preferences and the conditions of the moment involving a living patient or an exhumed body. Fortunately, the volume is much more than an uncritical manual of techniques since each chapter offers discussions of the principles on which the methods are based, and the applications to which they may be adapted in the laboratory. The author clearly explores the innumerable and interlinked reactions that determine, in part, at least, the chemical behavior of the *thing called man* reacting to accidental, suicidal or criminal poisoning.

> *"The body, for a time the unwilling sport*
> *Of circumstance and passion, struggles on;*
> *Fleets through its sad duration rapidly."*

I. NEWTON KUGELMASS, M.D., PH.D., SC.D., *Editor*

PREFACE TO THE THIRD EDITION

TREMENDOUS CHANGES in analytical methodology have taken place in the twelve years since the first edition of this book. In 1963, paper chromatography was the *sine qua non* with gas chromatography becoming a close second. In 1969, the time of the Second Edition, mass spectrometers were becoming an exciting new technique in addition to the favourites of thin layer chromatography, spectrofluorimetry, neutron activation analysis and atomic absorption spectroscopy.

The advent of the drug scene explosion sent toxicologists into the relatively new areas of radioimmunoassays and particularly into automated techniques designed for rapid screening procedures related to urine analysis of suspected abusers.

The changes involving very much more highly sophisticated instrumentation, and the special problems of drug addiction have increased the problems of writing what has so far been a comprehensive book on poison detection. To overcome these, it has been necessary to increase the sections dealing with the chemical principles involved in the extraction processes, and to assume a passing acquaintance with specialized instrumentation. It is recognized that the beginner may have only a little knowledge of the chemical properties of the drugs for which he is analyzing, but this must be acquired as rapidly as possible. In addition, the recognition of metabolic routes and the significance of tissue distributions of drugs are important, especially in attempting to interpret results. As far as instrumentation is concerned, the reader will recognize that it is unrealistic to try to describe the setting up of such instruments as gas chromatographs and atomic absorption spectrophotometers.

The format of the Second Edition has been retained in keeping an alphabetical list for the occasions when specific analyses are required. Enlarged is the section of the clinical biochemist who is asked to try and find the drug responsible for the condition of an unconscious patient. A separate section on screening for drug ad-

ix

diction has been added, and the various sections on interpretation of results have been enlarged.

The arrangements of references has been changed in this Edition so that all in one chapter appear at the end of the chapter. This also applies to Section II. To compensate the reader for the extra trouble, an effort has been made to give titles for each paper and to note authors in the text. References have occasionally been repeated to try and minimize potential searching problems

In writing this book I have been disappointed to find how little has been written in recent years on systematic toxicology which has the object of finding a poison whose presence is unsuspected. The literature is now full of papers dealing with the detection of barbiturates, amphetamines, opiates, methadone, etc. etc. by GLC, TIC, GC-MS etc. etc. and any analyst can find a suitable "specific" method for his purpose very easily. However, very nearly all this published work implies that the analyst knows what he is looking for—this book is meant to be different—it assumes that the analyst is pitting his wits against the criminal poisoner and that the capsules or medicine left by the side of the bed are *not* the ones taken in the accidental or suicidal overdose case.

I therefore make no apology for continuing to include what many consider to be "classical" references.

The basic aims of this book, to be of assistance in the treatment of the living patient and in the establishment of a correct cause of death, remain unchanged.

A. S. CURRY

INTRODUCTION
TO THIRD EDITION

CURRY's *Poison Detection*, originally written as one of an American Lecture Series in Living Chemistry has, in two editions in some ten years, become one of the most sought after laboratory handbooks, a little classic that no clinical or forensic laboratory analyst can afford to see borrowed or otherwise taken out of his reach. It was remarkably able in a short compass to answer all the practical problems that beset the clinical hospital and law enforcement laboratory analysts from day to day in a world that produces new synthetic drugs and puts them into clinical use almost before they have become registered and known as poisons.

English statistics in poisoning in the living and the dead have more than quadrupled in the last ten years; over 100,000 cases are treated in hospitals each year now, in 1973-4, and the spectrum of analysis becomes more complex every year. This is what makes a *Curry* so essential in every analytical laboratory. It has, in its first two editions, never failed to provide sound and very practical advice on techniques that put into use the sophisticated apparatus in chromatography and spectrophotometry, and perhaps in spectrofluorimetry, neutron activation and mass spectrometry also, that every self-respecting analytical laboratory must now have.

Home Office percipience, in creating an entirely new kind of research directorship for Alan Curry because of his outstanding flair for technical advance, has indeed been repaid most handsomely as this book again shows. Like Isaac Walton's classic, it is a complete guide to angling in most difficult waters that will help many a competent analyst look even more competent than he is. Poisons analysis is, indeed, a job for the expert, and Curry's particular expertise is, in this new third edition, once more available for all as if he himself were at one's elbow.

KEITH SIMPSON, C.B.E., M.D., F.R.C.
PATH., M.D. (GHENT) F.R.C.P.
*Emeritus Professor of Forensic Medicine
to the University of London*

xi

ACKNOWLEDGMENTS

I AM DEEPLY INDEBTED to several colleagues for many helpful discussions, in particular to Dr. H. M. Stevens and Dr. A. C. Moffat. Dr. J. V. Drayton has also been most helpful in relation to mass spectroscopy.

I am fortunate that in the six years since the last edition I have continued to be in the employment of the Home Office as Director of the Central Research Establishment, and as such I have been involved in the setting up of a computerized data bank in forensic science and toxicology. Because of this, the toxicological literature has come my way, and it has considerably eased the writing of this edition. To Mr. M. Swain and Mr. C. Brown I express my thanks for their help in this area.

Mrs. I. L. White has a special thank you for her efficient typing. Anyone who writes a book in his spare time must realize the great patience that his wife must have to endure and the months of spare time that have to be given up. I am most fortunate because my wife not only has such patience and provides me with the necessary encouragement, but she is also a biochemist and an excellent proofreader! Thank you, Venise.

I am also grateful to the editors of *Analyst, The Journal of Clinical Pathology, Clinical Chemistry, Clin Chim Acta, Forensic Science, The Journal of the Forensic Science Society, The Journal of Forensic Science, The Journal of Pharmaceutical Science, The Journal of Chromatography, The Journal of Pharmacy* and *Pharmacology and Nature* for permission to quote various methods verbatim from these journals.

The views expressed in this book are my own and do not necessarily reflect those of the Home Office.

A. S. CURRY

CONTENTS

PART II
ALPHABETICAL LIST OF POISONS

POISON DETECTION
IN
HUMAN ORGANS

PART I

Chapter 1

TOXICOLOGY:
GENERAL CONSIDERATIONS

I N CASES OF POISONING when the patient is still alive, two different sets of conditions can apply: first, those in which the poison agent is known or suspected; and second, those in which there is no reliable background information, and poisoning is suspected because of the clinical condition of the patient. In both circumstances the aim must be to provide information which will assist the clinician in his handling of the patient. It is axiomatic that the analyses must be finished in time to be of assistance, and that the results must be capable of intelligent interpretation.

These conditions constrain the hospital biochemist because, in many cases, the analyses will inevitably take too long, and the patient will either be dead or recovered by the time they are completed. Secondly, even if results can be obtained their interpretation is so fraught with alternative possibilities that the clinician still has to rely on his clinical judgement. Unfortunately, there seems to be a requirement for an analytical figure notwithstanding the constraints. This can lead to what may become a difficult situation, the physician not fully understanding the biochemist's position, and the biochemist being a little less tolerant on being called out at 3:00 A.M. to do a barbiturate blood level without a request for the particular drug to be identified. (Without the identification, the interpretation is impossible.) It is also unfortunately true that the treatment for the majority of poisons is mainly supportive, and in these cases, an analytical result will not have a major effect on treatment. However, in several instances, the result will lead not only to a correct diagnosis but also to a means of biochemical monitoring of treatment of the poisoning. In addition, there is increasing use of analyses in the treatment of patients on therapy for disease. There has been general recognition that blood, or sometimes urine analyses, can provide accurate information as to a particular person's required drug regime, and so considerably help clinicians in the treatment of their patients. This has been known for many years, but the ability of the analyst to fulfill these needs has only recently become possible.

The realization of the interaction on body processes when different drugs are given together has also grown rapidly, and this area is one of great importance to the toxicologist. The different formulation of drugs leading to alterations in rate of absorption and, consequently, differing blood levels are also areas in which analysis can produce significant results as to the effect of the varying doses. In all these latter cases the toxicologist has the advantage of knowing the drug which he is measuring, and a high degree of specificity is not required although the measurement of metabolites as well as unchanged drugs can require great skill and expensive instrumentation. In cases of suspected overdose of an unknown drug the situation almost always concerns an unconscious patient. The reader should turn to Chapter 3 where rapid screening procedures that can be completed in a few minutes are described. In requests for specific drugs, the reader should turn to Part II.

When the patient is dead there is also a need for rapid screening procedures, even when the circumstances of the death are apparently straightforward. The criminal poisoner is cunning; to quote Mr. Justice Diplock in the first murder trial involving injection of insulin, "poisoning is a cool, calculated, premeditated crime." Only systematic analysis can reveal such murders. A forensic toxicologist cannot hope to perform analyses for all known poisons in all cases that come to his attention, but he can perform a large number of very simple screening tests in addition to looking for the poison apparently involved in the case from circumstantial evidence.

It is the aim of this book to present the analyses in such a form that a sequence of tests is performed so that not only is there the greatest probability of detecting any poison, but also that the complications arising from different routes of administration (oral, injection, inhaled, through the skin, into orifices) as well as differing times between the onset of the illness and the taking of the samples are taken into account.

One aim of this book is to present a variety of techniques so that a choice can be made depending on the instrumentation available. Compromise has been inevitable, for although it has been found essential to continue to use test tube reactions for some simple screening procedures, several colorimetric procedures for less common poisons have had to be discarded. It is now more economical in time and money in reasonably populated areas for the toxicologist to drive or fly to the nearest centre with apparatus for atomic absorption spectrometry, mass spectrometry or nuclear reactions than to attempt *a priori* a new colorimetric procedure which takes several weeks to develop, and possibly more than a day to get a single result.

The tests are described in a rational operating sequence; simple spot tests and extraction routes are used wherever possible; paper, TLC and gas chromatography with infrared and ultraviolet spectrophotometry are considered to be simple procedures. When an improved, more sophisticated, test may be used, then this is noted and the detailed description is given with a quantitative method in the alphabetical list in Part II of this book. This has the advantage that both clinical biochemist and forensic toxicologist can utilize the same *modus operandi*. In cases where a specific analysis for a known poison is required, both the simple and more sophisticated methods may be found by reference to the index. It should be noted that inspired guesses are a waste of time and available material.

In clinical biochemistry the requests from physicians for toxicological investigations will have already taken account of the clinical condition of the patient, and the analyst will be expected to do what is required of him. Notwithstanding this caveat, the expert toxicologist will sometimes be able to suggest an alternative analysis if the original diagnosis is negative. Forensic pathologists and toxicologists see a different spectrum of patients from the majority of hospital physicians; in the last three years in the United Kingdom several cases of arsenic and thallium poisonings have been revealed after extensive hospital investigations only when forensic pathologists and toxicologists were consulted. Because of this, it is necessary for the toxicologist not to become an analytical automaton.

Analyses are often complicated and highly technical procedures, and it is prudent in all cases to ask the following question before undertaking a particular analysis which has been requested by clinician, policeman or lawyer: What will the result of this analysis tell you? In some cases the answer is so unsatisfactory that alternative procedures can be suggested by the poison expert which will save the toxicologist's time and provide the answer the questioner really needs.

Analyses in cases when the patient is dead have two main aims: first, to assist in establishing the cause of death, and, secondly, the collection of information which will further scientific knowledge.

Three questions will be asked of the toxicologist when he has completed his analyses of specimens in a case where poisoning has been suspected or where a postmortem examination by an experienced pathologist has failed to reveal an adequate cause of death. These are:

1. Did you find any poison—if so, what was it?
2. When and how was the poison taken into the system?
3. How much did you find and, hence, how much did the victim take?

It will be noted here that one question that should *not* be asked of the toxicologist at this stage is, "did the deceased die from poisoning?" This is because, at the time of his analyses, it is possible that he does not know all the circumstances. A mass of digitalis tablets in the stomach may have got there through the final actions of a desperate man fighting the symptoms of an oncoming coronary occlusion or the suicidal intent of a person may be so strong that, after taking 100 aspirin tablets, he shoots himself and then falls or jumps into a river. This type of intellectual, one-way street must also be avoided by the analyst, who, having found a low level of alcohol, may be tempted to infer the patient was sober, not having been told about or having analyzed for Librium,® Tofranil® and Tryptizol® that the patient had not disclosed he was taking.

In this context of interpretation of results it will be noted that in each section of this book will be found details of the blood, urine or tissue levels that have been found as a result of therapeutic, chronic high level or acute overdose administration of the drug or poison. The analyst must be careful to survey these critically before coming to his conclusion. To take a simple example, it is common to find blood levels in cases of acute poisoning that fall within the quoted therapeutic range either because death has occurred rapidly (when some tissue levels may be very high) or because death has occurred a considerable time after ingestion and metabolism has destroyed the bulk of the drug.

It is also being found that the same mg/kg doses of some antidepressants result in blood levels differing by a factor of perhaps thirty to forty-fold. This is because drugs are not necessarily equally distributed in body water—indeed for the vast majority they are not. The blood is simply a transport mechanism conveying drugs from one site to another. Concentrations occur sometimes at the site of action; this happens because of aqueous or lipid differential solubility properties of the drug in question. Similarly, the excretion of a drug into urine will depend on its protein binding, whether it passes the glomerulus and whether active or passive tubular secretion or reabsorption occurs. For some drugs, amphetamine for example, great changes in urinary concentration can occur because of changes in urinary pH.

There is sometimes a tendency to ask the toxicologist, "Is this a fatal level?" Often an unequivocal answer can be given; on other occasions only exposure to the drug or poison can be categorically assured. To deduce nonpoisoning from a low level is equally as bad as diagnosing acute suicidal poisoning from a high level when chronic high intake may be indicated. When there is a danger of this situation occurring, the toxicologist must be capable of suggesting alternative samples or procedures that will lead to a solution of the problem, and so provide the answer the clinician or pathologist requires.

In all cases a diagnosis should only be made after a consideration of all the facts of the case by the team of medical and scientific experts who have been concerned in its investigation. The toxicologist must be most careful not to try to extend his own function beyond its proper boundaries, but should be capable of providing reliable analyses and deducing useful information from them.

A. INFORMATION REQUIRED BY THE TOXICOLOGIST: THE COLLECTION OF SAMPLES, THEIR PACKING AND PRESERVATION

In order to answer the three questions posed above, adequate properly-preserved samples must be submitted to the laboratory. Although additional information may be not really essential, important results will be available more quickly if the details surrounding the circumstances of the incident are supplied. This could be vital in cases when the patient is still alive. A close liaison must be maintained therefore with the clinicians, pathologists and investigating authorities in the area.

1. Information Required by the Toxicologist

Anyone with experience asking busy professional personnel to fill in forms will look askance at the questions asked in the proforma detailed below. One occasionally comes across the wit who answers, "Yes, twice a week," to the sex question and the request, "Barbiturates, please," when the drugs available to the victim were noted as Tryptizol®, Nardil® and Valium®. However, notwithstanding such situations, in general, a little knowledge is not necessarily a dangerous thing, for otherwise the blind are leading the blind.

In analyses on samples from both the living patient and the dead, questions shown in Table I should be asked of the authority submitting the samples. It will be seen that the weight of the patient or deceased is asked as well as the obvious questions concerning name, age and sex. This is because calculations as to the ingested dose from tissue or blood concentrations depend on both weight and sex variables. Apart from the example of the differences between calculations concerning a twelve-month-old child and a 220-pound man, the minor variations in Widmark factors between men and women in reports on body contents of alcohol can be important. A defense attorney could pass comment if the toxicologist has ascribed male status to J. Smith who, it subsequently transpires, is a female.

The remaining questions have two aims: first, to set a time

TABLE I

REQUEST FOR CHEMICAL TOXICOLOGICAL EXAMINATION IN CASES
OF SUDDEN DEATH

Police Force:	*Name of Deceased*	*Date*
Sex:	*Age of Deceased:*	*Approx. Weight of Deceased:*

1. On what date and at approximately what time was the deceased last seen to have been in his usual state of health?
2. Time and date of death, if known.
3. If the time of death is not accurately known, when was the deceased found to be dead?
4. If deceased died suddenly give details and time of last-known meal, and his actions between this and the onset of symptoms.
5. Was the deceased admitted to hospital while still alive? If so, on what day and at what time?
6. Give details of the type and quantity of the substance thought to have been the cause of death. Give his occupation and details of his work.
7. Did the deceased take any medicine, pills, etc., in the three days prior to death? If so, give details.
8. Name of any medicine, pills, antibiotics, etc., given to deceased in hospital or elsewhere. If possible give quantities and times administered.
9. Please put a tick against any of the following symptoms that apply:

Diarrhoea	Constipation	Loss of weight	Eye pupils contracted
Vomiting	Blue tinge to the skin (Cyanosis)	Shivering	Delirium
		Hallucinations	Drunkenness
Thirst	Jaundice	Convulsions	Sweating
Blindness		Eye pupils dilated	Unconsciousness

10. When giving dates and times please be as exact as possible.
11. It would be appreciated if the pathologist could inform the laboratory of the findings of his postmortem.
12. Name and address of coroner/medical examiner.

framework, and, secondly, to elicit clinical information. The time framework is most desirable so that the analysis can be designed to search for poison in the sample in which it is likely to be in the highest concentration. The beginning of the incident is dealt with in question 1; the end, in questions 2 and 3. The clinical picture is asked in question 9 in which the investigating authority is asked to put a mark against salient features. Other questions enable the presence of drugs in therapeutic doses administered by way of treatment to be identified and quickly eliminated from the enquiry. The possibility of therapeutic accidents must also not be overlooked. There should be full cooperation between clinician and toxicologist as a matter of routine, but in some cases the samples may be delivered to the laboratory by a messenger who knows little or nothing of the case. In that position it is helpful to have duplicated copies of the form so that it can be returned to the responsible officer for subsequent retransmission to the laboratory.

2. The Samples

a. The Living Patient

As in other areas of clinical biochemistry the required samples must be of such a nature that valid conclusions can be drawn from the results. For example, no one would consider analyzing a partially hemolyzed blood sample for potassium. Similarly, in toxicology, the analogy is that of lead in blood when no one should analyze serum because lead is in the red cells. There are many examples of a corresponding nature and these will be noted under the particular drug or poisons involved.

In hospital work the case of the unconscious patient usually results in only a blood sample being taken because of the problems associated with collecting gastric lavage and urine. On such occasions as a general rule it is probably best to divide the sample into two parts, one being submitted with no additive whatsoever while to the other solid sodium fluoride is added to make a final concentration of about 1 percent. The fluoride acts as both a preservative and an anticoagulant. Each sample should be of at least five milliliters.

All urine that is passed should be collected. Most drugs are present in urine in much higher concentrations than in blood, and for many common substances positive tests will only be obtainable if urine is analyzed. A common example such as morphine (and a metabolite of heroin) serves to emphasize this point. Simple screening procedures can also be done on urine that are impossible on blood.

On those occasions when the patient is given a gastric lavage, *all* the aspirate and the wash should be submitted to the laboratory. It is not unusual to have only a one-ounce sample sent from a bucketful of stomach wash. This is useless—it is difficult enough to analyze for poisons under the best conditions; to be sent only one hundredth of the available sample is to make the task impossible.

Metal poisonings create their own problems, and in cases involving arsenic, hair should be plucked from the head. Full details are given on page 124. In analyzing blood samples for metals, special care is necessary to ensure that all sampling procedures are metal-free. Taylor and Marks (1973) found very large amounts of zinc leached from the rubber end cap of the piston of disposable plastic sterile syringes, and commented that the British standards for disposable syringes were unacceptable as far as heavy metals were concerned. Contamination by copper, zinc and magnesium from blood-collecting tubes was also found. They also found slight loss of mercury from urine in some plastic containers. Loss of mercury due to bacterial formation of volatile compounds has also been noted; this is referred to later.

Clearly, when the physician has reached the stage of considering poison he will have ideas as to its nature, and the analysis is much more likely to be concentrated on a firm line. Addiction to drugs poses a particular case; this is dealt with in Chapter 4.

In all situations the adequate labelling of the samples is imperative. This book may be mainly read by those who have not experienced the errors; hilarious examples could be quoted, but these are not so funny when an official inquiry is opened.

The patient *must* be identifiable; as indicated above, the hospital, ward, sex, initials, name, race, estimated weight of the patient and the specific analytical inquiry are so vital that if the doctor does not have the interest to fill in the details, then the toxicologists must weigh carefully the priority of the analysis. Conversely, the physician will have to face the fact that the laboratory may not be able to produce interpretable information for any one of a host of technical reasons.

b. The Postmortem Examination

The following samples should be sent in all cases; the emphasis is placed here on the submission of a full set of samples, even in cases where the circumstances are apparently straightforward, although often the time factor, coupled with the problems of the adequate provision of sample containers, places such a burden on the pathologist and his team that short cuts inevitably have to be taken. In previous editions of this book the ideal situation has been considered in depth, but some recommended procedures are clearly required for the routine poison case. In the writer's opinion, the stomach wall and contents, a sample of blood (vide infra), the liver *in toto* and any urine are essential. Let it be clearly understood that the writer is not advocating this selective sampling, but saying that if short cuts have to be made, they should be made in this direction.

In addition, experience has shown that, although it is common in an obvious case of carbon monoxide poisoning for only a blood sample to be submitted for analysis, the circumstances surrounding the death often do not become clear for several days. The investigating authority may then become very interested suddenly in a suggestion that the victim may have been drugged before being exposed to the gas. This is not an uncommon occurrence, and, in the writers opinion, it is far better for all the organs to be taken at the time of the original postmortem examination than for the body to be exhumed, or for the toxicologist to have to work on embalmed fluids. Samples should not be mixed but should be packed in separate jars. A kit of at least two large (2-litre capacity) and three medium sized jars (1-litre capacity) with four 25-ml bottles are required. The liver and intestines are put in the large jars; the stomach and contents, brain and kidneys are put in the medium-sized jars; the smaller bottles are for blood, bile and urine samples.

A special word is necessary about bile, because notwithstanding earlier promises, very few analytical studies have been made using this fluid. However, in studies relating to heroin, morphine and a few other drugs it is a useful material, and if the toxicologist is asked if he wants bile, the answer should be, Yes, please!

1. STOMACH WALL AND STOMACH CONTENTS. Even if the stomach is empty to the naked eye the wall should still be sent. Pathologists will no doubt wish to inspect the mucosa. Abernethy (personal communication) suggests that the stomach be tied off at both

ends, removed gently to a pan, slit lengthwise and carefully opened with examination for areas of color, tablets, etc., which can be removed with a spoon and preserved separately. The wall can then be unfolded to inspect the mucosa. This technique avoids disintegration of capsules and tablets due to disturbance and continued soaking. After inspection and the taking of samples for histology, the wall can be put in the same jar as the gross contents.

Increasing attention has been paid by toxicologists to the microscopic examination of stomach contents for tablet filler materials, for example, starch which is usually of the maize (corn) variety.

Such evidence is very easily obtainable and alerts suspicion that subsequent analyses for drugs should be positive. Many tablets are surprisingly resistant to gastric juices and the microscopic procedure is to be recommended. Analysis for dyes from tablets has not received serious study to date.

2. THE INTESTINES AND CONTENTS. The toxicologist will wish to work on the contents of the intestines, and the pathologist can greatly help by either separating them at the time of his examination or submitting the intestines in a continuous separated length so that the contents can be easily squeezed out at the time of the analysis. Not only is it much easier for the pathologist to cut off adherent fat, but the task can be unpleasant when done under laboratory conditions instead of in the mortuary. The analysis of the intestine contents is often necessary when death occurs many hours after the ingestion of poison, or when it is desired to establish how long before death ingestion occurred.

It should be normal practice for the intestines to be tied at about two-foot lengths to minimize mixing of the contents during submission of the samples to the laboratory. In one of the writers cases the coincidence of drug with the lunch-time meal in the stomach contents was of vital importance—the separate submission of stomach, duodenum and tied-off small intestines amply repaid the pathologist the small amount of extra trouble at the autopsy. In another case the differential distribution of two barbiturates in the alimentary tract was of great assistance in deciding the formulation of the ingested drug. The *routine* submission of intestines is recommended; there are several tablets which have an enteric coating, and when these dissolve they cause sudden and unexpected collapse of the patient. The inspection of the intestine contents often reveals whole undigested tablets.

The technique for removing the contents from the alimentary tract varies slightly with individual preference. When the intestines have been separated into a continuous easily handleable length by dissection, the analyst can either squeeze from one end, forcing the content out at the other end into a previously-weighed beaker, or he can cut open the wall longitudinally and, by means of a spoon, transfer the content to the beaker. In either case the wall is subsequently inspected for damage to the mucosa, then washed well with water and the weighed washings added to the contents. The writer's preference is for the squeezing technique if the wall is intact.

It must be recognized that the pathologist may not have inspected the intestinal wall, and that if abnormality is noted, e.g. salmonella ulcers, that he will wish to do so, and may require sections for microscopic examination. Clearly, close liaison is essential.

The increasing abuse of drugs by the intravenous route has decreased the significance of intestinal interpretations, but in a homicidal poisoning the oral route is still the preferred mode for the poisoner, and the importance of these analyses must not be forgotten. Many toxicologists do not like examining faeces in minute detail, but if a full search for an unknown poison is to be made it is unavoidable and must not be skimped.

Yellow phosphorus poisoning has gone out of fashion, but the coincidence of phosphorus and bran (from a commercial rat poison) in intestinal contents is written into English toxicological literature *(R. v. Wilson)*. The writer had a case in which examination for a chewed up gramophone record was important in a suspected murder by poison. Numerous other instances have convinced him, too, that this examination of the alimentary tract is well worthwhile. The *pica* phenomenon in young children will often result in amazing articles being found.

3. THE BLOOD SAMPLES. Two separate samples should be submitted, each 25 ml in volume. Both should be from different peripheral parts of the body and approximately 250 mg of sodium fluoride should be added to one sample. The subaxilla, neck veins and femoral artery are the usual sites for collection. Blood from the portal vein should be avoided because very high drug concentrations can be found in this blood immediately following ingestion, and this could give a misleading impression of the total amount of drug or poison in circulation. There is insufficient data to enable one to be dogmatic on the correlation between concentrations of drugs in peripheral blood and in heart blood, but, because the heart usually contains a relatively large amount of blood and concentrations often parallel peripheral levels, it is acceptable.* Because glucose diffuses from the liver into the right side of the heart after death, a similar phenomenon may occur with some drugs. Therefore, it is wiser for the pathologist to put left and right heart blood samples in separate bottles if for any reason sufficient peripheral blood cannot be obtained, in the case of young children for example. The reason for taking two blood samples is to provide by analysis a check on the uniform distribution of the drug throughout the blood in the body. This is especially important in cases involving alcohol determinations when no urine is available. Pathologists should be actively discouraged from sending large volumes of blood from body cavities taken at the end of the postmortem examination by means of a sponge. The *quality* of this blood, i.e. its authenticity as a circulating sample uncontaminated by other body fluids, is more important nowadays than the volume.

In narcotic addicts the victim is sometimes found dead in circumstances that suggest death occurred very shortly after he or someone else injected the drug. In such circumstances the analysis of tissue around the injection site and of blood from the injection arm, his other arm, heart and leg vein can often be most helpful in determining whether the supposition of a rapid death is correct.

4. THE LIVER. After removal of samples for histology, all the

---

*Gee and his coworkers have studied barbiturates comprehensively in this context.

liver should be sent for analysis. There are two reasons for re-
questing this large quantity. The first is seen from a consideration
of the toxic dose of many poisons, often less than a few milligrams
per kilo of body weight. At death the concentration left in the
body can be much less than this figure, and it is therefore necessary to analyze several hundred grams of tissue in order to obtain
the micrograms of poison required for detection and identification. The second reason depends on the fact that the liver as the
major detoxication organ has the power of concentrating many
poisons. This means that there may be a hundred-fold higher concentration in the liver than in the blood. This makes the liver one
of the most important specimens. Arsenic, barbiturates and
imipramine are three widely different examples which can illu-
strate this power of concentration.

5. THE KIDNEYS. In all cases both kidneys should be sent to
the laboratory. Analysis of the kidney is usually confined to cases
in which metal poisoning is suspected, investigations in a general
search for poison, and in cases in which histology has shown
crystals of calcium oxalate or a sulphonamide.

6. THE BRAIN. The lipoid tissue of the brain has the property
of retaining many poisons. Chloroform is said to be retained even
when the tissue is grossly putrified. Although it would be logical
to suggest that drugs that have an action on the brain are concentrated there, this premise unfortunately does not always hold.
Nevertheless, brain tisue and its extracts are technically easier to
handle than liver tissue, and, because a kilogram is normally
available, all the brain should be taken. In deaths of young children the relatively large bulk is especially valuable.

Analysis of the centre of the brain is particularly important
in cases of cyanide poisoning. Cyanide production has been noted
in postmortem samples, and unless the brain is analyzed the toxicologist may not be able to say whether a positive result for
cyanide in blood, liver or even gastric contents was from poison
alleged to have been taken or the result of putrefactive processes.

7. URINE. This is a most valuable fluid in toxicological analysis.
As well as being an excretory route which in many cases concen-
trates the drug or poison, urine provides a fluid which is suitable

for simple direct spot tests, enabling the toxic agent to be rapidly identified. This is important not only in clinical work, but also in systematic toxicological analysis in providing a rapid lead in the inquiry. As in the case of blood, urine provides an easy means of studying the metabolism of the body, and the tests normally employed by the clinical chemist must not be forgotten. In cases in which death occurs after a period of illness, prolonged perhaps for several days, traces of the toxic agent may be found in the urine when none is detectable in the viscera. Close inspection of the bladder by the pathologist is to be encouraged because as little as a single drop of urine may prove invaluable to the chemist. Urine is especially useful in screening for narcotics and stimulants.

8. BILE. The gallbladder should not be opened and the contents allowed to spill over the liver. Emulsions during the extraction may be traced to this particular autopsy technique which is to be avoided. Some poisons are concentrated in bile, for example glutethimide, ouabain and morphine.

These eight samples—stomach, intestines, blood, liver, kidneys, brain, urine and bile—will provide all the information that is necessary in the vast majority of cases where acute poisoning has occurred as a result of oral ingestion. Some toxicologists ask for other organs—spleen, heart, CSF, etc., and it is not intended here to discourage this procedure or to suggest that it is not desirable; anything that helps to answer the questions posed earlier in this chapter is to be encouraged. It may be that muscle will be more popular in the future as it constitutes a major proportion of the body; fat, too, may be considered necessary on occasions, for example in deaths involving anaesthetics and insecticides, but the samples discussed above are the ones for which the bulk of the literature relating concentration to dose intake will be found to apply.

9. OTHER SAMPLES. Special mention must be made of cases involving acute death from arsenic and thallium. Hair is especially valuable on these occasions for different reasons. In deaths from arsenic, neutron activation analysis of only a few strands will reveal the concentration pattern along the length of the hairs, easily and quickly determining whether the victim has ingested

a single fatal dose or whether other doses had been taken in the period of several months before death. Hair should be pulled, not cut, from the head, and it is desirable to send as large a quantity as possible. It should be tied in locks with cotton so that the toxicologist knows which ends are roots without the need for microscopy of individual hairs. In cases of thallium poisoning, the microscopic appearance of the hair root can be characteristic. In addition, on staining histological sections of formalin-fixed tissue with an alcoholic solution of iodine-potassium iodide for two days, brown granules, presumably of thallium iodide, may be seen in the medulla and the neurons of the cervical cord.

A relatively new feature of recent years has been the widespread abuse of drugs using the intravenous route. Reference has been made above to differential analysis of blood from different sites in the body. Another feature that may be found is the discovery under the microscope of particles of talc, fibres, etc., in the lungs resulting from the tablet excipient or adulteration of the abused drug. The lungs should be submitted also in a tightly closed glass jar (plastic bottles are not suitable) in cases where death is thought to have followed inhalation of poison. Gas chromatography is sufficiently sensitive for head-space analysis to reveal not only such gases as propane and butane, but other hydrocarbons such as acetylene which may be present in coal gas. The glue-sniffers also reveal their addiction when this simple procedure of sampling the air from the lungs is followed.

In cases possibly involving lead poisoning, bone samples should be taken. The femur is preferable. In inhalation berylliosis, lung lymph can give positive results ten years after exposure.

c. Preservation of Samples

Two special cases must be considered. These are the preservation of blood samples that are to be analyzed for alcohol and the preservation of urine samples for narcotic analyses.

The blood sample (including those taken from living patients) should be put into a container about 25 percent larger in volume than the volume of blood taken. It should be shaken immediately with an amount of solid sodium fluoride sufficient to make the final concentration at least 1 percent w/v. The cap should be of such a nature that the sample is airtight. Such samples should be analyzed within at least one week. Oxidation of ethanol by erythrocytes has been noted (Smalldon, 1973), and, at room temperature, loss of ethanol occurs at a rate of about 2 mg/100 ml per week. This can be inhibited by adding sodium nitrite (0.5% w/v) in addition to the fluoride. Attention is drawn to the necessity that the concentration of fluoride is at least 1 percent. Values of 0.5 percent are said to be worse than no fluoride at all because this concentration inhibits glycolysis, which provides extra sugar for unkilled bacteria to ferment.

Urine samples that have been collected for narcotic or drugs of abuse analysis also need to be preserved because they tend to produce interfering phenols and amines on even slight putrefaction. One-tenth percent w/v sodium azide has been found to be most satisfactory with the caveat that the formation of explosive metal azides must be avoided. Metal lids or inserts must not be used. Disposal of azide solutions can create hazards; explosions have occurred when plumbers have hit copper waste pipes in a laboratory where azide has been put down the sink.

The use of commercial kits containing drug-absorbent resin has become popular in that the collecting agency can pour the urine down the plastic tube containing the resin, discard the fluid and send the easily-packed container to the laboratory. Agitation of the urine with ion-exchange filter paper followed by posting of the paper has also been suggested. The writer has no personal experience of the efficiencies of these procedures and recommends careful appraisal. See Fujimoto and Wang 1970: Kullberg and Gorodetzky 1974: Montalvo *et al.* 1970: Mule, 1969.

It is often more acceptable to the toxicologist to add preservative to an aliquot of urine after the first analyses rather than to contaminate the whole sample before he has seen it. To the other samples nothing should be added; it is even desirable that the first stomach wash should be made with water, then submitted for analysis. Subsequent washes with bicarbonate, permanganate or other antidotes are best kept separate as their object is to destroy the poison and, hence, make it immune to detection.

In hot climates where some form of preservation is essential it is usual to use alcohol as a preservative. This is a procedure which has one disadvantage—it makes analysis for volatile poisons extremely difficult, and analysis for alcohol obviously impossible. There is, therefore, a strong case for a portion of the stomach contents and at least 100 g of blood, brain or liver tissue to be preserved separately with a nonvolatile preservative. Sodium fluoride solution may be suitable, but those with experience with this problem will find their own preferred solution. Undoubtedly refrigeration is the ideal. This will normally be employed for all samples when they arrive at the laboratory. Injection sites which are to be analyzed for insulin can be stored at 0 degrees C for several weeks without gross loss of hormone. Once deep frozen, the tissue must not be allowed to thaw before analysis.

d. Containers

It seems at first sight almost ridiculous that it is necessary to comment about containers for transference of the samples from the mortuary to the laboratory, but serious analytical difficulties can and do arise if incorrect packaging is used.

Any containers for the samples are suitable provided they are large enough, resist breakage and have air-tight caps to stop not only the loss of volatile gases, but also to prevent blood and faeces from spilling over the carrier. They must be clean and dry before use. In general, glass jars should be used. Plastic jars are convenient but, unfortunately, volatile poisons diffuse through them, and, in addition, contaminants from plastic pipes have been involved in cases of suspected poisoning. To date, no substitute for well-washed glass jars has been found. Rubber inserts should not be used under caps because this material can extract from the contents certain poisons such as chloroform and phenols.

As part of the normal working notes made by the toxicologist, a description of the containers and their contents is essential. Table II illustrates a *pro forma* which covers the main features. A mark is placed by the relevant description for each sample. Four copies of this form fit well on to one foolscap page.

A convenient system whereby suitable containers for the

TABLE II
DESCRIPTION OF CONTAINERS

Case No.		Date:	
Name:		Exhibit No.	
Sample:			
Quantity:			
Volume:			
Appearance:	Normal		
	Abnormal		
Preservative:	Fluoride, Oxalate, Phenyl Mercuric Nitrate, others.		
Container:	1 oz. (25 ml)	Screw cap	
	4 oz. (100 ml)	Metal	
	8 oz. (200 ml)	Bakelite	
	Medicine bottle	Cork	
	Buttock jar		
	½ size		
	Large		
	Squat		
Label:	Laboratory	Sealing:	Any
	Hospital		Nil
	Police		
	Written		
	Nil		

organs are readily available in the mortuary is also essential. One is for the toxicologist to replace jars when a case is received into the laboratory. In this way there is no possibility of accidental contamination with such substances as lysol, formaldehyde or alcohol because the jars will have come from the toxicologist's own laboratory.

e. Sealing of Containers

Adhesive tape makes a suitable seal under normal conditions with a signature across the join. An apparently straightforward suicide may eventually turn out to be a murder, and it is essential that this elementary medicolegal principle be followed routinely where the pathologist is not able to hand the specimens into the toxicologist's possession.

It is not possible to stress too strongly the adequate packaging, sealing and labelling of samples. A prosecution may be placed in serious jeopardy because evidential continuity cannot be established. If more than one body is being autopsied, a procedure in the mortuary must be established to ensure that the stomach of one does not go into the jar labelled for another. Familiarity breeds contempt, and all are potentially fallible. When such mistakes occur they are an object lesson, *but* they should not occur provided the dangers of mistakes are recognized beforehand, and positive action taken to counteract the remote possibility. Responsibility cannot be delegated in this area.

B. ANALYSIS OF EXHUMED AND DECOMPOSED BODIES

It is often thought that exhumations should be performed at midnight by the light of a policeman's torch so that secrecy can be maintained. This, however, is a fallacy—nothing is more likely to excite the population than a crowd of uniformed police officers watching digging in a graveyard in the dead of night. Daylight exhumation behind screens causes no abnormal suspicion, and, as well as providing much needed additional light, is to be recommended. Police officers should wear plain clothes. A twenty-four-hour delay, if the weather is inclement, is often of no consequence to the enquiry, but a great technical advantage to the professionals. The earth lifted from above the coffin should be placed well clear of the sides of the grave so that there is easy access to the coffin. Soil should be lifted from *below* the coffin so that the adhesion between the base of the coffin and the ground does not cause the bottom to fall out when lifting is attempted. Planks should be manoeuvered under the coffin and ropes placed around the coffin and under the planks. In this way a firm support is achieved before lifting begins. Some authorities refer to the dangers of infection from coffin dust—presumably, a rich source of bacteria. Forewarned is forearmed.

Photographs should be taken at all stages and legal identification of the coffin and body is essential. The mortuary to which the coffin is to be taken should be prepared in advance, and an ample supply of labelled glass jars ensured.

Sometimes the coffin will be full of water and pumping may even be necessary to keep the grave free from water. A generous supply of buckets should be available so that when a hole is drilled in the base of the coffin adequate collection facilities are ensured.

The basic problems associated with analyses of exhumed bodies are no different to those associated with analyses of reasonably fresh bodies. These cases can, however, be considered more interesting because of the production of artefacts during putrefaction, and because the interpretation of analytical results on the badly rotted body may sometimes be difficult. Because of the former it is necessary to collect at the time of the exhumation samples of soil from above, below and from each side of the coffin. Any fluid and debris in the coffin should be collected and portions of the shroud should also be taken. The samples obtained at the postmortem examination should be even more comprehensive than those indicated in section 1A2 because it may become necessary to make calculations on the ingested dose from tissue concentrations by simple arithmetic instead of making use of published data.

Exhumations are usually performed because a suspicion has arisen from circumstantial evidence that the cause of death was poisoning. In such cases it is also usual for the nature of the poison to be suspected, and analysis is immediately directed to that poison. In the writer's experience it is equally important that tests for other common poisons be performed as well. Poisoners display great cunning, and the toxicologist should be prepared for all eventualities. If, because of lack of time, manpower or equipment, or for any other reason, a full analysis has not been performed, arrangements should be made for the preservation of suitable samples for other analyses that may become necessary as the course of any subsequent trial unfolds the whole story. This applies in all cases of murder by poison; a negative result for one poison may eventually be as important as a positive for another (*R v Barlow*, 1957, when it was suggested that ergometrine and not insulin was injected; *R v Wilson*, 1958, when aphrodisiac pills containing yellow phosphorus and strychnine were produced by the defense, there was yellow phosphorus but no strychnine in the bodies). For a study on the detection of poisons in exhumed bodies see Weinig (1958).

The number of artefacts in exhumed bodies naturally depends on the decomposition reactions that have occurred; but in recent years a considerable amount of work has been done on the normal constituents of decomposing tissue. There is no doubt that cyanide is produced in toxicologically significant amounts—levels of up to 10 mg/100 ml of blood have been found in three-month-old blood, and most bacteria can produce ethanol. Only the belated realization that anaerobic bacteria in relatively good-looking muscle can do this has saved the author from erroneous conclusions in this field. However, blood ethanol levels are normally below 100 mg/100 ml when decomposition is involved, and values above this would arouse suspicion of alcohol intake.

The production of other higher alcohols can be expected during decomposition, and the gas chromatographic examination of the concentrated ether extract of a distillate of decomposing tissue always reveals a multitude of volatile components.

The apparent production of small amounts of carbon monoxide (less than 10%) in blood has been noted using spectroscopic methods Markiewicz (1967) and by gasometric analysis after the addition of ascorbic acid and hydrogen peroxide (Sjorstand, 1952). There is little experimental evidence on which to be dogmatic about the significance of elevated carbon monoxide in exhumed bodies. Undoubtedly, gas chromatography is the method of choice for analysis (see Part II).

Blackmore (1970) noted sporadic production of carbon monoxide production in stored blood although none was produced in twenty-one days at 40 degrees C following deliberate contamination of the samples.

An assessment of the distribution of these simpler molecules in the tissue, coupled with sufficient control experiments with incubated biological material, will often enable the toxicologist to reach firm conclusions, but, as with all scientific conclusions, they must be based on adequate experimental evidence.

A considerable amount of work has been done in recent years on the analysis of amines produced in putrefaction. Stevens and Evans (1973) and Kaempe (1969) have described their experiments and methods to recognize the amines that may interfere.

Nicotinamide can be expected to be present even in fresh liver, but as putrefaction proceeds, tyramine, then thymine followed by tryptamine and the phenylethylamines appear. In general, putrefactive bases tend to give reactions expected of simple primary and secondary aliphatic amines, and contrast considerably with the more complex tertiary amine structures found in alkaloidal drugs. For example, responses to potassium iodoplatinate tend to be less definite and give greyish or brownish-purple or blue spots. However, considerable amounts (tens of mg per 100 g) may be found, and clearly these substances can create considerable interference problems. Stevens and Evans (1973) recommend a TLC system using Merck precoated aluminum oxide plate F254 Type E with a mobile phase of the upper layer of methyl acetate 100: (880 ammonia, 2.5; water, 97.5); 50, giving a good separation between putrefactive bases and common alkaloids. The alkaloids generally ran faster than Rf 0.85 although morphine's Rf was only 0.60. The putrefactive amines ran below 0.7. Clearly this could be a useful preliminary separation procedure. Much useful analytical data on putrefactive bases are also given by Oliver and Smith (1973).

The presence of interfering phenolic substances can also be expected, and it behoves toxicologists to have such compounds as p-hydroxybenzaldehyde and p-hydroxy-β-phenylpropionic acid as control samples. The often recurring yellow compound found in decomposing liver tissue has been shown to be 4.4'-dihydroxychalcone (R.H. Fox, *et al.*, 1973).

Where tissues have been fixed in formalin it is still possible to extract several drugs and poisons from the tissue and the preserving fluid, and Tiess (1967) reports success for barbiturates, methaqualone, glutethimide, chloroquine and nicotine even after more than a year's storage. In cases where embalming has occurred and an autopsy has been ordered, the pathologist usually can still get plenty of unpreserved tissue, such as leg muscle, suitable for analyses of poisons affected by preserving fluid.

The problems associated with extracting poisons from formalin-fixed tissues are still not fully understood. In a case in which both fixed and fresh liver were available, barbiturate was shown to be present in the fresh tissue, but could not be isolated from the formalin-fixed tissue (Blackmore, personal communication).

Metallic poisons present their own difficulties; the incorporation and concentration of arsenic into hair from dilute solutions of the metal salts are the classic examples of this type of artefact, and it is for this reason that adequate soil samples must be taken from about the coffin. The soil may, however, also be useful in providing cultures for microbiological experiments.

C. THE WRITING OF REPORTS AND THE INTERPRETATION OF RESULTS

A positive report issued by a toxicologist usually consists of two parts: first, a statement of the poison that has been found and its concentration in the samples that have been analyzed; the second part deals with the interpretation of the figures for the benefit of other persons who are not toxicologists.

In the first part it is most desirable that the amount found in the tissues should be expressed as a concentration, and the form used in most parts of the world nowadays is milligrams (or micrograms) per 100 g (or millilitres) of sample.

It is, however, becoming increasingly common for the unit of volume to be reduced to 1 ml, and values in micrograms or even nanograms per ml to be used. In analyses involving levels of metal in tissue, one frequently finds units such as parts per million used, and one has to dig deep into a paper to discover what material was worked on; it can be fresh tissue, freeze-dried tissue or the ash from tissue incinerated at 500 degrees C. Approximate comparisons can be made by remembering that freeze-dried and ashed tissue make up approximately 16 percent and 1 percent of fresh liver tissue, respectively. When the contents of the alimentary tract are analyzed the total amount of poison as well as its concentration should be recorded. Concentration gradients in the alimentary tract can be most useful in providing estimates of the time since the ingested dose that caused death. This fact is often overlooked. It may well be found that in absolute amounts, the upper or centre portion of the small intestine contains a smaller amount of poison than the stomach, but that because this poison is contained in a small volume its concentration is many times higher. This would indicate that the poison had been taken at a longer period before death than considerations based on weight alone would indicate. Biliary secretion of drugs must, however, not be forgotten; in addition, the possible excretion of drugs from the circulation into the large intestine may be a complicating factor. It should be noted that reports which state the weight of poison isolated per whole organ are to a large extent useless for the purposes of comparative toxicology.

In the part dealing with the conclusions to be drawn from the analyses, efforts must be made to answer the questions posed earlier in this chapter. A simple statement on the toxicity of the poison in question can also justifiably be included so that the nonexpert can easily deduce whether a therapeutic dose or a small or large overdose has been involved in the particular case.

One factor that must not be forgotten in the analytical process is the quantitation of the recovery of the poison. Some extraction procedures are very inefficient, and in other cases the compound is very unstable so that what actually appears in the instrument used for quantitation may be very much less than the true concentration in the tissue. For a poison or drug which is met for the first time in a laboratory, it is prudent to perform experiments of adding the poison to tissue and measuring the recovery. Even when well-publicized methods are being followed, this is still an essential precaution. It has been shown that leaving some drugs in solvent overnight instead of using a freshly-prepared sample can materially affect the amount recovered because unsuspected reactions between drug and solvent can and do occur. It should be noted that increasing use of the *internal standard* technique is being made. In this technique a weighed or otherwise assayed quantity of another material chemically very similar to the drug being assayed is added to the fresh tissue, and, by subsequent comparative analysis after extraction, an accurate measurement of the drug can be made. Because it does not matter if, say, 78 percent of the drug and standard have been lost in extraction, provided both have been lost in the same proportion, comparison of the relative amount of drug to the known concentration of the internal standard enables the original concentration of the drug to be accurately measured. Examples where deuterium-labelled drug is added as the internal standard are already appearing in the literature, and clearly this is an ideal solution.

The problems associated with calculations of the probable ingested dose from the results of the analyses can only be fully resolved by comparing the concentrations in the blood and tissues with those in other cases in which the ingested dose was known. The toxicologist must therefore make extensive use of the published literature and of his own experience.

Tremendous changes have taken place in the availability of toxicity information in recent years. The need to coordinate analytical data in cases of therapeutic, chronic and large overdose cases has been widely recognized, and in many countries much of the information is co-ordinated using computers. Many major agencies have such data banks, and the *Register of Human Toxicology* organized by the American Academy of Forensic Sciences and a similar register maintained by the Home Office Central Research Establishment for British Forensic Science Laboratories are typical examples. In addition, there have been several books published containing such information (Sunshine, Clarke, Curry); the *Bulletin of the International Association of Forensic Toxicologists* now has data on levels found in fatal cases for nearly 200 drugs and poisons. Sunshine and forty-seven other contributors (1971) also give detailed experimental data for the analyses of seventy-two drugs. Clearly, this is an essential handbook in any toxicological laboratory. However, sometimes, when a new drug is involved, it may be necessary to take blood and urine samples from hospital patients receiving it in therapeutic quantities; if in these patients the concentration is twenty-fold lower than in the case under investigation, this implies that an overdose was taken. The control series should include patients who have received many therapeutic doses so that the possibility of accumulation will become apparent.

In other cases this may not be possible, and because self-dosing with, for example, a new insecticidal poison is not to be encouraged, the results on animals must be studied. In such cases it is also necessary to calculate the quantity of poison isolated from the viscera actually analyzed, and then, by inference, the amount in the whole body. If the concentrations in the blood, liver and kidney do not differ within themselves by a wide margin (say factor of 3 or 4), then the multiplication up to the whole body weight is relatively simple and acceptable. The result will certainly enable the toxicologist to deduce whether a single therapeutic dose or twenty times such a dose was taken.

When the poison is not evenly distributed and it is a completely new poison, the problem becomes acute, and occasionally the interpretation may have to be deferred until more data is available. However, in some of these cases, the mere presence of the poison is sufficient when all the other circumstantial evidence from pathologist and clinician has been taken into account to satisfy all concerned that death was from poisoning.

REFERENCES

Blackmore, D.J.: Interpretation of carboxyhaemoglobin found at post mortem in victims of aircraft accident. *Clin Aviation and Aerospace Med, 41:*757, 1970.

Clarke, E.G.C.: *Isolation and Identification of Drugs.* London, The Pharmaceutical Press, 1969.

Curry, A.S.: *Advances in Forensic and Clinical Toxicology.* Cleveland, CRC Press, 1972.

Fox, R.H., Scaplehorn, A.W., and Tonge, G.M.: The identification and removal of certain interfering substances encountered in the determination of barbiturates in human liver. *J. Forensic Sci Soc, 13:*107, 1973.

Fujimoto, J.M., and Wang, R.I.H.: A method of identifying narcotic analgesics in human urine after therapeutic doses: *Toxicol Appl Pharmacol, 16:*186, 1970.

Gee, D.J., Dalley, R.A., Green, M.A., and Perkin, L.A.: In Ballantyne, B.: *Forensic Toxicology.* Bristol, John Wright and Sons Ltd., 1974, p. 37-51.

Kaempe, B.: Interfering compounds and artifacts in the identification of drugs in autopsy material. In A. Stolman: *Progress in Chemical Toxicology.* New York and London, Academic Press, 1969, p. 1-57.

Kullberg, M.P., and Gorodetzky, C.W.: Studies on the Use of XAD-2 resin for detection of abused drugs in urine. *Clin Chem, 20:*177, 1974.

Markiewicz, J.: Investigations on endogenous carboxyhaemoglobin. *J Forensic Med, 14:*16, 1967.

Montalvo, J.G., Klein, E., Eyer, D., and Harper, B.: Identification of drugs of abuse in urine. 1. A study of the Dole technique. *J Chromatogr, 47:*542, 1970.

Mule, S.J.: Identification of narcotics, barbiturates, amphetamines, tranquilizers and psychotomimetics in human urine: *J Chromatogr, 39:*302, 1969.

Oliver, J.S., and Smith, H.: The interference of putrefactive bases in the analysis of biological materials, *J Forensic Sci Soc, 13:*47, 1973.

Sjöstrand, T.: The *in vitro* formation of carbon monoxide in blood. *Acta Physiol. Scand, 24:*314, 1952.

Smalldon, K.W.: Ethanol oxidation by human erythrocytes. *Nature, 245:*266, 1973.

Stevens, H.M., and Evans, P.D.: Identification tests for bases formed during the putrefaction of visceral material. *Acta Pharmacol Toxicol, 32:*525, 1973.

Sunshine, I.: *Methodology for Analytical Toxicology.* Cleveland, CRC Press, 1975.

Sunshine, I.: *Manual of Analytical Toxicology.* Cleveland, CRC Press, 1971.

Taylor, A., and Marks, V.: Contamination from syringes and blood container pots in trace element analysis. *Ann Clin Biochem, 10:*43, 1973.

Tiess, D.: Moglichkeitin toxikologisch—chemischer Analytik an gelargerten formaldehydefixierten Organasservation. *Z Anal Chem, 43:*43, 1967.

Weinig, E. Die Nachweisbarkeit von Giften in exhumierter Leichen. *Deut Z Gerichtl Med, 47:*397, 1958.

Chapter 2

THE ANALYSES

TOXICOLOGICAL ANALYSES are performed for many different reasons, and an algorithm indicating the appropriate action to be taken in relation to this book for some of them is shown in Figure 1. The most common occasions on which requests are made concern accidental or suicidal poisoning in the living or dead patient, cases involving drugs of abuse, and sudden deaths of no discoverable aetiology. The relevant sections of this book dealing with all these situations are given in Figure 1. It will also be noted that on several occasions the question is asked, Why do you require an analysis? This is not meant to be facetious—it is meant to cause the enquirer to reconsider his request and to realize that it may involve expenditure of several hundreds of pounds (or dollars) and many man/woman days of scarce expert labour. To be of use the results must be interpretable; if they are not, they can only be twisted to justify any conclusion the enquirer has preconceived.

It is not out of place here to consider specificity of identification in the context of the various analyses. For medicolegal purposes the analyst must be able to stand in the witness box and withstand all the slings and arrows that other scientists can throw at him. This also applies in many areas involving drug addiction where penal consequences can follow the discovery of a drug in a sample of urine. It is essential in such cases that the samples be identified and sealed in such a way that from collection to analysis there can be no mistake in identity. In hospital practice it is unusual to seal samples—indeed it is not necessary. It is necessary, however, to have adequate identification. In hospital work, because of the urgency of the situation, or because of the small quantity of sample available, it is often not possible to obtain a full identification of the poison; however, sufficient data can often be obtained from the analyses for them to be of clinical usefulness.

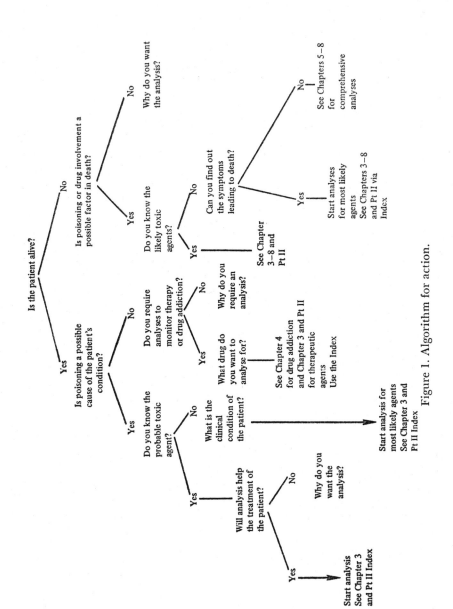

Figure 1. Algorithm for action.

Sometimes the borders between absolute identification and probable identification become a little blurred. It is very tempting to assume full identification of a drug from one or two chromatographic parameters, but only in the case of very simple molecules, for example carbon monoxide and alcohol, is this justified. Recent studies have investigated correlation coefficients as well as the ability of the system to separate one drug from another on paper and by thin layer and gas chromatographic methods in relation to basic drugs. These have emphasized that in the introduction of chromatographic systems into the laboratory it is very easy to do a lot of work using many chromatographic systems without significantly increasing the probability of identification over the first system that was used. It has been the practice for laboratories to settle a favoured system suitable for its own purposes. Clearly, this will continue, but rationalization is on its way, and due note of it has been taken in recommending systems in this book.

A. RATIONALE OF THE ANALYSES

The analyses have to be based on a chemical and not a clinical or pharmacological basis if success is to be achieved. In the living patient the clinician may have a good idea that a particular drug, for example a CNS depressant, has been taken, and often may make a very intelligent prediction that a phenothiazine or a tricyclic antidepressant is involved. However, it is becoming increasingly more common to find that many different drugs are taken simultaneously, perhaps with alcohol, and the clinical picture then becomes much more difficult to interpret. Sometimes, when this happens *dead men tell no tales!*

Apart from quaternary ammonium compounds, the vast majority of organic drugs and poisons can be extracted from aqueous solutions by such solvents as ether and chloroform. This very simple procedure forms the basis of their separation from blood, urine and tissue. Superimposed on this simple fact is an equally simple one which chemists learn in their first year of study,

$$Acid + Base = Salt + Water$$

Normally salts are water soluble whereas drugs may be acidic neutral or basic, but are soluble in organic solvent.

If the reader is unfamiliar with toxicological analysis he is advised at this stage to study the formulae of salicylic acid, phenobarbitone, meprobamate, strychnine and morphine. These five compounds represent five distinct classifications of drugs and poisons into which the vast majority of organic poisons can be slotted. The slots are as follows [pH changes using H_2SO_4–NaOH]:

1. *Strong acids (example—salicylic acid)*. These compounds can only be extracted into ether or chloroform *(the organic solvent)* from aqueous solution if the pH of the aqueous solution is less than 2. By pH 7 the *acid* has formed its sodium salt which is water soluble and insoluble in the organic phase.

2. *Weak acids (example—phenobarbitone)*. A glance at the formula and the knowledge that pKa's are between 7 and 8 will show that barbiturates will form sodium salts provided the pH of the aqueous solution is above 10. Thus, at pH 7 the barbiturate is still in its *acidic* form and will be extractable from the aqueous phase.

3. *Neutrals, (example—meprobamate)*. This class has neither acidic or basic groups and so can be purified by shaking a solution of them in organic solvents with aqueous acid, then alkali. What remains in the organic phase must be *neutral*.

4. *Basics (example—strychnine)*. The vast majority of tranquillizers, antianxiety drugs and nonbarbiturate hypnotics fall into this class. The reader should look at such diverse examples as all the phenothiazines, (e.g. Largactil®) the benzodiazepines (e.g. Librium®, Valium®, Mogadon®, Nobrium®), the triptylines (Tryptizol®, Nortrilen®) as well as the imipramines (Tofranil®, Pertofran®) to see that a tertiary amino group confers basic properties on these molecules. Examples of primary and secondary amines (e.g. amphetamine and ephedrine respectively) serve only as examples, indicating the very large number of other drugs that fall into this slot.

In general, these compounds form salts in acid solution and, hence, can be separated from the *acid, weak acid* and *neutral* drugs, all of which can be removed by an extraction by organic solvent at acid pH. The *basic* drugs can only be extracted by organic solvent if the pH of the aqueous phase is above 7, and in view of their widely differing pK_B's, it is usually made to 13 to 14.

Weak bases such as methaqualone can be isolated with *weak* acids like phenobarbitone in an intermediate zone if the pH of the aqueous phase is about 7; here organic solvents will remove both groups. This fact is not always recognized and the avoidance of slap happy alteration of pH is to be encouraged. By careful use of shuttling pH's and organic solvent one can be highly selective as to which class of drugs one selects, and, of equal importance, which group one pours down the drain.

Another factor sometimes complicates extraction procedures—this is the solubility of some base salts in organic solvents. Examples include such diverse compounds, as strychnine hydrochloride and amitriptyline hydrochloride which are soluble in chloroform. Sulphates seem to be relatively immune to this phenomenon and, hence, in analyses described in this book, sulphuric acid is used. Clearly, cross-contamination between organic and inorganic phases has to be avoided—very few basic drugs can withstand a hot sulphuric acid treatment which can easily occur if extracts are not well-washed prior to evaporation.

5. *Morphine group*. Morphine is almost unique in that it is amphoteric and only at its isoelectric point is it extractable into organic solvents. Preferred ones are given in the text. The only other drug that the writer has found to be extracted in this group is cephaeline, an alkaloid of ipecacuanha.

It is usual to use the amphoteric method of isolation, that is a preliminary extraction with organic solvents from acid, then basic aqueous solutions to remove other drugs and impurities, followed by a pH 9.4 extraction with special solvent to give a *purified* morphine extract.

6. *The quaternary ammonium compounds, (example, tubocurarine)* are water soluble, but by complexing with dyes or potassium iodide, depending on the size of the molecule, they can be extracted into organic solvent as the ion-pair. Purifica-

tion and concentration is then relatively easy.

7. *Special tests.* These cover areas not amenable to wide screening procedures and involve radioimmunoassays for digoxin and other cardiac glycosides and a few drugs which are lost in the extraction procedures used for general screening.

The need for a systematic approach is even more necessary if clinicians or pathologists turn to the toxicologists not for confirmation but for help. As was noted before in this book, the criminal poisoner is cunning in the extreme and some are highly intelligent and well read in the subject. Care, suspicion and considerable expertise are required to catch these criminals.

The physical properties of poisons most made use of in toxicological analysis are as follows:

1. Volatility, a simple distillation or diffusion, followed by color tests will detect such poisons as carbon monoxide, cyanide, fluoride, the alcohols and the halogenated hydrocarbons. *Head-space* gas chromatographic analyses are also most useful.

2. *Separation of inorganic poisons.* As far as anions are concerned these have to be separated by dialysis, concentrated in aqueous solution and tested for by spot tests. Examples are oxalates, silicofluorides and fluorides. Toxic cations are usually metals such as lead, arsenic, mercury, cadmium, etc., and have to be sought individually.

3. *Organic poisons.* As described above, these are isolated by solvent extractions at differing pH's.

B. ANALYSES IN THE LIVING PATIENT

1. Emergency Hospital Toxicology

The algorithm in Figure 1 shows that two sets of situations can occur—first, in which a specific request is made to the laboratory for analyses for a particular drug or poison, and, secondly, where the causative agent is unknown. The prior case is dealt with by looking in the index of this book, and the second by following the procedures in Chapter 3. It is a sad reflection of modern technology that since the first edition of this book in 1963 only one *simple* colour test (for paraquat) has been added to the spot tests that can be easily and rapidly performed in such cases. Clearly, if a battery of gas chromatographs is available on standby, or a mass spectrometer is available, the potential is greatly increased, but it is unrealistic to pretend that this situation exists generally in the Western World. It is much more usual for sophisticated instrumentation to be concentrated in area toxicological laboratories. In most cases the clinical picture will orientate the analysis, but it cannot be too strongly emphasized that tests should not be omitted because they do not seem to be pertinent—it is only by *not* believing all he is told and relying on his skill as an analyst that the toxicologist will uncover the poison murder. In such cases, premeditation and planning by the criminal lead to deliberate distortion of fact, and systematic analysis unclouded by circumstance is essential. Even in straightforward cases where the poison is strongly suspected and revealed by subsequent analysis it is good practice to perform as many additional tests for other poisons as possible. It is not uncommon in cases of the *accidental* taking of drugs or household commodities by young children to find completely unsuspected positive results for other drugs and poisons. In the writer's opinion, the use of a biochemical profile on all cases will become increasingly important in the future with the availability of fully automated clinical laboratories. The detection of poisoning must be sought not only in the demonstration of the poison, but also by the detection of the biochemical lesion that results in the illness or death of the patient.

The treatment of poisoning must also take account of metabolic disorders resulting from poisoning, and, indeed, in the majority of poisonings the measurement of the usual clinical biochemical parameters will be essential.

A large number of cases of acute emergencies involve the patient who has allegedly taken an overdose of one of the nonbarbiturate hypnotics, tranquillizers or antianxiety drugs. In the majority of these cases there is very little if anything the smaller laboratory can do. The extensive metabolism, low body fluid concentrations and chemical inertness of these drugs leads to an absence of suitable quick tests. Fortunately, mortality is low, and even sophisticated analysis leading to a result rarely leads to an alteration in treatment.

2. The Drug Addict

The specialist laboratory has an armoury of tests for screening very large numbers of urine samples for evidence of drug-taking. Clearly, details of such mass production laboratories is outside the scope of this book, but there exists in many countries the need for tests which can provide useful information to a clinician handling a relatively small number of persons suspected of being on the fringe of the drug problem, or in monitoring the truthfulness or otherwise of the addict he is treating. This is certainly so in many parts of the United Kingdom where, for example, the total number of addicts to opiates does not exceed 2000 at the present time. The smaller hospital does not have the throughput to justify relatively expensive automated drug-screening machines, and, hence the emphasis in Chapter 4 is on simple chromatographic procedures designed to handle only a few samples at a time.

It should be noted that urine is the essential fluid and that precautions are necessary to ensure that the sample in the bottle really is from the patient and is not drug-free urine from a container that he secretly brought with him to hospital!

C. ANALYSES OF THE DEAD

In the living patient every case is bound to be an analytical compromise, but, provided the pathologist has submitted adequate samples, in the investigation of a sudden death, the analyses can be systematic and comprehensive. In these cases spot tests, especially on urine, have great value, but they should not use more than a small proportion of the available sample. Blood drainings from the jar containing the liver can be used if the volume of the circulatory blood sample is small. The value of the spot test is that it provides a lead, and often a surprising one, early in the investigation. Simultaneously, with the spot tests, a start should be made on the analyses of the liver as described in Chapter 6. A large number of drugs and poisons concentrate in this organ, and by extracting 100 g quantities of tissue, the toxicologist can often isolate milligram amounts of poison. The ease of identification and assay of this order of magnitude amply repays extra time and cost involved in handling the larger weights of tissue. The greater quantity of poison one isolates, the less difficult the problems of identification become.

In addition to the tungstic acid, aluminium chloride and hydrochloric acid digestions, separate tests are made for arsenic and zinc phosphide.

In the first edition of this book, a test for yellow phosphorus was also done at this stage. This rodenticide was then on free sale in the United Kingdom and had achieved some notoriety as a murder agent. Since then its sale has been banned, and it can no longer be classed as a common poison. The continued inclusion in the book of the same test is now designed to detect zinc phosphide, another common rat poison. It behoves toxicologists to consider the most common rodenticide in their area (thallium compounds, for example) and to substitute tests for them at this place in the scheme.

After the relatively simple analyses on blood, urine and liver, a more prolonged and difficult stage is entered. It must include a full analysis of the contents of the alimentary tract for volatile poisons, for toxic metals, anions and organic solvent soluble poisons; treatment of liver for organic poisons; distillation of 100 g of brain for volatile poisons; and screening tests for numerous metals on liver and kidney. In addition, uncommon poisons not fitting into the general scheme must be sought.

Needless to say, on many occasions this full analysis can be shortened because sufficient reliable circumstantial evidence is available, but, when this is not so, short cuts are not recommended.

The purpose of each stage is basically different, and, although analyses for several poisons are duplicated or even triplicated, their function is not only to guard against mishaps in analysis, but also to detect different modes of administration of poisons, for example in a death from the inhalation of chloroform, a positive test may be found in the blood and brain but not in the stomach or urine.

It is the primary aim throughout this book to suggest means for the detection of poison. In many cases this will not be the most difficult part of the problem, but it is the most important stage and leads on to quantitative measurements. This is also considered in detail, and the emphasis is put on specificity, for it is essential for the toxicologist to realise that many tests developed for use on the pure compound are relatively nonspecific and useless for extracts from decomposed bodies.

When the analyses have been completed, all with negative results, the toxicologist will be able to report "no poisons detected" with the knowledge that he has satisfactorily eliminated the vast majority of toxic compounds that at the present time *can* be detected.

Chapter 3

EMERGENCY HOSPITAL
TOXICOLOGY

THE TOXICOLOGIST IN A BUSY hospital laboratory usually has to squeeze in the poisoning case along with the routine clinical biochemistry case load. Clearly, he cannot be expected to analyze for every possible poison, and, indeed, on many occasions there may not be a sample of gastric lavage or urine on which to work. However, something has to be done, and, if no positive information of the probable poison is forthcoming, then only rapid screening procedures can be used which will possibly provide a lead. The limitation is set by the available chemistry, the simplicity of apparatus and the requirement that results be available in time to assist in diagnosis and treatment.

It may be of some assistance to the reader if some indication is given of what tests a reasonably equipped laboratory should be expected to provide as an *urgent* service for clinicians. This subject was discussed at length at a Ciba Foundation Symposium in London in 1974, and the interested reader will find it reported in a book, *The Poisoned Patient—The Role of the Laboratory,* published by Elsevier (1974). In general it was agreed that guidelines were hard to define as every case was different, and, whereas in general, 3 A.M. requests for barbiturates were not necessary, no one would say they were never necessary. The major emergency requirements were for salicylates with the associated biochemical parameters, paracetamol and serum irons. These requests reflect the very few occasions where toxicological findings immediately affect the treatment of the patient. Decisions to dialyse following analyses for long-acting barbiturates were usually made during the working day and emergency requests for blood levels of the usual hypnotics, antidepressants and tranquillizers were considered to be treatment of the physician and not the patient!

43

See also Lundberg *et al.* (1974): Meade *et al.:* Wiltbank *et al.* (1974).

A. BLOOD

The order in which these screening tests will be done depends a great deal on the type of laboratory doing the work and the availability of instrumentation. One laboratory may use the rapid colorimetric screening method for barbiturate and a diffusion technique for ethanol while another may prefer extraction and ultraviolet spectrophotometry for barbiturate and gas chromatography for ethanol and other volatiles. The approach may vary even from case to case and day to day, depending on the availability of a particular instrument at a particular time. Tables III and IV give lists of the poisons and tests to be considered at this very first stage of the analysis and it is convenient to have a note of Table IV, with spaces for the results of the tests, attached to each set of case records. It is also convenient to perform the spot tests on urine at the same time (see p. 65).

The tests for alcohols, carbon monoxide, methylpentynol, cyanide, fluoride and halogenated hydrocarbons can be performed by the use of a simple diffusion apparatus such as the Cavett flask or the Conway unit. The poison is liberated from the blood, homogenised tissue or, where applicable, urine, and trapped by a reagent, the color of which is changed in the other compartment. The result can be seen by visual inspection. A half-hour is usually time for an obvious positive to be apparent. The other test for salicylate, which is even simpler, is also used to measure the concentration. The diffusion methods can all be adapted to give quantitative results as will be detailed below; at this stage, however, they are considered primarily as screening tests.

The tests have been placed in an order which reflects a possible compromise between the patient, clinician and laboratory scientist; they are by no means inflexible.

1. Blood Urea: Electrolytes: Blood Gases: Calcium and Magnesium

As indicated above, these should be routine in all cases of poisoning. Urea estimations are required to detect possible renal

TABLE III
RAPID SCREENING OF BLOOD

Poison	Volume of Blood Used	Details of Test	Quantitative Procedures	Interpretation of Results
1. Metabolic studies	Depends on apparatus available: separate arterial or capillary blood specimen for blood gases taken anaerobically. Usual clinical procedures.			
2. Insulin and oral hypoglycaemics	1 ml	Blood sugar	As preferred	Blood glucose below 40 mg/100 ml indicates poisoning
3. Salicylate	1 ml	Violet colour with ferric solution	See p. 47	See p. 47
4. Barbiturates and glutethimide	1 ml	Colorimetric	Titrimetic	See p. 192
4. Barbiturates and glutethmide	5 ml	Ultraviolet after protein precipitation	UV	See p. 192
4. Barbiturates and glutethmide	2 ml	Direct extraction then ultraviolet	UV	See p. 192
5. Paracetamol	2.5 ml	Colorimetric	See p. 57	See p. 58
6. Alcohols and Aldehydes	1 ml	Diffusion into acid dichromate	See p. 58	See p. 236
7. Carbon Monoxide	0.1 ml	Spectroscopic	Realing of ratios p. 60	See p. 212
7. Carbon Monoxide	1 ml	Diffusion into palladium chloride	See p. 61	See p. 212
8. Methylpentynol	1 ml	Diffusion into ammoniacal silver nitrate	See p. 61	See p. 283
9. Iron in serum	2 μl-5 ml	Colorimetric	See p. 62	See p. 62
10. Lithium	0.5 ml	Flame photometric	See p. 63	See p. 63
11. Organophosphorous pesticides	0.1 ml	Test papers	See p. 63	See p. 221

TABLE IV
EMERGENCY INVESTIGATIONS

1. Urea, electrolytes, blood gases, calcium and magnesium
2. Insulin and oral hypoglycaemics (blood sugar determination)
3. Salicylate
4. Barbiturates and glutethimide
5. Paracetamol
6. Alcohols and aldehydes
7. Carbon monoxide
8. Methylpentynol
9. Iron
10. Lithium
11. Organo-phosphorus pesticides
12. Gas chromatography

failure; electrolytes and blood gases are essential in aspirin overdoses; calcium and magnesium are frequently included on the request form in the case of an unconscious, twitching youngster. Phenothiazines and tricyclic antidepressants should also be sought on such occasions. Liver function tests may be required in cases of suspected paracetamol overdose.

2. Blood Sugar

This is such a well-known clinical procedure that experimental details will not be repeated here. The test is of little value on postmortem blood samples, but in the living, ill person its determination should be routine. Coma from suicidal, accidental or malicious administration of insulin or the oral hypoglycaemic agents is not uncommon, and this simple test will provide a rapid result of great value. Acetone in blood can also be conveniently tested, for at this stage by putting a drop of serum on an Acetest tablet,® scraping off the supernatant thirty seconds later and inspecting for a violet color. It can also be detected by gas chromatography or by a suitable dipstix for acetone bodies in the urine. Acetone is found not only in uncontrolled diabetics, but in starvation and as a metabolite of isopropanol, an ingredient of many dangerous synthetic intoxicant brews. A blood sugar determination must be considered as essential in all cases of coma.

3. Salicylate

SCREENING TEST AND ASSAY. Trinder (1954) Blood (1 ml) is mixed with 5 ml of reagent and centrifuged. A violet color in the supernatant indicates the presence of a salicylate. The reagent is made as follows: 40 g of mercuric chloride are dissolved in 850 ml of water with warming. After cooling, 120 ml of N hydrochloric acid and 40 g Fe $(NO_3)_3 9H_2O$ are added and the solution is made up to 1 litre with water.

For the quantitative assay, decant off the supernatant and read against standards and controls at 540 nm. [The calibration curve should be prepared with standards from 10 to 100 mg/100 ml, i.e. blood with 100 to 1000 μg/ml salicylic acid.]

IDENTIFICATION. Salicylamide, which is only rarely encountered, and salicylic acid from aspirin or methyl salicylate both give violet colors with ferric salts, but no other interfering substances have been noted. The screening test is simple and gives an accurate assay of salicylate within five minutes.

INTERPRETATION OF RESULTS. Levels greater than 30 mg/100 ml of salicylic acid in blood lead to an increasing probability of a major metabolic upset with a fatal outcome. Normally *headache cure* levels do not exceed 5 mg/100 ml, but in the treatment of rheumatoid arthritis with aspirin levels of 25 mg/100 ml are common. Such patients, however, have to be kept under observation and therapeutic accidents are not unknown if routine blood levels are not performed.

Excretion varies greatly with the pH of the urine.

Ingestion of methyl salicylate gives free salicylic acid as a metabolite with corresponding interpretation of toxic levels. Salicylic acid from ointment is readily absorbed through the intact skin.

4. Barbiturates and Glutethimide

Barbiturates are the most widely prescribed drugs and the most common poison in most western countries today. The toxicologist will, therefore, find them frequently in his analyses.

Two methods are described here and the choice of method

will depend on whether an ultraviolet spectrophotometer is available. If so, it is the method of choice.

a. Simple Colorimetric Procedure

Many hospital laboratories have found the need for a rapid screening procedure that can be set up in a corner of the laboratory or in a side ward. In the mortuary the test described below has proved of value in detecting unsuspected barbiturate deaths, (Gee and Dalley 1967) and, although not highly quantitative, it is useful to clinician, biochemist and pathologist as a do-it-yourself screening procedure. Its inclusion here reflects the widespread availability and misuse of these drugs.

It is essential to use this particular test for unchanged barbiturates in blood and not urine as several of the short-acting barbiturates are not excreted unchanged in the urine and false negatives could be so obtained. Stomach contents should not be used in this test because often they contain such large amounts of barbiturate that the glassware becomes overwhelmingly contaminated. The apparatus (see Fig. 2) is self-cleaning, and although the test is not specific for barbiturate and glutethimide, the only likely interfering substance to be met is bemegride. No significant difference exists between serum and whole blood barbiturate levels.

METHOD. (Curry, A.S., 1963, 1964 see also Clow and Smith. 1967) . Reagents are as follows:

1. *Phosphate buffer:* pH 6.95, M/15. Add 0.624 g of Na_2HPO_4. $2H_2O$ and 0.363 g of KH_2PO_4 to distilled water and make up the volume to 100 ml.
2. *Mercury reagent:* 0.5 g mercuric chloride is dissolved in 50 ml of distilled water to which three drops concentrated nitric acid have been added; 1 ml of this solution is diluted to 50 ml with distilled water, and 0.42 g sodium bicarbonate is added.
3. *Dithizone (diphenylthiocarbazone) solution:* Dithizone decomposes in light and old stock should not be used. A solution of 3.75 mg/100 ml in chloroform should be suitable. When one volume is diluted with two of chloroform, an

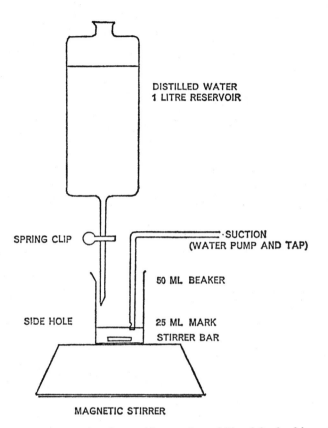

Figure 2. Apparatus for the rapid screening of blood for barbiturates.

optical density at 605 nm (1-cm cell) of approximately 1.0 should be obtained. The concentrated solution which is used for the test is stable for at least one week when stored in a dark bottle at 0 degrees C. (It is essential that both storage bottle and stopper, when first used, be well washed and stood with a concentrated solution of dithizone in chloroform to remove all traces of metallic impurity.)

Problems with this method of analysis for barbiturates in blood are nearly always traced to problems in making up this solution of dithizone in chloroform. Both the dithizone and chloroform are potential sources of problems. The solution should be bright green in color and, as indicated above, quite stable. The writer has seen freshly made solutions turn purple within a few minutes due to impurities present in a batch of chloroform, and, if this happens, the reagent is quite unsuitable. Perseverance is necessary to find suitably pure reagents, and this may involve testing those from several manufacturers.

The Test. Blood (1 ml) and phosphate buffer (3 ml) are magnetically stirred with chloroform (25 ml) for four minutes. After settling, the aqueous layer is removed by suction and discarded. The chloroform layer is washed with two 15-ml portions of water which are also discarded. By manipulation of the beaker, all but a drop of the aqueous layer can be removed. It is important at this stage to try not to remove a large amount of the chloroform layer; if a trace is inadvertently lost, it is made up by dropwise addition until the level again reaches the lower end of the suction tube. The chloroform layer is then slowly stirred for two minutes with mercury reagent (1 ml). After settling, as much as possible of the top layer is removed by suction. The chloroform layer must be free from aqueous droplets. Water (15 ml) is added, then immediately removed by the suction tube. It is essential to remove as much as possible of the aqueous layer. Dithizone solution (2 ml) is then pipetted into the beaker under the surface of the chloroform. If barbiturate is present, an orange color is seen; if none is present, the dithizone remains green. If the color is intermediate between orange and green, the barbiturate concentration is below 2 mg/100 ml. Before diagnosing barbiturate intoxication, repeat the test to remove any possible remaining traces of excess mercury reagent by washing with an additional 15 ml water before adding dithizone (1 ml). An orange color in the final dithizone solution then indicates relatively low levels of barbiturate, and the patient should be conscious in less than twenty-four hours.

It should be noted that blood samples from epileptics on phenobarbitone therapy and from other patients on long-term barbitone dosage are likely to give positive results; conversely, blood from patients with acute barbiturate poisoning, terminating in death in less than four to five hours may give a negative or doubtful positive result.

A more accurate estimate of the blood level can be made by titration, using the dithizone color from the orange to green as the end point; each millilitre of dithizone corresponds to 1 mg/ 100 ml of barbiturate in blood. It assists if, at the final stage, 3 ml of 0.5 N ammonia are added and very gentle stirring is used during the titration.

b. Ultraviolet Spectrophotometric Methods

There are two schools of thought concerning such methods— one prefers a direct extraction of blood with chloroform; the other likes a preliminary protein precipitation clean-up prior to extraction. The writer prefers the latter as it gives cleaner extracts, and levels of barbiturate below 1 mg percent can be detected. With the direct method this is sometimes difficult. In the case of short-acting barbiturates, patients may be deeply unconscious with blood levels below 1 mg percent, particularly if ethanol has also been taken. However, one has to recognize that this is an area where there is a clear division of preference, and both methods are described below. It must also be noted that in hot climates ether may be unuseable. In the middle of the night the hospital technician may not have a hot water bath readily available, and in these cases the final *evaporate* stages can be replaced by an extraction of the barbiturate into 5 ml 0.5N sodium hydroxide.

1. METHOD 1 (see Fig. 3). Blood, 5 ml, is mixed in a 100-ml beaker with 1 ml of 10% sodium hydroxide, 30.5 ml of water and 10 ml of 10% sodium tungstate (premixed in bulk if a number of analyses are done routinely) ; 3.5 ml of 10% sulphuric acid are then added with stirring. The beaker is immersed in a boiling water bath for ten minutes after which the precipitated protein is filtered off through a fluted filter paper; the filtrate is cooled and its volume measured. Because the original volume was 50 ml, the proportional recovery is therefore known, and the loss corrected for when quantitating. The filtrate is extracted with 50 ml of ether by vigorous shaking in a separating funnel. After

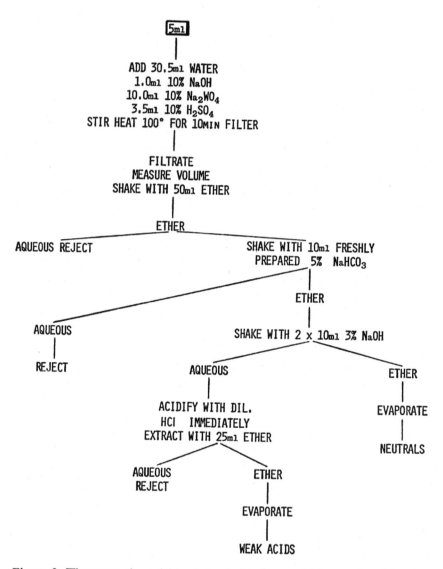

Figure 3. The extraction of blood for barbiturates which are found in the weak acid fraction. The neutral fraction can be retained for examination for neutral drugs such as meprobamate.

separation this ether is shaken with, first, 10 ml of 5% freshly prepared sodium bicarbonate which removes the strong organic acids, then with two portions of 10 ml of 3% sodium hydroxide which remove glutarimides and barbiturates.

The sodium hydroxide fraction is separated and acidified with dilute hydrochloric acid as rapidly as possible. It is even advisable to run the alkaline fraction into a separating funnel already containing the acid. Shake and check that the pH is acid; shake with 25 ml ether which is separated, dried with a spatula end of anhydrous sodium sulphate, decanted and carefully evaporated.

Care must be taken to ensure the purity of the organic solvent because of its relatively large volume compared to the quantity of drug (dioctyl phthalate is a common contaminant if the ether has been in contact with plastic) ; purified ether must not be stored and any antioxidant must be removed immediately before use. This warning especially applies to laboratories not using ether routinely. The ether should be shaken with freshly prepared ferrous sulphate solution immediately before use, and great care taken in subsequent evaporation to ensure the absence of lighted cigarettes, naked flames, electrical sparks and static. Evaporation must be done in a fume cupboard.

The evaporated ethereal extract is dissolved in 3 ml of 0.45N sodium hydroxide, and the ultraviolet absorption spectrum measured immediately from 220 to 320 nm. Any visible colors are noted—red indicates phenolphthalein, or phenothiazine metabolites, yellow, p-nitrophenol from parathion. After ten minutes at room temperature the readings are taken again. If there has been a change in reading at 235 nm α-phenyl α-ethyl glutarimide (glutethimide Doriden®) may be present. This compound has a maximum at this wavelength with $E_{1cm}^{1\%} = 1000$. Glutethimide, although it forms a sodium salt, is an extremely weak acid and is therefore not quantitatively extracted in the weak acid fraction. (If this drug is suspected, see Part II.) Hydrolysis in 0.45N sodium hydroxide is very rapid (50% loss in 5 min).

If the stimulant drug, β-methyl-β-ethyl-glutarimide (Megimide®), has been administered, an overriding peak at 230 nm will be present. This compound is also hydrolysed by alkali,

but much more slowly than glutethimide; 5,5-disubstituted barbiturates have an absorption maximum at 255 nm and salicylamide at 241 and 323 nm. Five-tenths ml of 16% ammonium chloride* is then added to both the sample and the compensating cell,
and the ultraviolet spectrum is reread from 220 to 320 nm at this
lower pH of 10. Interference from the glutarimides is removed,
and any barbiturate can be detected by a peak at 240 nm. Quantitative assay is achieved by adding a few drops of 50% sulphuric
acid to both cells to give pH 2 when the absorption of the barbiturates at this wavelength is reduced almost to zero. (The absorbance difference at 240 nm between pH 10 and pH 2 approximates
1.0 when 1 mg of barbiturate is dissolved in 45 ml of solution. See
Fig. 4.)

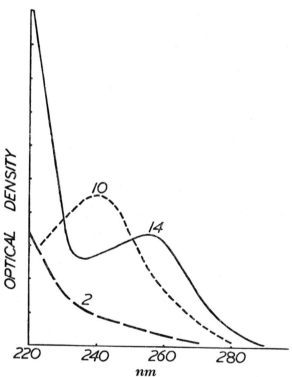

Figure 4. The ultraviolet curves of 5,5 disubstituted barbiturates at three pH
values.

*For each 3 ml of 0.45N sodium hydroxide.

When a clear barbiturate curve has been obtained, the approximate concentration present in the blood is calculated as follows: (N.B. If the concentration of barbiturate in the extract is high, then considerably more than 3 ml of 0.45 N sodium hydroxide may be necessary to bring the 255 nm peak within the range of the instrument. The addition of ammonium chloride to see the 240 nm peak shift should be in the ratio 3:0.5.)

$$\text{Concentration in mg/100 ml} = \frac{100 \times A \times V_1}{3 \times V_2}$$

Where A = absorbance difference reading at 240 nm between pH 10
　　　and pH 2
　　V_1 = volume of pH 10 buffer used to dissolve extract
　　V_2 = volume of tungstic acid filtrate

Glutethimide and megimide have no significant absorption at acid pH, but salicylamide shows peaks at 235 to 237 nm and 299 nm with $E_{1cm}^{1\%}$ values of 590 and 280 respectively.

The thiazide diuretic drugs will also be found distributed between the weak and strong acid fractions, and have absorption maxima at 264 to 300 nm in alkali and 310 to 315 nm in acid. They can be detected on paper chromatograms by a spray of 1.0N sodium hydroxide followed by a saturated solution of 1,2-naphthaquinone-4-sulphonic acid, sodium salt, in 50% aqueous ethanol. Red spots are observed in ten minutes. Pilsbury and Jackson (1966) report their separation using Street's well-known reversed phase system. A list of peaks that can be found in this fraction is shown in Table V, which also gives the names of drugs not showing significant absorption.

It is stressed that it is essential to read the ultraviolet spectra from 220 nm to 320 nm in every case at the three pHs, 13.5, 10 and 2. Normally no trouble will be experienced with clouding when the solution is acidified, but if this does occur, re-extraction into ether followed by evaporation after triturating with a little charcoal should overcome the problem. If a manual instrument is used, readings should be taken at 5-nm intervals. If a high background is found, then difference curves should be calculated and plotted for the readings pH 14—pH 2 and pH 10—pH 2. In old, decomposing blood, inflections at 240 nm not changing between pH 14 and pH 10 will be found. Leach (personal communication)

TABLE V
ABSORPTION MAXIMA OF WEAK ACIDS
(Solvent 0.5N NaOH)

225	Coumarin	260	Stilboestrol
226	Tolbutamide	265	Phenylbutazone
230	Bemegride	286	Phenols
235	Glutethimide	295	p-cresol
240	{Salicylamide, Chloroxylenols		Methyl-p-hydroxybenzoate
		296	Vanillic acid diethylamide
245	1,5,5-Trisubstituted barbiturates	305	Thiobarbiturates
		310	Warfarin
255	5,5-Disubstituted barbiturates	315	Dicoumarol
255	Paracetamol	325	Pentachlorophenol

(The figures shows absorption maxima in nm.)

Not Detected by uv
Hydantoins (e.g. phenytoin)

has also observed this following the administration of mustard as an emetic.

It is essential to identify the barbiturate that is present if the analysis is to be useful to the clinician. This part of the analysis is described on page 187.

Tompsett (1969) has described the spectra of substances that may interfere and indeed may be detected by an examination of this fraction. He notes particularly phenylbutazone, acetyl-p-amino phenol (paracetamol), dicoumarin, sulphatazole, p-cresol theophylline and phenytoin.

2. THE DIRECT METHOD OF EXTRACTION (Method 2). To 2 ml of blood in a glass-stoppered tube add 2 ml of phosphate buffer. [The buffer is made by dissolving 6.2 g $NaH_2PO_4 \cdot 2H_2O$ in 200 ml of water and mixing 47 ml of this with 4.0 ml of a solution of 7.1 g of $Na_2HPO_4 \cdot 12H_2O$ in 100 ml of water.] The buffered blood is vigorously shaken with 20 ml of chloroform for five minutes, then centrifuged. The upper aqueous layer is removed with a Pasteur pipette, and the chloroform layer is then filtered through a filter paper into a dry conical tube when it is carefully evaporated. This can be greatly facilitated by blowing an air stream on the surface. The extract is dissolved rapidly in 3 ml 0.45N sodium hydroxide, and the extract scanned from 220 to

320 nm rapidly, then again after five minutes. The procedure for altering the pH is followed as described on pages 54-55, and the curves obtained should be recognizable as shown in Figure 4. In this case the calculation is as follows:

$$\text{concentration in mg/100 ml} = 1.1 \times V \times A$$

where V equal volume of pH 10 buffer used to dissolve extract (normally 3.5 ml) where A equals the absorbance difference reading between pH 10 and pH 2 at 240 nm. It has been noted above that identification of the particular barbiturate involved is essential before the results can be interpreted. These aspects are dealt with on pages 187 and 192.

INTERPRETATION OF RESULTS. In the examination of the ultraviolet curves in the weak acid fraction, the toxicologist will soon learn to recognize an unusual peak or inflection. The identity of the drug responsible then has to be checked, and the results quantitated and interpreted for the clinician. Rather than try to do this at this stage each drug is considered in detail in the alphabetical list in Part II.

See also Plaa and Hine (1956); Plaa *et al.* (1958); Rehling (1967); Schreiner *et al.* (1958); Stone and Henwood (1967); Turner (1965).

5. Paracetamol: Acetaminophen

Because paracetamol is commonly taken in overdose and a rationale of treatment based on correcting the biochemical lesion it creates is available, the clinician will no doubt wish to have this drug included in a routine screen. A rapid spot test is described below (p. 67) for use on urine.

A blood and urine value can be obtained as follows:

METHOD (Tompsett, 1969).

Reagents

1. o-cresol 1% (w/v) in water.
2. 40 ml ammonia, sp gr 0.88, are diluted to 100 ml with water.
3. Standard solution of N-acetyl p-aminophenol (1 mg/ml) in ethanol.

Blood Serum. Into an 8 x 1-in glass tube are measured 2.5 ml of serum followed by 2 ml 10 N hydrochloric acid. The mixture is placed in a boiling water bath for one hour. After cooling, the mixture is diluted to 10 ml by the addition of water. The procedure is then continued as described for urine. Note—considerable frothing may be encountered on the addition of sodium hydrogen carbonate.

Urine. To 1 ml of urine contained in an 8 $\times$ 1-in tube are added 1 ml 10 N hydrochloric acid followed by 8 ml water. The tube is placed in a boiling water bath for one hour. After cooling, solid sodium hydrogen carbonate is added until neutrality has been achieved. This can be detected by the cessation of gas (CO_2) evolution and by the use of test papers. Forty ml chloroform are added and the mixture shaken vigorously for two minutes. The aqueous phase is separated and rejected. Anhydrous sodium sulphate is added to effect dehydration, after which the mixture is filtered.

Thirty ml of the chloroform extract are measured into a glass-stoppered 50 ml measuring cylinder and 10 ml N hydrochloric acid added. The mixture is shaken vigorously for two minutes.

Five ml of the acid aqueous extract are separated, and to this are added 0.5 ml o-cresol followed by 2 ml ammonia. The mixture is allowed to stand at room temperature for one hour, after which the absorbance of the blue color is read against an appropriate blank at 620 nm.

INTERPRETATION OF RESULTS. Plasma levels in overdose cases may be as low as 3 mg/100 ml, but may be higher than 30 mg/100 ml. Determination of plasma half-life can be a useful way of determining hepatic failure—in a healthy adult this can be as low as two hours. In liver failure it is sometimes over sixty hours.

Urinary excretion is high (over 30 g may be excreted in 24 hr) with a high proportion of conjugation, hence the need to do a preliminary acid hydrolysis on urine (see above).

Intravenous cysteamine is used in the treatment of severe overdosage (Prescott, *et al.,* 1974).

6. Alcohols and Aldehydes

This test depends on the reaction of the volatile poisons with a potassium dichromate/sulphuric acid solution. It can be performed in a Conway unit or Cavett flask; a positive result is seen by the change in color of the dichromate from orange to green. If positive, identification of the alcohol or aldehyde and its quantitative assay are necessary.

METHOD. Place 1 ml blood (or 1 ml urine, depending which is more readily available) with 1 ml saturated aqueous potassium carbonate solution in the base of a Cavett flask (assembly 2BC, Quickfit and Quartz). In the hanging cup put 0.5 ml of 0.1N potassium dichromate in 60% v/v sulphuric acid solution. Seal the flask with Ucon Lubricant®. Place in an oven at about 50 degrees C or on a hot plate at about 60 degrees C to 70 degrees C. A complete color change from orange to green is observed with 50 mg ethanol/100 ml fluid.

A green color, developing after half to one hour indicates ethanol, methanol, paraldehyde or possibly acetone. If positive, repeat with 0.2 ml blood. If still positive, ethanol is most probably present, but if the patient has been ill for several hours, suspect methanol. Metaldehyde may react similarly. (Extreme cleanliness of containers and purity of reagents is essential.)

Because ethanol is the most common volatile poison, it is probable that analysis will be directed to it first. Methanol, however, is often a cause of obscure acidotic coma which may not develop for several hours after ingestion of the poison. Although the metabolism of ethanol is relatively rapid, the rate of disappearance of methanol from the blood is so slow that appreciable amounts may be present over forty-eight hours after ingestion. It is therefore important that this test should be applied routinely.

The differentiation of the volatile reducing poisons is best made by gas chromatography. Quantitative color tests for methanol and paraldehyde are given in Part II. Ethanol is also considered in detail in Part II.

7. Carbon Monoxide

There are two basic methods for measuring the concentration of carbon monoxide in blood. The first depends on examining the visible spectrum of diluted blood to determine the relative amount of carboxyhaemoglobin to oxyhaemoglobin or total haemoglobin, while in the second the volume of gaseous carbon monoxide liberated from a measured amount of the total haemoglobins is determined.

The most rapid screening procedure for fresh blood is to make up a solution of 0.1 ml blood with 40 ml 0.4% v/v 880 ammonia solution and read absorbance ratios for 576:560 nm and 541:560 nm.

Ratios against percent carboxyhaemoglobin concentration are given in Figure 5. Blackmore (1970).

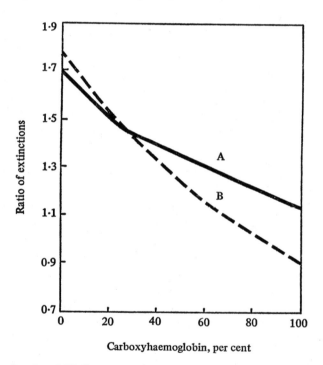

Figure 5. Graph of Heilmeyer extinction ratios determined on fresh blood mixtures of carboxyhaemoglobin and oxyhaemoglobin A, E541 to 560nm; and B, E576, to 560 nm. Courtesy of Blackmore, D.J., and the "Analyst."

It must be emphasized that fresh blood has to be used and that controls should be set up. Alternatively, adding 50 mg sodium dithionite to the diluted ammoniated blood and looking at the spectrum on the chart of a recording spectrophotometer is of great value. Oxyhaemoglobin is entirely converted to reduced haemoglobin by this treatment with a single peak at 555 to 557 nm whereas carboxyhaemoglobin is unchanged and retains two peaks at 538 to 540 and 568 to 572 nm. A laboratory can easily prepare spectra for comparative evaluation.

In these tests the blood must be from a living subject, taken to the laboratory and analyzed within about an hour. If these conditions do not apply, see Section II, for after all, the patient will be dead, will have recovered or will be suffering from irreversible cerebral anoxia.

Another rapid screening test involves the use of diffusion into a palladium chloride solution. This depends on the reaction

$$H_2O + CO + PdCl_2 = Pd + 2HCl + CO_2$$

One ml of blood and 1 ml of 10% sulphuric acid are put separately into one compartment of a Conway unit or into the base of a Cavett flask. Five-tenths ml of 0.001N palladium chloride solution is put into the other section of the diffusion vessel and the top sealed. The carbon monoxide is liberated by mixing the blood and the acid, and the liberated palladium can be seen as a black film within about thirty minutes if carbon monoxide is present.

This test is of value for general screening purposes; a positive result means that unsuspected carbon monoxide has been detected. If the clinician suspects carbon monoxide poisoning, then he will have requested a quantitative analysis, and suitable spectroscopic or gas chromatographic methods will already have been used.

The inclusion of a simple routine test such as the palladium chloride diffusion test is to be recommended in a routine screen. For interpretation of results see page 212.

8. Methylpentynol (methylparafynol)

Screening Test. Repeat the Cavett flask distillation using 1 ml blood with 1 ml saturated aqueous potassium carbonate in the base and 0.5 ml methylpentynol reagent in the hanging cup. Place on a hot plate at about 60 degrees C to 70 degrees C.

To obtain a known positive, dissolve the contents of one capsule of Oblivon (250 mg methylpentynol) in 10 ml ether. Shake with 10 ml water. Use 1 ml of water layer.

A white cloud in the methylpentynol reagent after about one hour indicates the presence of methylpentynol. Perform in parallel with negative and positive controls.

Reagent for Methylpentynol (Perlman and Johnson, 1952). To a 250 ml volumetric flask add 125 ml water, 2.12 g silver nitrate and, after solution, 15 ml 6N-sodium hydroxide. Add just sufficient concentrated ammonia (S.G. 0.880) to dissolve the precipitate. Fill it up to the mark with water. Store at 0 degrees C in the dark. Do not keep it for longer than one month.

For quantitative estimation, see Part II.

9. Serum Iron

Young children occasionally ingest tablets containing ferrous salts. These can be highly dangerous. Desferrioxamine is a chelating agent and is used in the treatment of iron poisoning. However, most clinicians prefer to use it only when analysis has shown it to be necessary, and an urgent serum iron determination is a common request in hospital laboratories.

METHOD (Ramsey, 1957).

Mix 2 ml of serum or plasma with 2 ml fresh 0.1M sodium sulphite and 2 ml 0.1% 2:2'-dipyridyl in 3% v/v acetic acid in a tube with a ground glass neck. Heat in a boiling water bath for five minutes and cool. Add 1 ml of chloroform, stopper and shake violently for thirty seconds. Remove the stopper and centrifuge. If not clear, repeat the shaking and centrifuging. Remove the supernatant and read at 520 nm. Standards are prepared from ferric ammonium sulphate in 0.005N hydrochloric acid.

An alternative method is given by D.S. Fischer (1967). He suggests that a serum iron level of $600\mu g/100$ ml is in the low part of the toxic range.

There are now many commercial kits available for this determination, and the reader is referred to the advertisements appearing in journals specializing in clinical chemistry.

10. Lithium

Lithium salts are widely used in psychiatric practice, and it is usual to monitor serum levels on medication. The following flame photometric method is suitable.

METHOD (Denswil and Detmers, 1972.) An EEL flame photometer working on natural gas is used with a 666-nm interference filter.

Reagents

1. Blank solution 8.18 g NaCl and 370 mg KCl in 1 litre water.
2. Stock solution 739 mg lithium carbonate + 5 ml conc HCl in 1 litre water.
3. Working standard lithium: dilute stock standard 1:10 with blank solution.
4. Acetone 20% v/v. Dilute 200 ml acetone to 1000 ml with water.

The serum from the living subject should be collected in sodium-heparin pots before the first morning dose of lithium. Dilute 0.5 ml serum and standard each with 5.0 ml 20% acetone. Use the flame photometer in the usual way. Lithium concentration $= \dfrac{\text{sample}}{\text{standard}} \times 2$. Results are in m moles/litre.

INTERPRETATION OF RESULTS. Usual therapeutic values are 0.6 to 1.5 m mole/litre. Toxic symptoms can be expected above 2 m moles/litre (Fry and Marks, 1971).

11. Cholinesterase

Because of the widespread availability of organo-phosphorus insecticides which have the property of depressing this enzyme, the routine inclusion of the following simple test is recommended.

Acholest® test papers can be used for the rapid roughly quantitative measurement of serum cholinesterase, or Wang's (1963) method can be used to prepare papers in the laboratory.

METHOD. A fresh 0.04% solution of bromothymol blue is prepared in glass distilled water. Acetylcholine bromide is added to this solution at a concentration of 100 mg/ml.

A piece of Whatman® No. 1 paper is impregnated with this

solution, transferred to a clean glass surface and allowed to dry at room temperature for about one hour. Cut into strips and store in tightly-closed bottles in a dessicator. Use within one month. Approximately two drops of plasma free from red cells is pipetted onto a glass slide, and a piece of test paper placed over the plasma with clean forceps; another clean glass slide is gently pressed on it to exclude air bubbles. The time is noted for the aquamarine color to change through green to match the pale yellow formed when a pH 5 buffer is put on another piece of test paper. Normal activity at 23 ± 3 degrees C takes about five minutes. Poisoning is readily recognizable as the change in color, if any, is delayed for as long as an hour (Churchill-Davidson and Griffiths, 1961 and Wang, 1963). See also Part II.

12. Gas Chromatography

Many area laboratories will have facilities to undertake gas chromatographic procedures for volatile compounds, barbiturates and possibly for antidepressants. These may be regarded nowadays as simple tests as indeed they are in experienced hands. However, the reader is referred to the relevant sections in Part II of this book if he wishes to incorporate them at this stage of the analyses.

B. URINE ANALYSIS

Hensel (1964) has provided much useful warning information on the need for care in the collection of urine samples. Most of this is pertinent to police investigations, but, as the hospital biochemist may be involved at an early stage in criminal cases, Hensel's points are worth repeating. They are for the collecting personnel (a) to use new, unused screw-capped wide-mouthed jars with a preservative; (b) to collect as much urine as is available; (c) to stay with the subject while he is providing the sample; and (d) to seal and label the sample properly. Finally, the analyst should be provided with as much information as possible concerning the circumstances and clinical history of the case.

A tremendous amount of information can be obtained very quickly from the analysis of a few millilitres of urine, and in a case of suspected poisoning the tests described below should be done at the very first stage of the analyses.

It is not often possible to interpret urine concentrations of drugs in terms of probable ingested doses, and the tests should be looked upon as merely providing evidence of ingestion. This, coupled with the clinical condition of the patient, is usually sufficient to assist in providing a firm diagnosis. In investigating a sudden death, the rapidity and ease with which the tests can be completed means that many of them are even suitable for use in the mortuary. The tests are described in detail below.

Note: Chapter 4 describes tests suitable for use in cases of drug abuse.

1. Spot Tests

Special Reagents (except where stated, these are stable at room temperature):

1. *Fluorescein reagent.* A saturated ethanolic solution of fluorescein sodium

2. *Gold chloride reagent.* A mixture of equal volumes of 20% w/v trichloroacetic acid and 0.25% w/v gold chloride

3. *FPN reagent* (Forrest and Forrest, 1960). A mixture of 20% v/v perchloric acid: 50% v/v nitric acid. 5% w/v ferric chloride (9:10:1, by vol)

4. *Reagent for imipramine* (Forrest *et al.*, 1960). A mixture of one volume each of 0.2% w/v potassium dichromate, 30% v/v sulphuric acid, 20% v/v perchloric acid and 50% v/v nitric acid

5. O-cresol reagent: 0.1 ml o-cresol in 3 ml 880 ammonia

6. Reagent for thioridazine (Forrest *et al.*, 1960). 1 vol 5% w/v ferric chloride added to 49 vol. 30% v/v sulphuric acid

7. Diphenylamine-sulphuric acid reagent. 0.5% w/v diphenylamine in concentrated sulphuric acid

8. Furfural reagent. A fresh 10% v/v solution of furfural in absolute ethanol

9. Sodium dithionite solution: add 0.1 g sodium dithionite ($Na_2S_2O_4$) to 10 ml 1N sodium hydroxide. Prepare fresh.

Urine
(Minimum volume required 8 ml)

Test	*Remarks*
1. Dip a Clinistix® briefly in urine and read after one minute.	Correlate with blood sugar results.
2. Dip a Phenistix® briefly in urine and read immediately. Alternatively, add one drop 5% w/v ferric chloride to one drop of urine.	A violet color indicates salicylate, salicylamide or chlorpromazine. If the color remains or is intensified by a drop of 50% v/v sulphuric acid, chlorpromazine is indicated. If the color disappears it is probably from salicylate.
3. Put a drop of urine on an Acetest tablet; observe the color after thirty seconds.	A violet color indicates acetone bodies.
4. Mix a drop of urine with a drop of gold chloride reagent on a white tile. To obtain a known positive for phenothiazines, grind one tablet of 25 mg chlorpromazine hydrochloride with 10 ml water. Use one drop.	A red color indicates chlorpromazine or other phenothiazine tranquillizer. A brown color indicates bromide; if positive, check for bromide by using the fluorescein test—0.2 ml urine is mixed with two drops of fluorescein reagent, four drops of glacial acetic acid and four drops of one hundred volumes hydrogen peroxide and heated to dryness in a boiling water bath: a red color is obtained if bromide is present.
Place 1 ml urine in each of six test tubes.	
5. To 1 ml of urine add 1 ml 20% w/v sodium hydroxide and 1 ml pyridine; heat in a boiling water bath for one minute. To obtain a known positive, grind one-half tablet of dichloralphenazone in 10 ml water. Take 0.1 ml diluted to 1 ml.	A red color in the pyridine layer indicates chloroform, chloral hydrate, dichloralphenazone or trichloroethylene. (Chlorodyne should also be considered as well as other medicines containing chloroform water.) Perform in parallel with negative and positive controls.
6. To 1 ml urine, add 1 ml FPN reagent. To obtain a known positive, grind one tablet of 25 mg chlorpromazine hydrochloride with 10 ml water. Use 1 ml.	A violet color indicates high dosage of chlorpromazine or other phenothiazine drugs. Pink colors may also be obtained—color depends on dose and metabolites.

Test	*Remarks*
7. To 1 ml urine add 1 ml imipramine reagent. To obtain a known positive, grind one tablet of 25 mg imipramine hydrochloride or 25 mg desipramine hydrochloride with 10 ml water. Take 0.1 ml diluted to 1 ml.	Green or blue colors indicate imipramine or desipramine ingestion. If the patient has hyperpyrexia, dilated pupils and is *drunk* or in coma, consider the possibility of imipramine interaction with a monoamine oxidase inhibitor such as phenelzine.
8. To 1 ml urine add 1 ml thioridazine reagent. To obtain a known positive, grind one tablet of 25 mg thioridazine with 10 ml water. Take 0.1 ml diluted to 1 ml.	A pink to blue color indicates thioridazine ingestion. The color depends on the dose and metabolites.
9. To 0.5 ml urine add 1.5 ml concentrated HCl and boil gently for at least two minutes; cool. Take 0.2 ml, add 0.8 ml water and 0.2 ml o-cresol reagent. Check to see if solution is alkaline.	A blue color developing in one to two minutes indicates phenacetin or paracetamol metabolites.
10. To 1 ml of urine add 1 ml of sodium dithionite solution.	A strong blue or green color indicates the presence of paraquat, diquat or both. The sensitivity can be improved by shaking the urine with alumina before adding the dithionite solution.
11. Consider tests for heavy metal poisoning.	See Index for arsenic, mercury, lead and thallium.

2. Extraction Procedures

In the acceptance of the fact that emergency toxicology has limitations, and that the major one of these is manpower, it is most probable that in the case of the unknown poison most laboratories will not undertake a full screen for all solvent extractable drugs in every case. It is much more likely that a specific suspected drug will be sought, and the attention of the reader is referred to Part II of this book. However, if the biochemist wishes to extend his search on urine for all extractable poisons he is referred to Chapter 4.

C. ANALYSES OF OTHER SAMPLES
FROM THE LIVING PATIENT
1. Stomach Wash and Aspirate

The examination of this material by the hospital biochemist should be compared with the analysis of the contents of the alimentary tract by the toxicologist which is described in detail in Chapter 6.

METHOD. Put aside one third of the stomach aspirate in reserve. The aspirate should be taken before washing out the stomach; it should be uncontaminated by administered antidote.

Test	*Remarks*
1. Smell the stomach aspirate; at this stage also carefully smell the urine.	Obvious smells such as those due to *Lysol®*, camphor and methyl salicylate should be noted. Methyl salicylate may indicate ingestion of surgical spirit. Phenelzine has its own peculiar odour, and this should be checked by smelling a crushed tablet. The drug is readily available and interaction of even therapeutic doses with imipramine, pethidine and dexamphetamine, etc., can cause serious reactions.
2. Measure the pH of the stomach aspirate with a piece of Universal Indicator paper. Note also the colour of the aspirate.	If neutral or slightly alkaline, ingestion of sodium barbiturate should be considered. Any color may derive from a tablet or capsule, or from a dye used to color a rat poison. Blue ferrous phosphate following ingestion of *anaemia pills* is usually obvious. Normal pH of aspirate is 3 to 4.
3. Perform the test for chloroform-like compounds described under urine test 5.	Tests 3, 4 and 5 are necessary on both body fluids as the concentration in each is altered by absorption and excretion factors, depending on the time which has elapsed between ingestion and obtaining the sample.
4. Perform FPN test for chlorpromazine as described under urine test 6.	

Test	*Remarks*

5. Perform imipramine test as described under urine test 7.

6. Put a quarter of the total stomach aspirate in a conical flask with an equal volume of 2N hydrochloric acid and a 0.5-cm square of copper foil. Boil for five minutes.

Observe color of the foil; a film of metallic mercury is obvious and arsenic, antimony and bismuth give black stains. Confirmatory tests are essential.

7. Treat a few drops of the aspirate with 1 ml concentrated ammonia.

Deep blue color indicates copper salts. Red indicates phenolphthalein.

8. Extract one third of the total stomach aspirate after acidification with 2N hydrochloric acid with four times its volume of chloroform. Separate and evaporate off the organic solvent. Dissolve the residue in 0.5 ml ethanol. Take about 0.01 ml and evaporate it on to a small spot on a filter paper. Superimpose 0.01 ml furfural reagent and allow to dry. Expose to the fumes of concentrated hydrochloric acid in a beaker.

To obtain a known positive, extract one tablet of 400 mg meprobamate with 5 ml chloroform. Separate, evaporate and dissolve the residue in 50 ml ethanol. As with the unknown, evaporate 0.01 ml as a small spot on a filter paper and treat with furfural reagent and hydrochloric acid fumes as described.

A purple-black color in about one minute indicates a carbamate, most probably meprobamate. A negative and a positive control on the same piece of filter paper are essential for purposes of comparison. Meprobamate is excreted in the urine and therefore 10 ml of urine can be used instead if the aspirate is very fatty or otherwise unsuitable.
(Furfural reagent—see p. 65)

9. Heat 0.01 ml of the alcohol extract obtained in test 8 to dryness on a white porcelain dish with two drops 2N sodium hydroxide using a microburner. Cool; add two drops fluorescein reagent, four drops glacial acetic acid and four drops 100 volume

A red color indicates carbromal or bromvaletone which are the most common bromoureides. The red color obtained is eosin.
(Fluorescein reagent—see p. 65)

Test	*Remarks*
hydrogen peroxide. Evaporate to dryness on a boiling water bath.	
10. To two drops of aspirate add two to three drops 2N hydrochloric acid and one drop 1% w/v potassium ferricyanide solution.	Blue precipitate indicates ferrous iron from anaemia pills and *female correctives*. Confirm by serum iron estimation—see Part II.
11. Repeat 10 using 1% w/v potassium ferrocyanide solution.	Blue precipitate indicates ferric iron —iron salts have been used as abortifacients. Confirm by serum iron estimation.
12. Add 1 ml diphenylamine-sulphuric acid reagent to two drops of aspirate.	A blue color indicates nitrite, chlorate or bromate. Nitrate ingestion will also give a positive result. (See page 65 for reagent.)
13. Treat a few drops of the aspirate or vomit with an equal volume of sodium dithionite solution as in urine test 11.	Blue colors indicate paraquat and/or diquat.

2. Faeces

Examination of faeces from the living patient is sometimes worthwhile. Mushrooms often resist digestion and excellent specimens have been found in faeces; this could be of great help in cases of suspected ingestion of toxic fungi and presumably for other botanical debris. For the identification of *Amanita phalloides,* see Part II.

Administration of powdered glass can be established by destroying all the organic material by a nitric-sulphuric acid digestion, dissolving any natural calcium sulphate and any barium sulphate that may have been given as an x-ray contrast medium in sodium ethylenediamine tetra-acetate and examining the centrifuged residue microscopically in polarised light to distinguish the glass from naturally occurring sand. Extreme precautions must be taken to exclude accidental contamination from laboratory glassware; normal faeces contain a few microscopic particles of glass, presumably from the glaze on cups and from cracked glasses and bottles. These, in experiments that the writer did, did not exceed eight per normal passage of faeces.

An x-ray examination of faeces often enables lead paint to be localized.

3. Hair and Nails

These are usually only examined in cases where it is desired to determine whether arsenical compounds have been administered to the patient over a period of time. The point of maximum concentration is related to its distance from the point of growth. In many cases the clinician will not want to arouse the patient's suspicions and will obtain samples of hair from a comb. There is insufficient hair obtainable in this way for classical analyses, but activation analytical techniques will provide the answer on as little as ten hairs.

The analyses are covered in detail in Part II.

4. Air from the Lungs

Exhaled air is a very convenient source for testing for volatile poisons. Several firms provide indicator tubes which are suitable for use in the context of emergency toxicology. Although several tubes are designed for testing industrial environments, they can easily be adapted, or indeed are designed, for testing exhaled air. Tubes for carbon monoxide and alcohol are obvious examples, and the latter are extremely useful in the middle of the night when a rapid, approximate answer is needed by a worried clinician.

Alcohol is a very commonly encountered poison, and a very rapid screen can be made by the use of such simple cheap devices as the Alcotest®. One litre of breath is forced through orange granules in a glass tube which turn green in the presence of alcohol. If the patient is unconscious and noncooperative, breath can be collected in the litre plastic bag, then forced through the tube. Such tests are nonquantitative, but of obvious value in excluding significant quantities of alcohol. Clearly it is not possible to give details of all the various commercial firms' instructions here; it is sufficient to say that toxicologists should consider their use and, in doing so, they may find that they get fewer disturbed nights.

REFERENCES

Blackmore, D.J.: The determination of carbon monoxide in blood and tissue. *Analyst, 95:*439, 1970.

Churchill-Davidson, H.C., and Griffiths, W.J.: Simple test paper method for the clinical determination of plasma pseudocholinesterase. *Br Med J, ii:* 994, 1961.

Clow, W.M., and Smith, A.C.A.: Rapid quantitative barbiturate estimation: A critical study of a bedside method. *Scott Med J, 12:*307, 1967.

Curry, A.S.: Rapid method of screening for barbiturate. *Br Med J, ii:*1040, 1963.

Curry, A.S.: Rapid quantitative barbiturate estimation. *Br Med J, i:*354, 1964.

Curry, A.S.: The Poisoned Patient, the Role of the Laboratory. Ciba Foundation Symposium, Elsevier, Amsterdam and New York, Associated Scientific Publishers, 1974.

Denswil, E.H., and Detmers, J.P.: Acetone as solvent in flame—photometric determination of lithium in serum. *Clin Chim Acta, 40:*129, 1972.

Fischer, D.S. A method for the rapid detection of acute iron toxicity. *Clinical Chemistry, 13:*7, 1967.

Forrest, I.S., and Forrest, F.M.: Urine colour test for the detection of phenothiazine compounds. *Clinical Chemistry, 6:*11, 1960.

Forrest, I.S., Forrest, F.M., and Mason, A.S. A rapid urine colour test for Thioridazine (Mellaril). *Amer J Psy, 116:*928, 1960—idem. ibid., A rapid colour test for imipramine (Tofranil) (Supplementary report with colour chart). *116:*1021, 1960.

Fry, D.E., and Marks, V.: Value of plasma lithium monitoring. *Lancet, 1:*886, 1971.

Gee, D.J., and Dalley, R.A.: Unsuspected poisoning. *Med Sci Law, 7:*56, 1967.

Hensel, E.: In Curry, A.S. (Ed): *Methods of Forensic Science.* New York, Interscience, 1964, vol. 3.

Lundberg, G.D., Walberg, C.B., and Pantlik, V.A.: Frequency of toxicology test-ordering (primarily overdose cases) and results in a large urban general hospital. *Clin Chem, 20:*121, 1974.

Meade, B.W., Widdop, B., Blackmore, D.J., Brown, S.S., Curry, A.S., Goulding, R., Higgins, G., Matthew, H.J.S., and Rinsler, M.G.: Simple tests to detect poisons. Technical Bulletin, No. 24, the Association of Clinical Biochemists, London.

Perlman, P.L., and Johnson C. The metabolism of Dormison, (3-methylpentyne-3 ol, methylparafynol) and methods for the estimation of Dormison in biological material. *J Amer Pharm Assoc, 41:*13, 1952.

Pilsbury, V.B., and Jackson, J.V.: The identification of the thiazide diuretic drugs. *J Pharm Pharmacol, 18:*713, 1966.

Plaa, G.L., and Hine, C.H.: A method for the simultaneous determination of phenobarbital and diphenylhydantoin in blood. *J Lab Clin Med, 47:* 649, 1956.

Plaa, G.L., Hall, F.B., and Hine, C.H.: Differentiation of barbiturates for clinical and medico-legal purposes. *J Forensic Sci, 3:*201, 1958.

Prescott, L.F., Swainson, C.P., Forrest, A.R.W., Newton, R.W., Wright, N., and Matthews, H.: Successful treatment of severe paracetamol overdosage with Cysteamine. *Lancet, 1:*58, 1974.

Ramsey, W.N.M.: The determination of iron in blood plasma or serum. *Clin Chim Acta, 2:*214, 1957.

Rehling, C.J.: Poison residues in human tissues (report of 150 barbiturate and 90 barbiturate/alcohol combinations). in Stolman, A. (Ed.): *Progress in Chemical Toxicology*, New York, Academic, 1967, vol. 3.

Schreiner, G.E., Berman, L.B., Kovach, R., and Bloomer, H.A.: Acute glutethimide poisoning. *AMA Arch Intern Med, 101:*899, 1958.

Stone, H.M., and Henwood, C.S.: The spectrophotometric determination of low levels of barbiturates in blood. *J Forensic Sci Soc, 7:*51, 1967.

Street, H.V.: The separation of barbiturates by reversed phase paper chromatography at elevated temperatures. *J Forensic Sci Soc, 2:*118, 1962.

Tompsett, S.L.: The detection and determination of phenacetin and paracetamol in blood, serum and urine. *Annals Clin Biochem, 6:*81, 1969.

Tompsett, S.L.: Interference from the presence of other substances in detecting and determining barbiturate in biological material. *J Clin Pathol, 22:*291, 1969.

Trinder, P.: Rapid determination of salicylate in biological fluids. *Biochem J, 57:*301, 1954.

Turner, L.K.: Some applications of acceleration thin layer chromatography in toxicology, *J Forensic Sci Soc, 5:*94, 1965.

Wang, R.I.H.: Determining cholinesterase activity in human plasma. *JAMA, 183:*792, 1963.

Wiltbank, T.B., Sine, H.H., Brody, B.B., Ross, D.L., McCarron, M.M., Walberg, C.B., and Lundberg, G.D.: Are emergency toxicology measurements really used? *Clin Chem, 20:*116, 1974.

Chapter 4

DRUG ABUSE SCREENING

THE PURPOSE OF THE ANALYSES described below is to assist the clinician in answering the question, "is the patient on drugs?" However, the question can be asked in such a variety of contexts that a systematic chemical approach is necessary. Clearly, the analyses can be selectively shortened depending on the clinical emphasis.

The tests described below are suitable for those cases that appear occasionally in the hospital or police laboratory. They are not to be read in the context of a mass screening programme in which perhaps thousands of samples per week have to be analysed.

Commercial kits are available for the radioimmunoassay and other immunological methods of some drugs, for example barbiturates, amphetamines, methadone and morphine. Clearly, if the laboratory is equipped to do these, the toxicologist has only to follow the instructions on the box. In general terms, immunological methods are never perfectly specific, and usually the tests are used to select the few urines from the thousands examined that require chemical screening.

If possible, a sample of at least 25 ml of urine should be used. Because the urine will contain metabolites of, or in addition to, unchanged drug, and because metabolites are usually more polar, the technique of examining urine must take this into account. It is stressed that the aim is to isolate and identify drugs; quantitative procedures, with few exceptions, are of limited value because of the difficulties of interpretation. It is well established that excretion of both acidic and basic drugs (e.g. salicylates and amphetamines) vary with the pH of the urine and little useful data is available to enable one to deduce the probable dose when only a single urine sample has been voided.

It is suggested that the spot tests described in the previous section are done first where they relate to possible drug involvement.

Head space gas chromatography is also useful to detect addicts of volatile solvents. Details of this technique are given elsewhere (see Chapter 5B1a.

A. EXTRACTION PROCEDURES

The schematic diagram for the isolation of the various extracts is shown in Figure 6.

Urine, 25 ml, is made acid to pH 2 with dilute sulphuric acid. and sufficient solid ammonium sulphate to make a saturated solution is added. The solution is extracted with 2×150 ml of ether which are separated. The aqueous phase is retained. The combined ether layers are washed with 10 ml of a freshly prepared solution of 5% sodium bicarbonate in saturated salt (sodium chloride) solution. This aqueous layer is rejected, and, if necessary, it can be examined for salicylates. Barbiturate and glutethimide metabolites are next extracted from the ether by 2×10-ml extractions with 3% w/v sodium hydroxide. The aqueous alkaline layers are combined, made acid with dilute hydrochloric acid to pH 2, saturated with solid ammonium sulphate, and re-extracted with 2×100-ml portions of ether. The ether layers are combined, dried with 2 g of solid anhydrous sodium sulphate, separated and evaporated. This gives the barbiturate extract, the *weak acid* fraction.

The ether fraction remaining after the bicarbonate and alkali extractions is dried with solid sodium sulphate, poured off and evaporated to give the *neutral* fraction.

The acidified aqueous urine remaining after the ether extraction above is made alkaline with 880 ammonia and extracted with 35 ml of ether. The ether is separated and dried by triturating with solid anhydrous sodium sulphate. It is then decanted and evaporated in two stages; first, to approximately a 3 ml volume by heating over a boiling water bath in a fume cupboard (beware cigarettes, etc.), and, secondly, the final stage is accomplished in a 15 ml Quickfit® test tube with a finely tapered base, at 40 degrees C on a water bath to reduce the volume to 40 μl; 10 μl of ethanol are then added. The extract must *not* be allowed to dry. The tube should be glass-stoppered.

As far as morphine is concerned, the sample will contain about

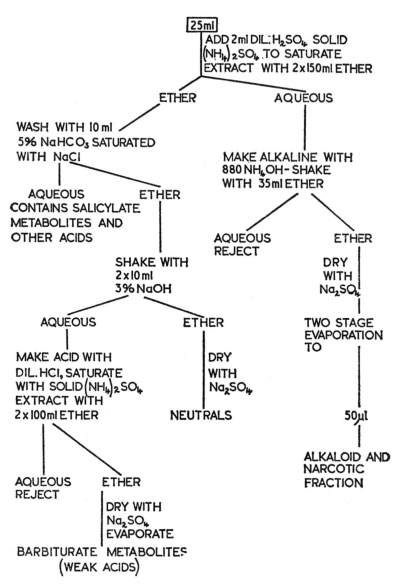

Figure 6. Extraction procedure for urine.

ten times as much morphine glucuronide as free morphine. The conjugate can be efficiently hydrolysed by autoclaving a separate portion of the urine sample at 125 degrees C for thirty minutes with hydrochloric acid. The optimium concentration is achieved by adding 1 ml concentrated acid to 10 ml of urine. Alternatively, 5 ml concentrated acid is added to 10 ml of urine and refluxed for thirty minutes. After cooling, it is made to pH 14 with alkali and extracted with ether which is rejected. Morphine is then extracted after the pH has been adjusted to pH 9.4. Many solvents have been used for extraction, but shaking with a volume of chloroform: isopropanol (4:1 v/v) equal to that of the urine is efficient. After separating, the organic phase is run through a fluted filter paper to remove last traces of moisture and evaporated. Analysis of this morphine extract then proceeds following the general methods described for the alkaloid and narcotic fraction. It should be noted that the morphine extract tends to be intractable, and repeated solution with warm ethanol is the best treatment prior to chromatography.

1. Examination of the Extracts

a. Acid Extracts

Provided it is required to detect toxicologically significant amounts of glutethimide or barbiturate, the weak acid extract can be examined directly by ultraviolet spectrophotometry at three pH's as described for blood see (Chap. 3, A4b.). Metabolites retain the chromophoric ring intact, and an obvious positive can be obtained. When it is required to detect the residues of therapeutic doses, a high background absorption interferes, and the prior purification of the extract by a paper chromatographic separation as described on page 187 is necessary. Absorbing spots under 254 nm light are cut out, eluted with 0.45N sodium hydroxide and individually read from 220 to 320 nm at not more than 5-nm intervals. A piece of blank paper from the same chromatogram is similarly eluted and put in the reference beam. Normally, 3.5 ml of sodium hydroxide are used for elution, but if the absorption under 254 nm is only weakly seen, then a microcell and 0.7 ml can be used. Identification of the particular barbiturate or barbiturates from the metabolic excretion chromatographic pattern may be possible if only one drug is involved. Experience with barbitone, phenobarbitone (and p-hydroxyphenobarbitone), amylobarbitone (which gives 3-hydroxy-amylobarbitone) is readily acquired. Other barbiturates tend to give complex patterns.

Glutethimide (Doriden®) gives 2-phenylglutarimide in the urine which is slowly hydrolysed at pH 13 to 14, losing its 235 nm peak. The procedures described above for ultraviolet spectrophotometry should, therefore, be closely followed.

As far as the neutral fraction is concerned, no doubt that unless large quantities of visible crystals can be seen, the routine procedure of choice is to sublime this extract at 100 degrees C at 10^{-2} mm for two to three hours. The appearance of beautiful sublimed crystals from an extract that would otherwise have been consigned to the sink indicates that this must be done routinely in systematic toxicology. Carbromal, phenacetin and meprobamate are but a few examples. Identification can proceed by a determination of micro melting points, (Table XVII) a TLC examination, (see p. 112) or, best of all, by infrared spectroscopy comparing the curve with knowns.

b. Narcotics and Bases (including morphine)

There are two approaches which can be used to screen these two fractions for basic drugs of abuse. The first uses gas chromatography, the second, paper or thin layer chromatography.

1. GAS CHROMATOGRAPHY. Although gas chromatography is the method of choice for rapid screening of urine for amphetamines, there is a grave doubt whether it is yet the best method for detecting and identifying unknown alkaloids in urine or tissue.

It would be highly satisfactory if gas chromatography could be classed as a procedure suitable for deciding whether there was a toxic alkaloid present or not present in the extract, but two difficulties arise—first, the fact that normal urine can contain bases which give peaks of no toxicological significance, and, secondly, some alkaloids either decompose on the column or have such long retention times that even with temperature programming each urine analysis can take over an hour. If a peak is obtained, its identification becomes a matter of inspired guesswork even if a good reference map has been previously made before one can decide on the best potential derivative formation. If gas chromatography-mass spectrometry is available, this is clearly the method of choice, although, as far as the amphetamines are concerned, it is often advisable to do mass spectroscopy on derivatives giving better fragmentography patterns.

As a consequence of this philosophy it is therefore advisable, as far as amphetamines are concerned, to inject 2 to 5 μl of the ethereal-ethanol extract obtained as described above or to use a separate aliquot of urine (for full details see Part II).

2. PAPER CHROMATOGRAPHY AND THIN LAYER CHROMATOGRAPHY. The literature is full of suggested systems for use in toxicological analysis, but until recently very little systematic work had been done to decide which were the best.

Moffat and Smalldon (1974) have now published an appraisal of thirty-seven paper and thin layer systems using one hundred most common basic drugs. The best discriminating systems with minimum correlation and most practical usefulness form the basis of the recommendations given below. Paper chromatography is rarely used nowadays, but as it is convenient, easy and separates dirty extracts much better than TLC, the preferred system is still that of Curry and Powell (see below).

In order to get good chromatographic spots it is necessary to test a 1-μl portion of the 50-μl extract to estimate, roughly, the aliquot that is to be put on a chromatogram. This is done by running the 1 μl on a piece of filter paper. A microdrop of potassium iodoplatinate reagent is run onto it, and the depth of any deep purple colour observed. Experience soon enables one to judge the required volume to put on the chromatogram. The inexperienced analyst can prepare 1, 5, 10 and 50-μg standards (say 1, 5, 10 and 50 μl of a 0.1% solution of quinine in alcohol). This test will *not* detect amphetamine and here the analyst is in something of a dilemma. The 50-μl extract must be put onto a chromatogram before the ether evaporates and it must be divided in such a way that there is the maximum chance of detecting a wide variety of drugs; at the same time, overloading the chromatogram must not occur so that the results become uninterpretable. It is for this reason that a GLC screen (see Part II) on a 1-μl injection is so valuable. Submicrograms of amphetamines can be detected within a few minutes, and the very high sensitivity ensures detection of therapeutic doses even on 1 ml samples of urine. However, a TLC screen for amphetamine-type drugs on 10 μl takes only little longer, but care in stoppering the extract and storing it in the refrigerator must be observed.

A cautionary word must be interposed concerning the stability of drugs in solvents. Tertiary amines are very prone to attack by chloroform, dichloromethane and ethylene dichloride. In addition, other highly reactive halogenated hydrocarbons are present as impurities in these solvents. Total loss of basic drugs can occur if such solvents are used and it is for this reason that ether, *which must be peroxide-free,* is recommended in the extraction described above.

CHROMATOGRAPHIC METHODS FOR IDENTIFICATION. PAPER (Clarke, 1967). Whatman No. 1 paper is dipped in 5% sodium dihydrogen citrate solution (see p. 113), blotted and dried. It can be stored. The solvent is 2.4 g citric acid in 65 ml of water with 435 ml of n-butanol. About 10 to 20 μg spots are applied to the paper. Detection is achieved by spraying with iodobismuthate or iodoplatinate. It is useful to note that with the latter reagent, amphetamine gives a slowly developing white spot at Rf 0.45. It is impossible here to give a complete list of Rf values for about 1,000 alkaloids and basic drugs that can appear in this fraction, and identification can only be achieved by inspection of the chromatogram under 254 nm light before spraying, the colour and Rf of the coloured spots, elution and ultraviolet or infrared spectrophotometry, and comparison of all the results with published or self-determined data.

Reagents for Alkaloids and Bases:

1. *Potassium iodobismuthate (Dragendorff's spray).* (a) 2.0 g bismuth subnitrate and 25 ml glacial acetic acid in 100 ml water. (b) 40 g potassium iodide in 100 ml water. Before use, mix 10 ml of (a), 10 ml of (b), 20 ml of glacial acetic acid and 100 ml of water. The spots on TLC plates can be enhanced by overspraying with 5% sodium nitrite solution.

2. *Potassium iodoplatinate spray (for paper chromatograms).*

Add 10 ml of 5% platinum chloride solution to 240 ml of 2% potassium iodide solution, and dilute with an equal volume of water.

Iodoplatinate solution (acid, for thin layer chromatograms)
Add 10 ml of 5% platinum chloride solution and 5 ml of concentrated hydrochloric acid to 240 ml of 2% potassium iodide solution.

Tables VI gives Rf values for one hundred very common basic drugs in alphabetical order; Table VII gives them in ascending order of Rf.

TABLE VI

RF VALUES OF 100 BASIC DRUGS IN THE CURRY-POWELL SYSTEM

Data from Moffat, A.C., and Smalldon, K.W., *J. Chromatogr., 90*:9, 1974.

Drug	Rf × 100	Drug	Rf × 100
Acetophenazine	23	Diazepam	89
Ametazole	8	Diethylpropion	58
Amethocaine	48	Dimethoxanate	54
Amitriptyline	77	Diphenhydramine	62
Amphetamine	51	Diphenylpyraline	46
Antazoline	74	Dipipanone	85
Atropine	37	Ephedrine	45
Benzocaine	90	Ethoheptazine	52
Benzphetamine	75	Ethopropazine	72
Bromodiphenhydramine	69	Fluphenazine	36
Buphenine	80	Guanethidine	3
Butacaine	78	Hydroxyzine	67
Butethamine	51	Hyoscine	23
Caffeine	65	Imipramine	63
Carbetapentane	76	Iproniazid	75
Carbinoxamine	46	Isocarboxazid	94
Chlorcyclizine	74	Isothipendyl	58
Chlordiazepoxide	82	Levallorphan	73
Chlorpheniramine	45	Lignocaine	62
Chlorpromazine	68	Lysergide	47
Cinchonine	47	Meclozine	92
Clemizole	77	Mephentermine	62
Cocaine	38	Mepivacaine	62
Codeine	16	Mepyramine	32
Cyclizine	55	Methadone	74
Cyclopentamine	64	Methapyrilene	32
Desipramine	65	Methaqualone	94
Dextropropoxyphene	75	Methotrimeprazine	65
Diamorphine	33	Methyl phenidate	63

TABLE VI — (Cont'd)

Drug	Rf × 100	Drug	Rf × 100
Methylamphetamine	56	Piperocaine	68
Morphine	14	Pramoxine	61
Naphazoline	51	Procaine	31
Nialamide	78	Procyclidine	84
Nicotine	7	Promazine	58
Nicotinyl alcohol	16	Promethazine	65
Nikethamide	86	Propiomazine	77
Nitrazepam	92	Prothipendyl	55
Nortriptyline	74	Pyrrobutamine	84
Orphenadrine	67	Quinine	46
Papaverine	49	Strychnine	30
Perphenazine	23	Thenyldiamine	27
Pethidine	0	Thiopropazate	53
Phenelzine	38	Thioridazine	76
Phenindamine	63	Thonzylamine	52
Pheniramine	27	Tranylcypromine	45
Phenmetrazine	49	Trifluoperazine	34
Phenylpropanolamine	44	Trimeprazine	70
Phenyramidol	52	Tripelennamine	35
Pipamazine	50	Triprolidine	59
Piperidolate	76	Yohimbine	54

TABLE VII
RF × 100 VALUES OF 100 BASIC DRUGS IN THE CURRY - POWELL SYSTEM

Drug	Rf × 100	Drug	Rf × 100
Guanethidine	3	Diamorphine	33
Nicotine	7	Trifluoperazine	34
Ametazole	8	Tripelennamine	35
Pethidine	9	Fluphenazine	36
Morphine	14	Atropine	37
Codeine	16	Cocaine	38
Nicotinyl alcohol	16	Phenelzine	38
Acetophenazine	23	Phenylpropanolamine	44
Hyoscine	23	Chlorpheniramine	45
Perphenazine	23	Ephedrine	45
Pheniramine	27	Tranylcypromine	45
Thenyldiamine	27	Carbinoxamine	46
Strychnine	30	Diphenylpyraline	46
Procaine	31	Quinine	46
Mepyramine	32	Cinchonine	47
Methapyrilene	32	Lysergide	47

TABLE VII — (Cont'd)

Drug	Rf × 100	Drug	Rf × 100
Amethocaine	48	Piperocaine	68
Papaverine	49	Hydroxyzine	67
Phenmetrazine	49	Orphenadrine	67
Pipamazine	50	Bromodiphenhydramine	69
Amphetamine	51	Trimeprazine	70
Butethamine	51	Ethopropazine	72
Naphazoline	51	Levallorphan	73
Ethoheptazine	52	Antazoline	74
Phenyramidol	52	Chlorcyclizine	75
Thonzylamine	52	Methadone	74
Thiopropazate	53	Nortriptyline	74
Dimethoxanate	54	Benzphetamine	75
Yohimbine	54	Dextropropoxyphene	75
Cyclizine	55	Iproniazid	75
Prothipendyl	55	Carbetapentane	76
Methylamphetamine	56	Piperidolate	76
Diethylpropion	58	Thioridazine	76
Isothipendyl	58	Amitriptyline	77
Promazine	58	Clemizone	77
Triprolidine	59	Propiomazine	77
Pramoxine	61	Butacaine	78
Diphenhydramine	62	Nialamide	78
Lignocaine	62	Buphenine	80
Mephentermine	62	Chlordiazepoxide	82
Mepivacaine	62	Procyclidine	84
Imipramine	63	Pyrrobutamine	84
Methylphenidate	63	Dipipanone	85
Phenidamine	63	Nikethamide	86
Cyclopentamine	64	Diazepam	89
Caffeine	65	Benzocaine	90
Desipramine	65	Medozine	92
Methotrimeprazine	65	Nitrazepam	92
Promethazine	65	Isocarboxazide	94
Chlorpromazine	68	Methaqualone	94

THIN LAYER CHROMATOGRAPHY. Two systems are recommended, the first being directly comparable to the paper system described above.

METHOD. Cellulose 20 × 20 cm × 100-μ plates are dipped in 5% sodium dihydrogen citrate solution, drained and dried at 80 degrees C for twenty minutes. The plates are run in n-butanol:citric acid:water (435 mls:2.4 g:65 mls). Detection is as for paper, and the Rf values shown in Tables VI and VII apply.

The second system is chloroform:methanol (90:10) run on a Merck® Silica gel 60 plate sprayed with 0.1N NaOH and dried. Rf values are shown in Table VIII. Table IX shows these arranged in ascending order of Rf.

TABLE VIII

RF VALUES OF 100 BASIC DRUGS IN A TLC SYSTEM
SILICA GEL — CHLOROFORM — METHANOL (90:10)
Data from Moffat, A.C., and Clare B., *J. Pharm. Pharmacol., 26*:665, 1974.

Drugs	Rf × 100	Drugs	Rf × 100
Acetophenazine	47	Dipipanone	61
Ametazole	01	Ephedrine	08
Amethocaine	60	Ethoheptazine	43
Amitriptyline	59	Ethopropazine	69
Amphetamine	19	Fluphenazine	50
Antazoline	13	Guanethidine	05
Atropine	06	Hydroxyzine	77
Benzocaine	87	Hyoscine	67
Benzphetamine	93	Imipramine	57
Bromodiphenhydramine	67	Iproniazid	49
Buphenine	29	Isocarboxazid	95
Butacaine	62	Isothipendyl	57
Butethamine	51	Levallorphan	46
Caffeine	81	Lignocaine	94
Carbetapentane	40	Lysergide	68
Carbinoxamine	34	Meclozine	98
Chlorcyclizine	74	Mephentermine	15
Chlordiazepoxide	74	Mepivacaine	87
Chlorpheniramine	37	Mepyramine	52
Chlorpromazine	63	Methadone	40
Cinchonine	24	Methapyrilene	55
Clemizole	89	Methaqualone	97
Cocaine	73	Methotrimeprazine	65
Codeine	39	Methyl phenidate	64
Cyclizine	67	Methylamphetamine	28
Cyclopentamine	33	Morphine	24
Desipramine	21	Naphazoline	10
Dextropropoxyphene	80	Nialamide	36
Diamorphine	64	Nicotine	62
Diazepam	94	Nicotinyl alcohol	40
Diethylpropion	88	Nikethamide	85
Dimethoxanate	43	Nitrazepam	74
Diphenhydramine	58	Nortriptyline	23
Diphenylpyraline	58	Orphenadrine	63

TABLE VIII — (Cont'd)

Drug	Rf × 100	Drug	Rf × 100
Papaverine	91	Promethazine	78
Perphenazine	01	Propiomazine	84
Pethidine	63	Prothipendyl	52
Phenelzine	20	Pyrrobutamine	78
Phenindamine	82	Quinine	50
Pheniramine	30	Strychnine	29
Phenmetrazine	42	Thenyldiamine	61
Phenylpropanolamine	08	Thiopropazate	91
Phenyramidol	77	Thioridazine	73
Pipamazine	32	Thonzylamine	68
Piperidolate	03	Tranylcypromine	68
Piperocaine	62	Trifluoperazine	75
Pramoxine	94	Trimeprazine	80
Procaine	64	Tripelennamine	63
Procyclidine	64	Triprolidine	18
Promazine	65	Yohimbine	76

TABLE IX

RF VALUES × 100 OF 100 BASIC DRUGS IN A TLC SYSTEM
SILICA GEL — CHLOROFORM — METHANOL (90:10)

Drug	Rf × 100	Drug	Rf × 100
Ametazole	1	Pipamazine	32
Perphenazine	1	Cyclopentamine	33
Piperidolate	3	Carbinoxamine	34
Guanethidine	5	Nialamide	36
Atropine	6	Chlorpheniramine	37
Ephedrine	8	Codeine	39
Phenylpropanolamine	8	Carbetapentane	40
Naphazoline	10	Methadone	40
Antazoline	13	Nicotinyl alcohol	40
Mephentermine	15	Phemetrazine	42
Tripolidine	18	Dimethoxanate	43
Amphetamine	19	Ethoheptazine	43
Phenelzine	20	Levallorphan	46
Desipramine	21	Acetophenazine	47
Nortriptyline	23	Iproniazid	49
Cinchonine	24	Fluphenazine	50
Morphine	24	Quinine	50
Methylamphetamine	28	Butethamine	51
Buphenine	29	Mepyramine	52
Strychnine	29	Prothipendyl	52
Pheniramine	30	Methapyrilene	55

TABLE IX — (cont.)

Drug	$Rf \times 100$	Drug	$Rf \times 100$
Imipramine	57	Thioridazine	73
Isothipendyl	57	Chlorcyclizine	74
Diphenhydramine	58	Chlordiazepoxide	74
Diphenylpyraline	58	Nitrazepam	74
Amitriptyline	59	Trifluoperazine	75
Amethocaine	60	Yohimbine	76
Dipipanone	61	Hydroxyzine	77
Thenyldiamine	61	Phenyramidol	77
Butacaine	62	Promethazine	78
Nicotine	62	Pyrrobutamine	78
Piperocaine	62	Dextropropoxyphene	80
Chlorpromazine	63	Trimeprazine	80
Orphenadrine	63	Phenindamine	82
Pethidine	63	Propiomazine	84
Tripelennamine	63	Nikethamide	85
Diamorphine	64	Benzocaine	87
Methylphenidate	64	Mepivacaine	87
Procaine	64	Diethylpropion	88
Procyclidine	64	Clemizole	89
Methotrimeprazine	65	Papaverine	91
Promazine	65	Thiopropazate	91
Bromodiphenhydramine	67	Benzphetamine	93
Cyclizine	67	Diazepam	94
Hyoscine	67	Lignocaine	94
Lysergide	68	Pramoxine	94
Thonzylamine	68	Isocarboxazid	95
Tranylcypromine	68	Methaqualone	97
Ethopropazine	69	Meclozine	98
Cocaine	73		

It is emphasized that inspection in 254 nm light is of great value in that it provides a separation of the bases into those which absorb ultraviolet light and appear as dark spots on a pale background, those which fluoresce and those which show as a positive iodoplatinate spot and do not show up in 254 nm light. After inspection in the ultraviolet, the iodoplatinate spray is used. From a comparison of these results with controls, a tentative identification can often be made.

Ultraviolet spectrophotometry and mass spectrometry can be used to further the identification. To recover the base from the sprayed paper or thin layer plate the relevant area is cut out or scraped off and put into a warm solution of 0.1N sulphuric acid (1 ml). One drop saturated sodium sulphite is added and after alkalinisation with 880 ammonia the liberated base is extracted into 2 ml ether. For mass spectrometry the ether extract is evaporated and the residue transferred to the probe of the instrument; for ultraviolet spectrophotometry it is re-extracted into the smallest volume of 0.1N sulphuric acid suitable for the microcells used in the laboratory and the curve read from 230 to 350 nm.

Table X includes absorption maximum for those compounds in Tables VI and VIII that have $E_{1cm}^{1\%}$ values over 20. Below this value it is very doubtful if an ultraviolet examination is worthwhile. Table XI shows these in wavelength order.

c. Morphine

The alcoholic solution containing the morphine extract is tested according to the procedure described on page 79 to assess the probable amount of morphine present in the total extract. An estimated 5 to 10 μg is put onto a citrated TLC plate and run as described above for basic drugs. After a run of about 15 cm the plate is removed from the tank and dried in an oven at 100°C. When dry it is cooled and carefully dipped in 2% formaldehyde in concentrated sulphuric acid (Marquis reagent). Control spots (5-10 μg) of morphine and codeine are put on the same plate. Clear differences in Rf and colour shade are easily obtained to discriminate between these substances, and it must also be noted that codeine will be found in the base extract, not in the morphine extract.

It can be seen from Table XII that no interfering compounds have been noted. The test can also be applied in the study of the basic drug identification, and it is for this reason that the table contains such a diverse number of compounds.

d. Interpretation of Results

In general, the relevant section of Part II of this book will give a good lead as to whether a particular drug is being abused. However, the abuser is cunning. He or she may take sodium bicarbonate with his amphetamine to reduce the amphetamine concentration in the urine, or swear that the morphine in the urine specimen is

TABLE X

ULTRAVIOLET CHARACTERISTICS OF 71 COMMON BASIC DRUGS

Courtesy A.C. Moffat

Drug	Peak Maximum in N/10 H_2SO_4	Shift* after making solution strongly alkaline	Drug	Peak Maximum in N/10 H_2SO_4	Shift after making solution strongly alkaline
Acetophenazine	243	0	Methapyrilene	237	+ 4
Amethocaine	312	—10	Methaqualone	234	+30
Amitriptyline	240	0	Methotrimeprazine	252	+ 7
Antazoline	241	+ 6	Morphine	284	+13
Benzocaine	272	+12	Naphazoline	281	0
Benzphetamine	258	0	Nialamide	265	+40
Bromodiphenhydramine	230	0	Nicotine	260	0
Buphenine	274	—32	Nicotinyl alcohol	260	0
Butacaine	278	+ 4	Nikethamide	264	— 2
Caffeine	272	0	Nitrazepam	279	+86
Carbinoxamine	264	— 2	Nortriptyline	238	0
Chlorcyclizine	232	0	Orphenadrine	264	0
Chlordiazepoxide	245	+15	Papaverine	250	—13
Chlorpheniramine	265	— 2	Perphenazine	254	+ 2
Chlorpromazine	255	+ 3	Phenindamine	259	+ 4
Cinchonine	235	+55	Pheniramine	262	0
Clemizole	274	—21	Phenyramidol	237	+ 4
Cocaine	233	+37	Pipamazine	255	+ 3
Codeine	284	0	Piperocaine	232	+39
Cyclizine	263	— 5	Pramoxine	285	0
Desipramine	251	0	Procaine	279	+ 6
Diamorphine	279	+19	Promazine	252	+ 2
Diazepam	241	+ 9	Promethazine	249	+ 4
Diethylpropion	253	— 8	Propiomazine	241	+ 5
Dimethoxanate	254	0	Prothipendyl	242	+ 8
Ethopropazine	249	+16	Quinine	250	+30
Fluphenazine	254	+ 2	Strychnine	255	0
Hydroxyzine	232	— 2	Thenyldiamine	239	+ 7
Imipramine	251	0	Thiopropazate	256	+ 2
Iproniazid	267	+37	Thioridazine	263	+12
Isothipendyl	245	+ 5	Thonzylamine	235	+10
Levallorphan	278	—39	Trifluoperazine	256	+ 2
Lysergide	315	— 5	Trimeprazine	251	+ 5
Meclozine	230	0	Tripelenamine	239	+ 9
Mepyramine	238	+10	Triprolidine	289	—56
			Yohimbine	272	+ 8

*Values in nm

TABLE XI
UV CHARACTERISTICS OF 71 COMMON BASIC DRUGS

Drug	Peak maximum in N/10 H$_2$SO$_4$	Shift* after making solution strongly alkaline	Drug	Peak maximum in N/10 H$_2$SO$_4$	Shift* after making solution strongly alkaline
Bromodiphenhydra-mine	230	0	Perphenazine	254	+ 2
Meclozine	230	0	Chlorpromazine	255	+ 3
Chlorcyclizine	232	0	Pipamazine	255	+ 3
Hydroxyzine	232	— 2	Strychnine	255	0
Piperocaine	232	+39	Thipropazate	256	+ 2
Cocaine	233	+37	Trifluperazine	256	+ 2
Methaqualone	234	+30	Benzphetamine	258	0
Cinchonine	235	+55	Phenindamine	259	+ 4
Thonzylamine	235	+10	Nicotine	260	0
Methapyrilene	237	+ 4	Nicotinyl alcohol	260	0
Phenyramidol	237	+ 4	Pheniramine	262	0
Mepyramine	238	+10	Cyclizine	263	— 5
Thenyldiamine	239	+ 7	Thioridazine	263	+12
Nortriptyline	238	0	Carbinoxamine	264	— 2
Tripelennamine	239	+ 9	Nikethamide	264	— 2
Amitriptyline	240	0	Orphenadrine	264	0
Antazoline	241	+ 6	Chlorpheniramine	265	— 2
Diazepam	241	+ 9	Nialamide	265	+40
Propiomazine	241	+ 5	Iproniazid	267	+37
Prothipendyl	242	+ 8	Benzocaine	272	+12
Acetophenazine	243	0	Caffeine	272	0
Chlordiazepoxide	245	+15	Yohimbine	272	+ 8
Isothipendyl	245	+ 5	Buphenine	274	—32
Ethopropazine	249	+16	Clemizole	274	—21
Promethazine	249	+ 4	Butacaine	278	+ 4
Papaverine	250	—13	Levallorphan	278	—39
Quinine	250	+30	Diamorphine	279	+19
Desipramine	251	0	Nitrazepam	279	+86
Imipramine	251	0	Procaine	279	+ 6
Trimeprazine	251	+ 5	Naphazoline	281	0
Methiotrimeprazine	252	+ 2	Codeine	284	0
Promazine	252	+ 2	Morphine	284	+13
Diethylpropion	253	— 8	Pramoxine	285	0
Dimethoxanate	254	0	Tripolidine	289	—56
Fluphenazine	254	+ 2	Amethocaine	312	—10
			Lysergide	315	— 5

*Values in nm

TABLE XII
ALKALOIDS LISTED AS GIVING STRONG REACTIONS WITH MARQUIS
REAGENT*

		Alkaloid	
Alkaloid	*Rf*	*λ Max*	*Colour with Marquis*
Pseudomorphine	0.02	231 262	Red
Morphine	0.14	285	Purple
Codeine	0.16	284	Purple
Dihydromorphine	0.16	283	Red-purple
Apocodeine	0.18	280	Purple
Neopine	0.18	284	Blue-purple
Norcodeine	0.18	N/A	Blue-purple
Dihydrocodeine	0.20	283	Purple
Boldine	0.23	282, 301	Green-purple-green
Methyldihydromorphine	0.23	281	Purple
Mescaline	0.24	269	Orange
Protopine	0.24	240, 288	Blue-green
Prochlorperazine	0.24	253	Purple
Sinomenine	0.26	263	Orange-green-blue
Cryptopine	0.27	236, 283	Blue-green
Meparine®	0.27	279, 222	Bright yellow
Thenyldiamine	0.27	239 315	Black-violet
Tripelennamine	0.28	239, 315	Red brown
Ethyl morphine	0.30	285	Yellow-purple-black
Heroin	0.30	279	Purple
Apomorphine	0.32	273	Purple-black
Methapyrilene	0.32	237, 313	Black-violet
Thebaine	0.32	284	Red-orange
Desomorphine	0.35	277	Purple
Harmine	0.38	247	Orange-grey
Lachesine	0.39	258, 261, 251	Orange-green-blue
α-allo cryptopine	0.40	N/A	Purple
Pipamazine	0.40	255 306	Purple
Narcotine	0.42	312 290	Blue-purple (fading)
Methyldesorphine	0.44	283	Purple
Narceine	0.46	276	Brown-green
Pipenzolate	0.46	258, 252	Orange-green
Benzyl morphine	0.47	284	Red-purple
Chloropyrilene	0.49	238, 314	Purple
Diphenylpyrilene	0.50	258, 253	Yellow
Detigon®	0.55	260	Red-purple-brown
Diphemanil	0.56	231	Orange-red
Ethyl narceine	0.57	277	Brown-green-blue
Piperoxane	0.58	274	Deep purple
Pyridium®	0.58	405 238, 277	Red
Phenindamine	0.59	260	Grey-green

TABLE XII — (Cont.)

Alkaloid			
Alkaloid	*Rf*	*λ Max*	*Colour with Marquis*
Dimenoxadol	0.60	259, 263, 270	Orange-greenish blue
Dimethythiambutane	0.60	281, 269	Purple-brown
Bephenium	0.62	269, 263, 275	Red-purple
Linadryl	0.62	258, 252	Yellow
Neobenodine	0.62	259, 264	Yellow
Phenyltoloxamine	0.62	269, 276	Purple
Antadril	0.63	220	Yellow
Medrylamine	0.63	273	Yellow
Diphenhydramine	0.64	258, 253	Yellow
Bromodiphenhydramine	0.65	230	Yellow
Chlorpromazine	0.65	255	Purple
Methotrimeprazine	0.65	250 301	Blue-purple
Promethazine	0.65	250 297	Purple
Reserpine	0.65	270	Blue-grey-green-brown
Diethylthiambutene	0.67	287, 269	Purple-brown
Phentolamine	0.67		Yellow
Allylprodine	0.69	258, 252, 264	Blackish-blue
Pecazine	0.69	252, 301	Purple
Ethylmethylthiambutane	0.71	268, 285	Purple-brown
Captodiamine	0.73	266	Bright purple
Octaverine	0.75	248 321, 357	Green-brown
Alphameprodine	0.75	257 251, 263	Brown-red
Diethazine	0.75	250	Purple-brown
Ethylisobutrazine	0.82	250	Purple
Trimetozine	0.84		Red-brown
Oxethazaine	0.87	258 252, 264	Red-brown
Bisacodyl	0.88	233, 288	Purple-brown
Clomiphene	0.90	264	Purple

Solvent 0.1N H_2SO_4 for uv spectrophotometry.

N/A Sample not available for uv spectrophotometry.

Rf values in Curry-Powell system.

*Clarke, E.G.C.: In Lundquist, F. (Ed.): *Methods of Forensic Science*, vol. 1, Interscience, 1962, and personal communication.

from codeine intake, and indeed he may also take codeine with his morphine or heroin to support the lie.

In some areas quinine is used to dilute heroin, and the presence of this base in urine is considered to be indicative of narcotic abuse. This is clearly unsafe if the patient has been drinking gin and tonic as the tonic usually contains about 6 mg of quinine per 100 ml. Abuse of all sedatives, hypnotics, tranquillisers, antianxiety drugs and stimulants is to be expected, but the toxicologist must also look out for aspirin, phenacetin, propoxyphene and paracetamol as well as the addictive analgesics such as morphine and heroin.

Unfortunately, while the majority of patients will be from the general population, the ready availability of capsules and tablets in hospitals carries with it the probability that many samples will be from this environment. The caveat expressed on page 64 that the physician ensures that the sample really came from the patient is emphasized.

REFERENCES

Clarke, E.G.C.: *J Forensic Sci Soc, 7*:46, 1967. Based on Curry, A.S. and Powell, H.: *Nature, 173*:1143, 1954.

Heaton, A.M., and Blumberg, A.G.: Thin layer chromatographic detection of barbiturates, narcotics and amphetamines in urine of patients receiving psychotropic drugs. *J Chromatogr, 41*:367, 1969.

Fujimoto, J.M., and Wang, R.I.H.: A method of identifying narcotic analgesics in human urine after therapeutic doses. *Toxicol Appl Pharmacol, 16*:186, 1970.

Kullberg, M.P., and Gorodetsky, C.W.: Studies on the use of XAD-2 resin for detection of abused drugs in urine. *Clin Chem, 20*:177,1974.

Moffat, A.C., and Smalldon, K.W.: Optimum use of paper, thin-layer and gas-liquid chromatography for the identification of basic drugs. Pt. II, paper and thin-layer chromatography. *J Chromatogr, 90*:9, 1974.

Montalvo, J.G., Klein, E., Eyer, D., and Harper, B.: Identification of drugs of abuse in urine. 1. A study of the Dole technique. *J Chromatogr, 47*:542, 1970.

Mule, S.J.: Identification of narcotics, barbiturates, amphetamines, tranquilizers and psychomimetics in human urine. *J Chromatogr, 39*:302, 1969.

Chapter 5

INVESTIGATIONS
IN THE DEAD

THE OBJECT OF THIS SECTION and the next three chapters of the book is to try to provide a rationale to poison detection which should help the toxicologist trying to unravel those deaths that cause worried frowns on the faces of policemen, clinicians and pathologists.

In the first and second editions of this book this object was a primary feature, and it is solely a reflection of the increasing concern of the toxicologist in clinical biochemistry involving the use of drugs in therapy and the detection and treatment of drug addiction that has somewhat altered the format in this edition. Notwithstanding these alterations the primary object still remains, and it must be emphasized that if society believes that a true death certificate is desirable and that the criminal poisoner should be at least detected, then it must be prepared to train expert toxicologists and give them time and materials to do the job.

It must be realized that this is an area in which success is proportional to the effort applied. Policemen, clinicians and pathologists can provide shortcuts, but when the chips are down only systematic analysis can succeed. It only needs a cursory glance at the history of toxicology to realize the continued truth of this statement.

A. RATIONALE OF THE ANALYSES

The sequence of analyses in a systematic look is most important. Every case is different, but it is essential that the poisons covered in each area are tested for and efficiently eliminated or found. Each analyst must be satisfied that his test will detect the residues of a toxic dose. In some cases this is still impossible, but the ultimate aim must be maintained.

The sequence, as the writer sees it, must first involve rapid screening tests on blood and urine, followed by simultaneous tests on extracts from the liver and the relevant portion of the alimentary tract. In addition, there is an increasing armoury of *special tests* which defy systematic inclusion in other than the sense they must be done one after the other.

The next sections in this book are perhaps the most tedious to read, expensive in time to carry out and obnoxious in practice to perform. If the toxicologist chooses to short-cut them, he carries the responsibility of failing to detect the criminal poisoner.

B. THE SYSTEMATIC APPROACH

1. Blood

The tests detailed in Chapter 3 must be followed by the tests described below:

a. Head Space Analysis for Volatiles

A 1.0-ml sample of blood is sealed in a closed vial of about 10-ml capacity. The vial is warmed to 60 degrees C, and a 5-ml air sample from above the blood sample is injected into the gas chromatograph with a commercially available gas-tight syringe.

(The test should be repeated after the addition of an equal volume of 6N H_2SO_4 which will liberate acetaldehyde from paraldehyde.) A column of five feet of 10% PEG 400 on 100 to 120 Celite at 70 degrees C is used with a flame ionisation detector. Volatile poisons are revealed, and the retention time gives a lead as to identity. This simple test will reveal not only the common poisons such as methanol and ethanol, but also as Table XIII shows, a large number of toxicologically important compounds. It should be noted that if an electron capture detector is available, it is possible to selectively detect the halogenated hydrocarbons.

The accurate determinations of ethanol in 10 μl of blood by gas chromatography is described in Part II.

This air space test can also be applied at the same time with a urine sample, but it should be noted that at high sensitivity settings several compounds can be found in *normal* urine, for example acetone and sometimes traces of ethanol. A profile of urines *not* containing poison should be examined before red herrings are chased.

TABLE XIII

RETENTION TIMES FOR VOLATILES USING 5 FEET OF
10% PEG400 ON CELITE AT 70° C

Order of Elution	Approximate Time in Minutes
Ether	1
Acetaldehyde	1.5
Tetrachloroethane	
Acetone	
Diacetonealcohol	3
Carbon tetrachloride	
Ethyl acetate	4
Methyl-ethyl ketone	
Dichloromethane	5
Benzene	
Methanol	6
Trichloroethylene	7
Isopropanol	
Methyl n-propyl ketone	
Perchloroethylene	8
Ethanol	
Chloroform	
Methyl-isobutyl ketone	9
Toluene	10
Dichloroethane	11
Butyl acetate	13
Paraldehyde	15
Amyl acetate	18

It is also worth taking an 5-ml air sample from the container holding the liver at room temperature. This will readily show the presence of petrol in fire victims if they were breathing the fumes of accelerant at the time of the incident.

Ethchlorvynol can also be detected by the head space method, but with a column at 70 degrees C it has a long retention time. Finkle (personal communication) uses a 2% SE30 column at 150 degrees C for the detection and assay of this compound (see also Part II). Bonnichsen *et al.* (1966), using GLC methods as well as paper chromatography and TLC, report on thirty-five cases (26 fatal) involving benzene, toluene, xylene and nitrobenzene and found tissue levels of the order of 0.1 to 2 mg/100 g. They used 20% Apiezon on Chromosorb at 190 degrees C.

Methanol

The inclusion of a colorimetric test here depends on the sensitivity of the flame ionisation detector used for head space analysis for volatiles. This is often not sufficiently high for this poison to be detected with certainty. If experiments show that a least 10 mg% of methanol can be detected by gas chromatography, then the colorimetric test described below can be omitted.

Methanol is detected by controlled oxidation to formaldehyde, and determination of this compound with chromotropic acid or with Schiff's reagent under conditions specific for formaldehyde. Omission of the oxidation step makes the method suitable for formaldehyde. It is essential to perform exact controls with methanol added to blood.

METHOD (Feldstein and Klendshoj, 1954). Sulphuric acid (2.2 ml of 10%) is pipetted into the centre well of a Conway cell. In the outer compartment is placed 1 ml of saturated aqueous potassium carbonate solution. Sealing of the ground glass plate is made with Vaseline®.

Half a millilitre (0.5 ml) of sample is introduced into the outer compartment, the cell sealed and tilted several times to thoroughly mix the sample and carbonate. Diffusion is allowed to proceed for two hours at room temperature. At the end of this period 1 ml of the sulphuric acid is pipetted into a 25-ml test tube, one drop of 5% aqueous potassium permanganate is added and the tube shaken. After five minutes at room temperature, drops of a saturated aqueous solution of sodium bisulphite are added until the permanganate is decolorised. After the addition of 0.2 ml of freshly prepared 0.5% aqueous chromotropic acid, the tube is cooled in ice and 4 ml of concentrated sulphuric acid added. The tube is shaken and then immersed in a boiling water bath for fifteen minutes after which it is cooled to room temperature. After making up to exactly 10 ml, reading at 580 nm are taken for the test and controls. Suitable standards are in the range 0 to 80 μg of methanol.

Schiff's reagents can be used to test for methanol by adding it to the permanganate oxidized distillates made up to 10 percent with sulphuric acid. Acetaldehyde does not then interfere, and estimates of concentration can be made by comparison with standards.

b. Cyanide

The ability to smell cyanide is hereditary, and if the policeman, pathologist and toxicologist all do not have sensitive noses, its presence will be missed unless routine chemical screening is performed. Inhalation and injection of cyanide can also be easily missed, and even absorption through broken or burnt skin may have to be considered. This screening test is the one least often performed routinely; the "cyanide is obvious" philosophy is strongly entrenched, but it is fallacious and it should be re-emphasized that, in the case of a full screen for poisons, cyanide must not be missed.

SCREENING TEST AND ASSAY: METHOD (Gettler and Goldbaum, 1947) see Fig. 7. Nitrogen is blown through water in the bubbling Tube A which acts as a flowmeter, and then through 2 ml of blood placed in the tube B with 3 ml of water, two drops of saturated lead acetate solution and 5 ml of 10% trichloroacetic acid. Tube B is then immersed in a water bath at 90 degrees C. The liberated hydrogen cyanide is slowly blown through a ferrous hydroxide paper held by the Gutzeit holder (Fig. 8) at the exit of B; ten minutes is sufficient, and the flow rate should be held constant. The paper is prepared by soaking a Whatman No. 50 paper in

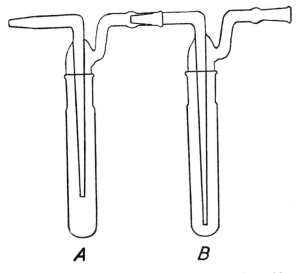

Figure 7. Apparatus for the determination of cyanide.

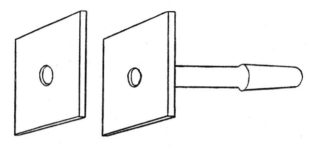

Figure 8. A simply made holder for use in the apparatus shown in Figure 7.

10% ferrous sulphate for five minutes, drying, immersing the dried paper in 20% sodium hydroxide and quickly blotting. The cyanide reacts with the ferrous hydroxide and can be seen as a stain of Turnbull's blue by immersing in 25% v/v hydrochloric acid. The stain is quantitative: 1 to 5-μg are convenient standards.

Cyanide can be produced in blood that is stored, probably both by enzyme action and by bacteria; the addition of 1% sodium fluoride prevents this. If cyanide is found in the above test then 5 g from the centre, undecomposed area, of the brain should be excised and analysed. In fatal cases of cyanide poisoning, levels in the brain are usually very much lower than blood levels—as low as 10 μg/100 g—but a positive finding, even of this low concentration, can be extremely useful in confirming the cause of death and excluding cyanide production. Cyanide is bound to red cells, and the concentration in the spleen is usually high. Cyanide is very toxic, but blood from healthy adults can contain up to 15 μg/100 ml. In death from inhalation of the gas, blood levels of about 100 μg/100 ml or more are found. Rapid loss of cyanide from postmortem blood not preserved with fluoride can occur and, in any case, the analyses should be done as quickly as possible. In deaths from large overdoses by oral ingestion, blood levels are often much higher—sometimes of the order of mg/100 ml.

Recovery has been noted in victims whose cyanide level in the blood reached 750 μg/100 ml. For references see page 224.

c. Halogenated Hydrocarbons

IDENTIFICATION AND ASSAY. There are many halogenated aliphatic hydrocarbons which the toxicologist must consider. These include chloroform, carbon tetrachloride, ethylene dichloride, trichloroethylene, perchloroethylene and methylene dichloride. In addition, chloral hydrate is still in widespread use, and tablets containing a chloralphenazone compound may be encountered. Most of these can be detected by head space analysis (see Table XIII), but a colorimetric method is included here in case this apparatus is not available. The halogenated hydrocarbons can be separated from blood or a tissue slurry by microdiffusion and selectively absorbed into an organic solvent. Alternatively, the blood can be shaken with the solvent.

METHOD (Fujiwara Reaction). Shake 1 ml of blood with 2 ml of ether, pipetting off into a test tube 1 ml of the supernatant, and after adding to it 1 ml of pyridine and 1 ml of 20% w/v sodium hydroxide, immerse the tube in a boiling water bath for one minute.

Red colours in the pyridine show a positive result provided a full *blank* determination has been done at the same time.

Some measure of differentiation of the various compounds can be achieved by varying the condition of the reaction and noting those for maximum colour development; Table XIV shows some of those together with the recommended isolations.

For the routine screening in blood, the diffusion technique described in Reference 1, Table XIV is also recommended.

The carbon tetrachloride test requires amounts of the order 0.1 mg of the poison, and the test is therefore only applicable in this form to distillates of at least 100-g quantities of tissue or stomach contents which may be expected to contain this amount.

Moss and Rylance (1966) have investigated the red complex formed from different halogenated compounds, by spectrophotometry and TLC (using ethyl acetate saturated with water on Merck® Kieselgel GF254). They give absorption maxima for the normal reaction as follows: chloroform, chloral hydrate, trichloroacetic acid and chlorbutanol, 365 and 530 nm; trichlorothylene, 365 and 540 nm; trichloroethanol, 365 and 430 nm.

TABLE XIV

CONDITIONS FOR THE FUJIWARA REACTION

Ref.	Volume of Blood	Method	Reagents	Time of Heating	Compound
1	1-4 ml	Diffuse into 1 ml toluene at 37°C for 2 hours.	0.5 ml toluene 2.5 ml 20% NaOH 5 ml pyridine	5 min at 100° C	chlorform
2	5 ml	Cool, add 1 ml 30% KOH, shake for 1 minute. Add 6 ml heptane, shake 2 minutes	5 ml heptane. 2 ml 30% KOH 4 ml pyridine.	10 min at 80° C	chloroform chloral
3	3 ml	Shake with 7 ml acetone and centrifuge	2 ml acetone 7 ml pyridine 3.5 ml 20% NaOH	2.5 min at 100° C	carbon tetrachloride
4	—	—	10 ml pyridine 0.4 ml 0.1N NaOH	15 min at 100° C	carbon tetrachloride

References

[1]Feldstein, M., and Klendshoj, N. C.: *J Forensic Sci*, 2:39, 1957.
[2]Kaye, S., and Goldbaum, L.: *Legal Medicine*. St. Louis, Mosby, 1954, p. 620.
[3]Klondos, A. C., and McClymont, G. L.: *Analyst*, 84:67, 1959.
[4]Burke, T. E., and Southern, H. K.: *Analyst*, 83:316, 1958.

Jain and his co-workers (1967) add an equal volume of 50% aqueous ethanol solution containing 5 μg/ml chlorbutanol as an internal standard to blood or tissue homogenate supernatants, and inject 1 μl on to 5 feet x $\frac{1}{8}$-inch 15% FFAP on 60-80 acid washed Chromosorb W at 105 degrees C and 120 degrees C using an electron capture detector to separate and assay chloral and trichloroethanol.

For the differential determination of chloral hydrate, trichloroethanol and trichloroacetic acid in tissues and urine by the use of the Fujiwara pyridine-alkali reaction and by gas chromomatography, the reader is referred to the list of references.

INTERPRETATION OF RESULTS. A major problem exists in interpreting tissue levels of halogenated hydrocarbons because there is a progressive loss of the volatile compound between death and analysis. Fortunately, in the majority of cases, the presence of the poison coupled with the pathologist's findings are sufficient to account for death. In general, it is obvious that lower concentrations of the highly toxic carbon tetrachloride are more significant than the less toxic perchloroethylene. It is sometimes necessary to distinguish between a therapeutic dose and an overdose of chloral hydrate, and although this may be difficult, levels in the blood of 10 to 20 mg/100 ml will indicate that considerably more than a single therapeutic dose has been taken.

Jain and his co-workers report a trichloroethanol level of 0.9 mg/100 g in the blood of a fatal overdose of chloral. They confirm the very rapid *in vivo* conversion of chloral to trichloroethanol.

In the case of chloroform, 7 mg/100 ml in the blood indicates a condition associated with light surgical anaesthesia, and by the time 15 to 25 mg/100 ml has been reached, the patient is in a state of fourth-plane anaesthesia. Gettler and his co-workers have also shown that the concentrations of chloroform in the brain are similar to those in the blood as far as interpretation is concerned, and that the poison could be detected in this organ even after several months storage. Weinig, in a review, says that chloroform has been detected at exhumation 103 days after death.

Manning (personal communication) reports a death from trichloroethylene in which the blood level was only 10 μg/100 ml; liver and urine concentrations were 0.2 and 0.5 mg/100 g respectively. Hall and Hine (1966) report two cases of fatal trichloroethane poisoning by inhalation with blood levels of 13.0 and 72 mg/100 g respectively. Bonnichsen and Maehly (1966) report on six chloroform, twenty-three trichloroethylene (3 survivors) and three chloral hydrate poisonings. These results clearly show that the detection method should be capable of showing the presence of 0.1 mg/100 g of blood if the involvement of these compounds is to be demonstrated.

Trichloroethane findings in fatal cases have been reported by Stahl *et al.* (1969). Gas chromatography was used, and values varied from 0.15 mg/100 ml in blood to 59 mg/100 g in brain. (See Bonnichsen and Maehly, 1966; Cabana and Gessner, 1967; Garrett and Lambert, 1966; Gettler and Blume, 1931; Gettler, 1956; Hall and Hine, 1966; Jain *et al.*, 1967; Kaplan *et al.*, 1967; Moss and Rylance, 1966; Rehling, 1967; Stahl *et al.*, 1969; Turner, 1965; Weinig, 1958.)

d. Fluoride

Fluoride is not a common poison, but it is available to the general public in several forms—as a remover of iron mould as a liquid and paste; as solid sodium fluoride for use as a pesticide; and as hydrofluoric acid as an etching fluid or as a glass cleanser in horticulture.

The promise of a rapid quantitative screening procedure using diffusion from acidified blood directly into alizarin complexone reagent has not been fully realized because of the difficulty of diffusing the hydrofluoric acid within the stability life of the colour reagent. However, as a screening test, i.e. to detect unsuspected fluoride poisoning, the procedure has proved itself to the author.

SCREENING TEST AND ASSAY (Frere, 1961 and Frere and Rieders, 1961). Blood, 1 ml, and 1 ml of 80% v/v sulphuric acid containing 0.25% Tergitol are put without mixing in the outer compartment of an Obrink polypropylene diffusion vessel.* Into the centre compartment are mixed 0.25 ml each of an aqueous solution of cerous nitrate (43.2 mg/100 ml Ce $(NO_3)_3.6H_2O$) and alizarin complexone (38.5 mg/100 ml in pH4.3 acetate buffer: 4.2 ml glacial acetic acid + 2.2 g anhydrous sodium acetate or 5.3 g of trihydrate). The sealing compartment is filled with 1.5 ml of 80% sulphuric acid containing 0.25% Tergitol, and the blood and liberating acid are mixed. Diffusion at room temperature of the hydrofluoric acid into the color reagent is complete in about three hours. The color of the reagent is blue if fluoride is present. This test should be done in parallel with positive and negative controls at the same time so that direct comparison of the colours is possible. The positive control should be a blood sample containing 1 μg/ml of fluoride.

A specific fluoride electrode is also available, and clearly it is

---

*Otainable from Arthur H. Thomas, Philadelphia. Catalogue No. 44725.

most useful for monitoring for fluoride in serum and urine (see Part II).

2. OTHER TESTS

Because these involve analyses on different specimens—liver, alimentary tract, brain and kidney—they are described in separate chapters, but analyses must be proceeding at the same time.

REFERENCES

Bonnichsen, R., and Maehly, A.C.: Poisoning by volatile compounds; chlorinated aliphatic hydrocarbons. *J Forensic Sci, 11:*495, 1966.

Bonnichsen, R., Maehly, A.C., and Moeller, M.: Poisoning by volatile compounds, aromatic hydrocarbons, *J Forensic Sci, 11:*186, 1966.

Cabana, B.E., and Gessner, P.K.: The determination of chloral hydrate, trichloroacetic acid, trichloroethanol and urochloralic acid in the presence of each other and in tissue homogenates. *Anal Chem, 39:*1449, 1967.

Feldstein, M., and Klendshoj, N.C.: Determination of methanol in biological fluids by microdiffusion analysis. *Anal. Chem., 26:*932, 1967.

Frere, F.J.: Specific microdiffusion method for the determination of fluorine based on lanthanum-alizarin complexone colour system. *Anal Chem, 33:* 644, 1961.

Garrett, E.R., and Lambert, H.J.: The gas chromatographic analysis of trichloroethanol, chloral hydrate, trichloroacetic and trichloroethanol glucuronide. *J Pharm Sci, 55:*812, 1966.

Gettler, A.O.: The Historical Development of Toxicology. *J Forensic Sci, 1:* 15, 1956.

Gettler, A.O., and Blume, H.: Chloroform in the Brain, Lungs and Liver Quantitative Recovery and Determination. *Arch Path, 11:*554, 1931.

Gettler, A.O., and Goldbaum, L.R.: Detection & Estimation of Microquantities of Cyanide. *Anal Chem, 19:*270, 1947 (modified.).

Hall, F.B., and Hine, C.H.: Trichloroethane poisoning, a report of two cases. *J Forensic Sci, 11:*404, 1966.

Jain, N.C., Kaplan, H.L., Forney, R.B., and Hughes, F.W.: A rapid gas chromatographic method for the determination of chloral hydrate and trichloroethanol in blood and other biological materials. *J Forensic Sci, 12:*497, 1967.

Kaplan, H.L., Forney, R.B., Hughes, F.W., and Jain, N.C.: Chloral hydrate and alcohol metabolism in human subjects. *J Forensic Sci, 12:*295, 1967.

Moss, M.S., and Rylance, H.J.: The Fujiwara reaction: Some observations on the mechanism. *Nature, 210:*945, 1966.

Rehling, C.J.: Poison residues in human tissues (17 cases of chloral hydrate poisoning). In Stolman, A. (Ed.): *Progress in Chemical Toxicology.* New York, Academic, 1967, vol. 3.

Stahl, C.J., Fatteh, A. V., and Dominguez, A.M.: Trichloroethane poisoning:

Observations on the pathology and toxicology in 6 fatal cases. *J Forensic Sci, 14*:393, 1969.

Turner, L.K.: Searching for drug metabolites in viscera. In Curry, A.S. (Ed.): *Methods of Forensic Science.* New York, Interscience, 1965, vol. 4.

Weinig, E.: Die Nachweisbarkeit von Giften in exhumierter Leichen. *Deut. Z Gerichtl Med, 47*:397, (1958).

Chapter 6

THE ANALYSIS OF LIVER

IN THE UNITED KINGDOM four tests are conveniently done early in the investigation because they are designed to detect poisons common in that geographical area. These will be considered first. They usually follow the simple tests on blood and urine, and precede the tests on the alimentary tract described in Chapter 7. The second stage in the analysis of the liver (p. 130) follows the tests on the tract, although it is often convenient to cut the portions of tissue required for all these analyses at one time.

In all, the following weights are required: 2 g, 2 × 10 g, 2 × 50 g, 2 × 100 g and 250 g. It is also a convenient moment to weigh the whole organ. The tissue and any fluid in the jar should be macerated together before the weights are taken. This applies for all analyses on liver.

The weight amounts to approximately one third of a normal liver, and the same proportion should apply in the case of young children. If acute necrosis has been noted, the liver should be examined by x-ray to determine whether the damage is from Thorotrast which was used about 30-40 years ago as an x-ray contrast medium and which causes death by the radiation from thorium dioxide. The pathologist will usually have remarked on the macroscopic appearance of the liver, but the toxicologist should be capable of recognizing gross pathological changes and of searching first for those poisons which interfere with the metabolism of this very important organ.

A. THE FIRST STAGE

A firm recommendation should be made here as to which method to use for the general extraction of organic compounds from liver, but there is no universal panacea, and if negative tests result from one method, then all the following three methods must be done in sequence. The testing of acid and basic extracts is the same in each case. It is the variable efficiency between methods that causes this problem. Certainly the hydrochloric acid method must be done. Aluminum chloride can also be used and tungstic acid is an old well-proven method.

1. The Sodium Tungstate Precipitation

METHOD (Fox, R.H.: Personal communication). Tissue 100 g, 430 ml water and 100 ml 25% w/v sodium tungstate solution are thoroughly homogenised in an electric blender. The contents of the blender are washed into a 2-litre stainless steel beaker with a further 300 ml of water. The beaker is placed in a boiling water bath; 100 ml of 50% w/v sodium bisulphate solution are added and rapidly stirred electrically for ten minutes. This gives an excellent precipitation of granular material which can be easily removed by filtering through a 40-cm Whatman No. 114 paper. No suction is required, and about 850 ml (85% recovery) of filtrate is obtained in only two to three minutes.

After cooling, the filtrate is extracted with 1 litre of ether which has previously been freed from antioxidant and stored over ferrous sulphate solution. The subsequent treatment of this ether and the acid aqueous solution for the strong acid, weak acid, neutral, alkaloid and morphine fractions follows that described in Figure 6 and Chapter 4 with the volumes of extracting and re-extracting solutions suitably scaled up to deal with the larger volumes. For the morphine fraction, for example, 240 ml chloroform and 60 ml isopropanol are suitable volumes. It is again emphasized that the evaporation of ether in such large volumes requires the greatest care and laboratory discipline. Amphetamine is not lost to a significant degree if evaporation of the alkaloid fraction is done in two stages—first, reduction of the 500-ml volume to 5 ml by normal evaporation, and secondly, from 5 ml to 50 μl in the special tube with drawn-out base on a 40 degree C water bath. The 5-ml volume is redried with solid anhydrous sodium sulphate before the second evaporation. The extracts from the acidic extractions should be allowed to cool, then carefully inspected for any crystalline product. Examination follows the general procedure suggested for the blood and urine samples described in Chapters 3 and 4 in addition to the notes given below.

THE ALUMINIUM CHLORIDE METHOD (alternative to sodium tungstate). Stevens and Bunker. (personal communication)

METHOD. To 100 g liver add 200 ml water followed by 250 ml of 2N hydrochloric acid containing 10% w/v aluminium chloride and 10% w/v citric acid and macerate. Heat to 60 to 65 degrees C in a boiling water bath and filter immediately. The extraction and separation of extracts follow exactly as described for the tungstic acid precipitation stage.

The extracts are examined as follows:

a. Strong Acid Fraction

This is dissolved in 5 ml (more if necessary) of 0.45N sodium hydroxide and its ultraviolet absorption spectrum measured from 220 nm to 320 nm. Control spectra are essential in any toxicological laboratory, but the most common poison in this fraction is salicylic acid with an absorption peak at 295 nm and $E_{1cm}^{1\%} = 250$. A rapid spot test for salicylate is to test an aliquot of the extract, evaporated to dryness on a filter paper with ferric chloride solution with which it gives a violet color.

Even if the screening test for salicylate has proved negative the isolation of this fraction should not be ignored. Besides acting as a means of separating interfering acids from the other fractions, sometimes unusual poisons appear; 2,4-dichlorophenoxyacetic acid is one example which has an absorption maximum at 280 nm with $E_{1cm}^{1\%} = 110$. However, mandelic acid may be found if Mandelamine® has been taken, and succinic acid is commonly found as a natural product.

For this fraction, the weak acid fraction and neutral fraction, references to Tables X, XV and XVI to identify ultraviolet peaks will be useful.

b. The Weak Acid Fraction

The way this is examined depends on the instrumentation available. Mass spectrometry on a very small aliquot will give identification in a few minutes. If enough poison is present, infra-

TABLE XV

ABSORPTION MAXIMA OF "STRONG ACIDS"

(Solvent 0.5N NaOH)

226	Acetylsalicylic acid	273	{ Hydrochlorthiazide / Bendrofluazide
228	Chlorpropamide		
233	Benzoic acid	274	Hydroflumethiazide
235	p-chlorbenzoic acid		
238	β-p-hydroxphenylpropionic acid	280	{ p-hydroxybenzoic acid / 2,4-dichlorophenoxyacetic acid
255	2.4-dinitrophenol		
263	Nicotinic acid	292	Chlorthiazide
265	p-aminobenzoic acid	295	Salicylic acid

(The figures shows absorption maxima in nm)

No Absorption Peak

succinic acid

red spectroscopy is also most useful while sublimation and mixed melting point measurements (Table XVII) are still not archaic. However, ultraviolet spectrometry is a very good rapid method for identifying all the barbiturates and many other drugs that appear in this fraction (see Table V). A similar statement can also

TABLE XVI

ABSORPTION MAXIMA OF NEUTRALS

(SOLVENT ALCOHOL)

220	α-Naphthyl thiourea	265	Methaqualone
236	DDT	269	Phenylindanedione
240	(Methyltestosterone*	270	Approx: many sulphonamides; Benzocaine
	(Ethisterone*		(Mephenesin
	(Santonin	273	(Chloromycetin
241	Acetanilide		(Caffeine
245	(Progesterone*	275	Theophylline
	(Testosterone*	276	Parathion
	(Prednisolone*	288	α-Naphthyl thiourea
250	(Phenacetin		
	(Khellin		

(The figures shows absorption maxima in nm)

Not detected by UV

Meprobamate	Methyprylone
Bromvaletone*	Sedormid*
Carbromal*	Sedulon
Mephenesin carbamate	Styramate
Methylpentynol carbamate	

*Unlikely to be present in blood but relevant to tissue extracts.

TABLE XVII
MELTING POINTS

Melting Point (°C)	Substance	Melting Point (°C)	Substance
41- 43	Phenyl salicylic acid	163	Rotenone
46	Trimethadione	165	Methyl testosterone
48- 50	Urethane	165	Sulphanilamide
51	Thymol	169-172	Stiboestrol
		168	p-Acetamidophenol
69	Coumarin	170-173	Santonin
72	Antabuse	175	Sulphathiazole
74- 76	Sulphonethylmethane	171	Isonicotinyl hydrazide
75	Noludar	179	Camphor
87	Glutethimide	184	Sulphacetamide
91	Persedon	185-187	Succinic acid
97	Chlorbutanol (sublimes)	185-188	Hexestrol
97	Ethinamate	186	Hexachloroethane
100-102	Aldrin	190-191	Pentachlorophenol
103	Isopropylphenazone	190	Sulphaguanidine
104-106	Meprobamate	191	Oxalic acid
109	DDT	192	Sulphapyridine
109-110	TDE	193	Pregnelone
111-113	Antipyrine	194	Sedormid
113-115	Acetanilide	198	α Ethylcrotonyl carbamate
114	Hexachlorcyclohexane		
116-118	Carbromal	199	Sulphamethazine
122	Benzoic acid (sublimes 100)	203	Picrotoxin
		209	Phenylacetyl urea
124-126	Sulphonmethane	212-216	Phenurone
130	Nicotinamide	219	Irgafen
131	Progesterone	228	Saccharin
134-135	Phenacetin	237	Nicotinic acid
135	Aspirin	238	Caffeine (sublimes 178)
136-137	Methylphenylethyl hydantoin	238	Sulphamerazine
140	Salicylamide	256-257	Digitoxin
145-153	Bromvaletone	258	Phenolphthalein
148	Cholesterol	262	Sulphadiazine
151	Chloramphenicol	265	Digoxin
153	Khellin	270-274	Theophylline
155	Testosterone	295-298	Diphenylhydantoin
157-159	Salicylic acid (sublimes)	357	Theobromine (sublimes 290-295)
161	Warfarin		

be made for gas chromatography, but it must be emphasized that at this stage the purpose of the analysis is to find the poison. Accurate quantitation follows later, although rough estimates can be made if recovery factors in the protein precipitation stages are known. Barbiturates are the most common group of poisons found, but glutethimide and paracetamol are probably the closest runners-up. However, red colors during the alkaline extraction may indicate phenolphthalein while yellow colors indicate nitrophenols. The ultraviolet scan is best performed by dissolving the extract in 10 ml ether and taking a 1-ml aliquot. After evaporation, this is dissolved in 0.45N sodium hydroxide.

The volume of solvent used for spectrophotometry depends on the amount of drug present; therapeutic amounts need only 5 ml of sodium hydroxide or even less, but toxic doses may take over 100 ml to bring the reading within the range of the instrument. Visible examination of the extract gives a rough guide of the volume to be used, but it must be found by experiment. $E_{1cm}^{1\%}$ values for the common barbiturates are shown in Table XXVII. The values shown are for the maxima; when an optical density difference between pH 10 and pH 2 is to be taken, the $E_{1cm}^{1\%}$ values are slightly less. The characteristic absorption maxima illustrated in Figure 4 are found if barbiturate is present. As was indicated in relation to blood in Chapter 3B4b, glutethimide must also be sought by observing the reading at 235 nm in 0.45N sodium hydroxide (pH 13.5) for several minutes. A diminution in reading indicates the opening of the glutarimide ring. Bemegride gives a peak at 230 nm at this pH. The amount in the extraction, and then by simple arithmetic the amount in 100 g of liver can be calculated roughly at first by using an $E_{1cm}^{1\%}$ value of 450 at 240 nm for pH 10 − pH 2, then exactly when full identification of the barbiturate or barbiturates has been achieved.

The method for altering the pH is to add saturated ammonium chloride to the 0.45N sodium hydroxide solution in the ratio 3:0.5 (NaOH/NH₄Cl). This changes the pH to 10. Microdrops of 20% v/v sulphuric acid are added to the cuvette to change it to pH 2.

For identification and interpretation of results, see "Barbiturates" in Part II.

Paracetamol is another very common drug that will be found in this fraction. It will be detected by a peak at 255 nm.

(See also Algeri and Walker, 1952; Bladh and Norden, 1958; Bogan *et al.,* 1965; Bogan and Smith, 1967; Comstock *et al.,* 1967; Curry, 1957; Curry and Sunshine, 1960; Curry, 1961; Olsen, 1967; Pilsbury and Jackson, 1966; Plaa and Hine, 1956; Plaa *et al.,* 1958; Rehling, 1967; Schreiner *et al.,* 1958; Stone and Henwood, 1967; Street, 1962; Turner, 1965) .

c. Neutral Fraction

This is examined by ultraviolet spectrophotometry using alcohol as solvent (see Table XVI) and then by the spot tests for carbamates. On many occasions sublimation can provide crystalline products suitable for melting points, infrared spectroscopy and gravimetric assay. In deaths from bromo-ureides, the corresponding compound with a hydrogen replacing the bromine atom may be found.

The spot test for carbamates is to take a 10-percent aliquot of the extract in ether and evaporate it onto a small spot on a filter paper. A drop of 10% furfural in alcohol is allowed to run carefully onto the spot and dried. The pap eris then exposed to fumes of hydrochloric acid in a beaker for several minutes when any carbamate will reveal its presence as a blue-purple spot.

The carbamates, 3-carbamoyloxy, 3-methylpentyl, 1-carbamyloxy-methyl 2-o-tolyloxyethanol, 2-2-dicarbamoyloxymethylpentane, and 1-ethynyl cyclohexyl carbamate are the most commonly sought drugs in this fraction. A paper chromatographic separation enables identification to be achieved while the acetylenic linkage in ethinamate and methyl pentynol carbamate provides another centre for attack by ammoniacal silver nitrate. Solvent systems recommended for this fraction are (a) isoamyl alcohol:water (190:10) ; (b) glacial acetic acid:water (100:100) on Whatman No. 1 paper that has been impregnated with 20% olive oil in acetone and dried; (c) methanol:water (180:20) also on olive oil paper.

Detection is achieved by exposing the paper to chlorine gas for ten minutes, then spraying with a 2% starch solution containing 1% potassium iodide after a period of aeration sufficiently long so that the background is nearly colorless.

THIN LAYER CHROMATOGRAPHY. The thin layer chromatography of neutral drugs has been reported by Haywood, Horner and Rylance (1967) using three solvent systems—ethyl acetate; dioxan:methylene chloride:water (1:2:1); and chloroform:acetone (9:1). Detection is achieved by inspection in 254 nm light or by the chlorine-starch-potassium iodide reaction. Several drugs, notably meprobamate, methylpentynol carbamate, methylprylone and Sedulon® are not detected in ultraviolet light. The procedure for the chemical detection is as follows.

The plates are exposed to chlorine gas for a few seconds, left in air for fifteen minutes and sprayed with 2% starch solution containing 1% potassium iodide. In ethyl acetate solvent using Merck Kieselgel GF254, TLC plates the following Rf values are found:

Meprobamate 0.48	Glutethimide 0.68
Methylpentynol carbamate 0.66	Mephenesin 0.48
Amidopyrine 0.25	Mephenesin carbamate 0.50

See also "meprobamate" in Part II.

A color test for meprobamate is to heat an aliquot of the evaporated extract with 3 ml of a solution of 2% hydroquinone in 85% v/v sulphuric acid for twenty-five minutes at 100 degrees C. A rose fluorescence is seen on inspection under Wood's light (365 nm).

Another useful test is Folin-Ciocalteau reagent which gives blue colors with methyprylone (Noludar®) when a 10% aliquot of the extract is tested with 0.5 ml reagent, then made alkaline with an equal volume of 2N sodium hydroxide.

Methaqualone may be found in this fraction if the first ether extraction was made from an acidic aqueous filtrate that was not at least 2N with sulphuric acid.

Any positive test will alert the toxicologist, and identification will probably be best achieved by isolation of milligram quantities from the alimentary tract unless, of course, sufficient is present in the liver or sophisticated instrumentation is available.

Cholesterol is frequently found in this liver extract, but

fortunately it has no significant contribution to make to the ultra-violet spectrum.

d. Alkaloids and Bases

As was noted above, the extraction by ether from ammoniacal solution is done in two stages, finishing with a final volume of 50 μl. The rationale of the examination of this fraction has been discussed in relation to the urine fractions, and there is no difference in principle here. The preferred method is to use paper or TLC using the butanol citric acid system on either buffered paper or cellulose TLC plates. Rf values are the same whichever system is used; TLC gives higher sensitivity and can be conveniently used as a relatively rapid screening procedure.

The total extract is divided into three 15-μl alcoholic aliquots which are run separately on the chromatogram. The solvent system consists of n-butanol:water:citric acid (435:65:2.4g) . The paper is Whatman No. 1 which has previously been dipped in 5% sodium dihydrogen citrate solution (23.5 g $Na_3C_6H_5O_7$. $2H_2O$ + 30.4 g citric acid dissolved in 1024 ml of water) and dried at 60 degrees C for twenty minutes. Merck Cellulose TLC plates can also be used. (When 100 g of liver has been processed, the writer's preference is for the paper system) . Control spots of nicotine, morphine, strychnine, quinine, phenazone and any other alkaloid that may be involved in the enquiry are also applied to serve as comparison spots; 2 μl of 2% solutions are suitable for these standards. After running and drying, the paper is inspected in 254 nm light; one extract is sprayed with Dragendorff's or iodo-platinate reagents leaving the other two extracts for other tests. If a positive reacting spot is obtained on spraying with iodoplatin-ate, elution of the spot from the chromatogram for ultraviolet spectrophotometry is probably the next simplest approach. When a base has been localised by iodoplatinate or Dragendorff reagents, it can be eluted by shaking the cut-out spot with ether (2 ml) after wetting the paper with 880 ammonia and adding a drop of 5% sodium sulphite and one drop of 10% barium chloride. Separation and evaporation of the ether, after filtering through a fluted filter paper, gives a clean extract suitable for ultraviolet spectrophotometry in 0.5 ml 0.1N H_2SO_4.

This extract is also suitable for examination by mass spectrometry. In the writer's opinion this latter procedure is the best way at the present time of identifying basic drugs. Many workers use gas chromatography-mass spectrometry for the examination of this extract, but the detection by gas chromatography of all bases is uncertain if only one system is used; then one is at the mercy of the separator between the gas chromatograph and the mass spectrometer. The elution of iodoplatinate positive reacting spots and the introduction of the recovered base (alkaloid) into the probe of the mass spectrometer has many advantages in that a chromatographically-purified compound is transferred with minimum loss to the mass spectrometer. Iodoplatinate positive spots must be treated as probable poisons whereas peaks on a gas chromatograph can be obtained from the most innocent liver. For those without mass spectrometers, analysis has to proceed on the basis of ultraviolet spectrophotometry and color tests. The ultraviolet maximum of bases to be found in this fraction are shown in Tables X and XI. The most useful color tests involve FPN reagent (p. 65) and Marquis reagent (p. 87). Very often a combination of these approaches will lead to a tentative identification being made especially when an Rf value and appearance in 254 nm light are taken into account. Final judgment of proof of identity rests with the toxicologists. As for quantitation, all the tests carry with them an exploitation as far as amount is concerned.

The purification of the unknown alkaloid by paper, TLC, or GLC can also be followed by an infrared examination. GLC is the best purification system, and excellent infrared curves can be obtained on 10 μg of trapped effluent. Using 0.5-mm discs, curves on as small a quantity as 200 nanograms can be obtained. In this technique a 1:10 splitter is used and the larger effluent trapped in a small glass tube to which it is carried by means of a heated line. The tube is cooled in liquid nitrogen and the geometry is important to avoid fog formation. The trapped extract is dissolved in 25 μl chloroform which is taken up into a repeating Hamilton Syringe; 0.5-μl aliquots are dispensed onto 0.5 mg potassium bromide allowing the chloroform to evaporate between each dispensation. When all 25 μl have been transferred, the microdisc is made with the KBr in the usual way. This method is most useful for nonvolatile acidic, neutral and alkaloid fractions (Curry *et al.,* 1968).

The paper or TLC chromatogram, on spraying with Dragendorff's solution or iodoplatinate, will show a positive reacting spot at Rf 0.05; it does not absorb or fluoresce in ultraviolet light. This alkaloid serves as an internal marker and should be obtained from all livers. Tables VII and XI give the Rf values and ultraviolet maxima for a number of common alkaloids, and Table XII gives Rf values for alkaloids reacting with Marquis reagent.

This particular examination is only one of the three designed to detect alkaloids in the liver in a comprehensive analysis. The other two, using hydrochloric acid digestion and continuous extraction with alcohol, are described below. Each has its separate function; none must be missed in a complete analysis.

e. Morphine Fraction

Morphine may be found in the alkaloid fraction because it can be salted out into ether. It is for this reason that the extract is redissolved in ethanol prior to chromatography. An extraction with chloroform : isopropanol (4 + 1) serves to complete the extraction. Morphine is detected by the use of paper chromatography or TLC on the evaporated extract. The solvent system of butanol/citric acid on citrated paper, as described above, will separate morphine not only from codeine and other opium alkaloids, but also from nalorphine which may have been given to counteract the poisoning. When 2% formaldehyde in concentrated sulphuric acid (Marquis reagent) is poured onto the dried paper chromatogram side by side with control spots of morphine, the beautiful violet spots that appear, coupled with the Rf value, provide criteria of identity that, as far as the writer is aware, are not paralleled by any other compound. However, further criteria can be obtained by the use of crystal tests on the eluate when even 0.025 μg will give characteristic-shaped crystals with potassium cadmium iodide solution. This reagent is made by mixing 1 g of cadmium iodide with 2 g of potassium iodide in 100 ml of water.

The volume of alkaloid and reagent solutions can be made as low as 0.1 μl by using the capillary rod technique for transfer (Clarke and Williams, 1955).

It is striking that reference is still made to a paper that is twenty years old in this context, but, again, it is a fact of life that in many parts of the world a crystal test is useful in that it is simple and cheap. Unfortunately, most sophisticated tests cost a great deal of money and not everyone can afford them. Therefore, included here is this now classic test.

f. Interpretation of Results

Tungstic acid and aluminum chloride are capricious in that they result in a nil recovery for many basic drugs. However, a sufficient number of drugs do appear in the extract that the extra effort following the look for acidic and neutral drugs is worthwhile. The following method (hydrochloric acid) is more efficient generally, and is rapid to perform, but it must be considered as complementary to the other methods rather than competitive.

For a general review of the efficiency of protein precipitation methods see Stevens, H.M., and Bunker, V.W. (In press). Their recoveries for basic drugs added to blood are shown in Table XVIII.

2. Hydrochloric Acid Digestion

Phenothiazines are very popular in the field of psychiatric medicine and severe side effects following therapeutic doses as well as poisoning following large overdoses have been noted for most, if not all, of the members of this group. Their popularity results in a need for consideration at this early stage of the analysis.

Normal extraction procedures do not recover the phenothiazines from blood or tissues samples, but Dubost and Pascal (1953, 1955) found that a strong hydrochloric acid treatment would release bound chlorpromazine and the other phenothiazines will respond to the same treatment. This preliminary hydrolysis also often gives greatly increased yields of other alkaloids, for example the tricylic antidepressants, quinine and imipramine, over more

TABLE XVIII
PERCENTAGE RECOVERIES OF DRUGS ADDED TO BLOOD USING DIFFERENT PROTEIN PRECIPITANTS

Name of Compound	λmax (nm)	$E_{1cm}^{1\%}$	μg per ml added to blood	% Recoveries of Added Substance							Special Remarks
				H_2WO_4	$(NH_4)_2SO_4$	$AlCl_3$	5N HCl (w)	8° (u)	TCA	$HClO_4$	
Amitriptyline	240	500	50	2	NIL	27	32	32	NIL	8	Chloroform used as extractant
Amitriptyline	240	500	50					NIL			
Amphetamine	257	15	200	62	27	35	35	82			Amphetamine is soluble 1 part in 50 parts of water
Antazoline	241	570	25	8	4	29	29	67			
Antazoline	241	570	8	11	NIL	31 (u)	50	60			
Caffeine	272	470	50	NIL	NIL	NIL	NIL	NIL			} Chloroform used as extractant
Caffeine	272	470	500	<1	<1	<1	<1				}
Caffeine	272	470	10	4	8	21		9			One ether extraction gives 66% recovery for $AlCl_3$
Chloroquine	343	496	20	2	10	50	69	87			
Chlorpromazine	255	1280	20	5*	7*	60*	43	43	17*	23**	Recovered as sulphoxide λmax 239nm, $E_{1cm}^{1\%} = 1120$
Chlorpromazine	255	1280	20				NIL				Chloroform used as extractant
Cocaine	233	470	20	5	11	24	NIL*	NIL*			*Probably decomposed by hot acid. Chloroform used as extractant
Codeine	284	52	125	17	21	83	90	90			Chloroform used as extractant
Colchicine	247	730	15	12	NIL*	NIL*	NIL*	NIL*			*Probably hydrolysed. Chloroform used as extractant
Cyclizine	262	28	250	9	22	43	68	68			
Dextropropoxyphene	257	12	350	9	NIL	40	d*	d*	6	30	d* = decomposed giving product λmax 252nm, $E_{1cm}^{1\%} > 200$

TABLE XVIII — (Cont'd)

Name of Compound	λmax (nm)	$E^{1\%}_{1cm}$	µg per ml added to blood	% Recoveries of Added Substance							Special Remarks
				H_2WO_4	$(NH_4)_2SO_4$	$AlCl_3$	5N HCl 8° (w)	5N HCl 8° (u)	TCA	$HClO_4$	
Ephedrine	257	12	460	55	35	17(w) 57(u)	14	90			Ephedrine is soluble 1 part in 36 parts of water
Imipramine	251	238	40	5	2	32	36	36	NIL	10	
Imipramine	251	238	50			11		NIL			Chloroform used as extractant
Lignocaine	262	13	340	40	24	44	60	71			
Mepyramine	239	633	15	16	32	34	26	48			λmax shift from 239 → 231nm by 5N HCl at 80°
Mescaline	268	39	150	45	34	47	55	55			
Methadone	259	18	300	NIL	NIL	35	33	41			Loss of peak λmax 292nm from hot 5N HCl method
Methaqualone	234	1300	25	6	7	7(w) 12(u)	10	38			No acid clean-up given. $2NH_2SO_4$ used to extract base
Methylamphetamine	257	10	600	30	36	30	61	71			
Morphine	251	255	200	38	35	35		72	46	50	
Morphine	251	255	20	39	52	41			49	26	
Nicotine	259	490	30	40	61	47	80	95	55	28	
Nicotine	259	490	6	48	71	56	80		50	30	
Opipramol	255	734	20	2	7	28	70	70	4	20	λmax shift from 255 → 259nm by $(NH_4)_2SO_4$ and TCA
Orphenadrine	264	24	230	12	NIL	21	NIL	NIL			
Papaverine	250	1830	5	4	<1	10	11	11			Chloroform used as extractant
Paraquat	257	693	25	8	2	2					
Pentazocine	278	112	60	9	NIL	37	64	64			
Pentazocine	278	112	30	15	NIL	47	73	73			
Perphenazine	254	833	20	3*	17*	43*	30	36			*Recovered as sulphoxide using chloroform as extractant. Figures are approximate

	1	2	3	4	5	6	7	8	Notes
Pethidine	257	8	870	27	34	60	93		Chloroform extracts dried with Na$_2$SO$_4$ and taken to dryness
Phenazone	230	588	30	20	57	NIL	NIL		
Quinine	250	1005	8	4	49	29	44	13	Chloroform used as extractant
Strychnine	255	315	15	15	52	61	61	22	Chloroform used as extractant
Thioridazine	263	1240	16	NIL	15*	NIL	NIL	44	Chloroform used as extractant. *Possibly sulphoxide (λmax 275nm)
Thioridazine	263	1240	25	NIL	12*	10	10		*Possibly sulphoxide (λmax 275 nm) so figure is approximate
Tranylcypromine	264	16	325	45	50	32	40	36	*Recovered as sulphoxide, so figures approximate
Trifluoperazine	256	739	25	3*	37*	20	20	30	
Tryptamine	278	349	25	22	8	13	56		Putrefactive base which sometimes interferes in analysis
Tyramine	275	110	50	3	2	18	55		Putrefactive base. NH$_3$ used to make 5NHCl digest alkaline

Symbols: (w) Solvent extract washed with water; (u) Solvent extract dried with anhydrous Na$_2$SO$_4$ without washing with water.

General: All weights and recovery percentages refer to free base. Unless otherwise stated extractions were made with ether and were water-washed.

Courtesy of Stevens, H.M., and Bunker, V.

conventional extraction procedures such as those using ethanol, and detection following isolation should include tests not only for the phenothiazines, but also for other alkaloids.

METHOD. 10 g of liver are macerated with 10 ml of water, and 13.5 ml of concentrated hydrochloric acid are added. If the test is being done by the clinical chemist, 10 g of blood are mixed with 2 ml of water and 8 ml of hydrochloric acid. The acid digest is then heated in a beaker in a boiling water bath for five minutes after which time it is removed and placed in an ice bath; 12 ml of 60% potassium hydroxide (previously washed with ether) are added with stirring, and the pH is checked to ensure alkalinity. If acid, more alkali is added. When cool the solution is shaken with 150 ml of purified ether. Any emulsion is broken by centrifuging and the ether is removed. A further portion of 50 ml of ether is used for extraction and the ether extracts are combined. These are shaken with 10 ml of 2.5% sodium hydroxide, followed by 10 ml of water and 5 ml of water. Finally, the ether is extracted with 5 ml of 0.1N sulphuric acid which is separated, and, after blowing off the ether, is examined by ultraviolet spectrophotometry from 220 to 320 nm.

It is absolutely essential to use peroxide-free ether and not halogenated hydrocarbons such as chloroform or ethylene dichloride in the extraction process. Most phenothiazine sulphoxides are converted back to the parent drug by the hydrochloric acid digest. Stevens and Bunker (vide supra) noted that, of thirty-six common drugs studied, only orphenadrine and phenazone were undetectable after this procedure.

Tungstic acid isolation methods will convert most phenothiazines to their sulphoxides; strong hydrochloric acid treatment usually results in the phenothiazines themselves being isolated.

Provided the hydrochloric acid is distilled before use and adequate precautions are taken about the purity of the other reagents, the background absorption from normal blood and brain can be made very low. Liver extracts have a small maximum at 250 nm. The detection and estimation of toxic doses of the phenothiazines in such samples by ultraviolet spectrophotometry therefore is possible, and, in any case, the detection of other alkaloids and basic drugs with high absorption is also ensured. The phenothiazines show an absorption maximum at approximately 255 nm with $E_{1cm}^{1\%}$ values about 1,000. Any chlorpromazine sulphoxide present is converted to chlorpromazine by the strong acid treatment. The sulphoxide with absorption peaks at 240, 275, 300 and 340 nm will be found in the urine.

Amitriptyline and nortriptyline are two common drugs that will also be found in this fraction. (Their recovery using the tungstic acid procedure is nil.) They give no colours with FPN reagent but have λ max at 238 to 240 nm unchanged by the addition of alkali to the acid solution (Table X).

Nikethamide, with a maximum about 260 nm, may often be encountered. The background absorption in liver extracts, however, tends to rise about the wavelength maximum shown by the phenothiazines, and even if a good curve suggestive of a phenothiazine is obtained, further confirmatory tests must be applied. The quickest of these is to re-extract the alkaloid fraction into ether after making the sulphuric acid solution alkaline with ammonia. Dry with a little sodium sulphate and evaporate to about 0.1 ml. About 1 μl is then allowed to dry on a filter paper, and a drop of FPN reagent is allowed to flow into it. Positive results in the form of red, purple, blue or green colors indicate the presence of a phenothiazine. These compounds can be rapidly separated from impurities by paper electrophoresis on Whatman 3-mm paper at 200 volts in 6% acetic acid in about two hours. A strongly reacting aliquot is applied to the paper which is exposed to 254 nm. light for three minutes after partially drying off the acetic acid on completion of the chromatogram. It is finally sprayed with FPN reagent. Color comparisons with standards give estimates of quantity. Further results are obtained by paper chromatography, and Table XIX shows the results with a number of common phenothiazines.

It is also worthwhile testing an aliquot of the extract with Dragendorff's reagent because of the increased yield of many alkaloids in this extraction process. If positive, paper or TLC chromatography is used as described in Chapter 4.

If blue colors are noted on exposure to ultraviolet light or

TABLE XIX
PAPER CHROMATOGRAPHY OF PHENOTHIAZINES

Compound	Rf Value*	Colour of Spot** on Exposure to 254 nm Light	Colour with FPN Reagent
Perphenazine	.50	yellow/grey	red
Prochlorperazine	.50	—	red
Trifluoperazine	.55	—	orange
Fluphenazine	.64	—	orange
Promazine	.71	orange	orange
Notensil	.72	—	orange-red
Thiopropazate	.73	—	red
Pecazine	.74	salmon	orange
Veractil	.77	violet	violet
Chlorpromazine	.77	yellow/green	red
Promethazine	.78	—	pink-red
Trifluopromazine	.81	—	orange-yellow
Ethopropazine	.81	—	red
Diethazine	.81	—	orange-red brown
Imipramine	.81	—	turquoise
Thioridazine	.81	green	blue

*In butanol 100: water 100: citric acid 2 g top layer on Whatman No. 1 paper impregnated with 5% sodium dihydrogen citrate and dried.
**After electrophoresis

with the spray, thioridazine or imipramine are indicated (see Part II for quantitative assay).

The TLC separation of forty phenothiazines and their sulphoxide derivatives has been studied by Kofoed and his co-workers. Silica-Gel GF 254 (Merck) is used with a solvent of 1.5 g ammonium acetate; water, 10 ml; methanol to 50 ml. The phenothiazine is converted to the sulphoxide by treatment on the plate with 10 to 20% hydrogen peroxide with hot air to dry the spot. Elution with water is followed by ultraviolet spectrophotometry. Their results are shown in Table XX.

These authors have also used 60 cm $\times$ 7 mm 3% SE30 on Gas Chrom Q 80/100 mesh at 210 to 250 degree C for the separation of phenothiazines.

INTERPRETATION OF RESULTS. If a phenothiazine can be detected in a 10-ml sample of blood using ultraviolet methods, then considerably more than a normal therapeutic dose has been in-

TABLE XX
TLC OF PHENOTHIAZINE SULPHOXIDES

Generic Name	Rf Value		λMaxima of the Sulfoxides Obtained in the Manner Described
	Original Drug	Sulfoxide	
Acetophenazine	0.69	0.16	251-274S-310
Acetopromazine or acetylpromazine	0.58	0.39	251-272S-310-343
Aminopromazine or proquamezine	0.60	0.28	232-266-295-333
Carphenazine	0.71	0.16	264-277S-310
Chlorpromazine	0.62	0.48	238-273-298-340
Chlorproethazine	0.69	0.49	238-250S-273-298-340
Chlorprothixene	0.66	0.45	255-302
Cyamepromazine	0.61	0.39	243-274S-304-340
Diethazine	0.69	0.44	233-268-293-338
Dimethoxanate	0.56	0.41	240-274-295
Ethopropazine or prophenamine	0.70	0.47	233-267-292-336
Fluphenazine	0.75	0.59	232-273-304-343
Isopromethazine	0.63	0.39	233-267-291-336
Isothipendyl	0.64	0.41	238-273-336
Levopromazine	0.87	0.59	250-276S-296-333
Mepazine	0.58	0.39	231-272-299-342
Methdilazine	0.64	0.43	232-272-298-342
Methopromazine or methoxypromazine	0.67	0.35	244-274S-294-330
Methylpromazine	0.62	0.40	238-272-299-340
Perphenazine or chlorpiprozine	0.65	0.45	240-250S-274-342
Phenothiazine or fenethazine	0.69	0.37	232-266-294-334
Pipamazine	0.83	0.53	239-274-300-342
Prochlorperazine	0.55	0.15	238-274-300-340
Promazine	0.51	0.37	231-271-299-342
Promethazine	0.66	0.38	232-270-297-340
Propiomazine	0.77	0.54	246-265S-304-360
Prothipendyl	0.69	0.48	238-276-340
Pyrathiazine or pyrrolazate	0.64	0.43	232-269-295-336
Thiazinamium	0.53	0.33	232-269-294-336
Thiethylperazine	0.47	0.28	238-272-301-350
Thiopropazate	0.77	0.25	238-274-300-340
Thioproperazine	0.43	0.26	245-262S-275-304-342
Thioridazine	0.71	0.45	237-273-302-340
Transergan	0.53	0.33	225-266-291-330
Trifluoperazine	0.63	0.41	233-273-302-343
Triflupromazine	0.69	0.50	233-274-301-343
Trimeprazine or alimemazine	0.71	0.50	232-297-340
No. 6710 Rhöne-Poulenc	0.63	0.46	251-273-298-332
No. 9260 Rhöne-Poulenc	0.85	0.59	240-274-305
No. 7261 Smith Kline & French	0.78	0.27	233-272-302-340

*J. Kofoed, C. Fabierkiewcz and G. H. W. Lucas: A study of the conversion of phenothiazine derivatives to the corresponding sulfoxides on thin-layer plates. *J Chromatogr, 23:*410, 1966.

gested. As indicated above, concentrations in liver may be much higher than those in blood. In a case in which 2 g of thioridazine had been taken, the blood level was only 0.18 mg/100 ml, although 8 mg/100 g were found in the liver (author). In general, levels in excess of 0.1 mg/100 ml in the blood indicate large doses. A single dose of 1 g of chlorpromazine can be expected to lead to blood levels of about 0.1 to 0.2 mg/100 ml. Imipramine (Tofranil) and desipramine (Pertofran), when taken in gram quantities, also give concentrations in the blood of about 0.1 mg/100 ml, although the liver may contain several milligrams/100 g.

Many psychotic patients take very considerable doses of these drugs—sometimes of the order of grams per day. Withdrawal symptoms when these are suddenly stopped may be alarming, and tests on the urine will indicate the probable dosage.

The toxicological literature is full of papers on the metabolism of the antidepressant drugs. Probably the phenothiazines hold the record for the number of products that may appear as a result of the body's detoxication mechanisms. The reader who wishes to study these must go to the literature. The purpose of this section is to detect overdoses. Detailed references for each phenothiazine are given in Part II.

(See also Algeri *et al.,* 1959; Anders and Mannering, 1962; Bramlett, 1966; Dubost and Pascal, 1953; Dubost and Pascal, 1955; Forrest and Forest, 1960; Kofoed, *et al.,* 1966; Turner, 1963).

3. Tests for Arsenic

Arsenious oxide is one of the classic poisons in the long history of toxicology. In many parts of the world it is still a common poison although it is slowly being displaced by chemotherapeutic agents or by insecticides. Because it holds a foremost place in the minds of most clinicians and some murderers, its inclusion in a systematic search for poison is obvious. Blood levels are low even in cases of acute poisoning, and it is more convenient to take a 2-g sample of liver at this stage in the analysis. In the living patient, however, analysis of vomit, blood and urine are all often undertaken; 10 ml of urine is a convenient volume.

In the United Kingdom in the last few years there have been

several murders involving arsenic, and it is emphasized again that toxicologists must not think that arsenic is now an antique poison. In any routine screen, tests for it *must* be included.

So as to emphasize that the test must be done at this stage in the analyses the analytical details are given here.

METHOD 1. In a Kjeldahl flask, 2 g of liver (5 ml of blood or 10 ml of urine) are evaporated with 10 ml of concentrated nitric acid and 2 ml of concentrated sulphuric acid. As soon as charring is seen, more nitric acid is added. Charring carries with it the possibility of reduction of arsenic to the trivalent ion and its loss by volatility. The heating and addition of nitric acid is continued until all organic material has been destroyed. This takes about a quarter of an hour; 20 ml of water are then added and the volume is reduced by boiling to about 4 ml; 10 ml of a saturated solution of ammonium oxalate are then added, and the boiling is continued until white fumes appear. After cooling, the digest is transferred with washing from the Kjeldahl flask into a suitable Gutzeit apparatus.

This is so well known that a complete description will be omitted; 4 ml of concentrated hydrochloric acid, 5 ml of 15% sodium iodide and 0.4 ml of 40% stannous chloride in 50% hydrochloric acid with 10 g 16-22 mesh zinc are added and the liberated arsine and hydrogen passed through a plug of cotton wool soaked in lead acetate, then through a filter paper which has been previously soaked in a saturated solution of mercuric bromide in alcohol and dried. The filter paper is held in an accurately machined metal or glass holder with a center hole 5 mm in diameter (see Fig. 8). After one hour or less, if control experiments so indicate, the filter paper, now stained yellow, or brown if large quantities are present, is removed and placed in a cardboard or metal frame for insertion in a spectrophotometer. This frame is fixed so that light from the spectrophotometer is made to pass through the area of filter paper showing the stain on to the photocell where optical density readings at 400 nm and 500 nm are taken.

Calibration graphs are prepared for stains from 0 to 1 μg at 400 nm and 0 to 10 μg at 500 nm. Any subsequent stain from 0 to 10 μg can therefore be accurately measured. The great advantage in using this method of assay is that standard stains do not have to be prepared every day as they do if visual comparison is used; in addition, a black cardboard or metal holder for the spectrophotometer can easily be made to give an accuracy of ±5 percent even in the 0 to 1μg range. Black is used to prevent errors from reflectance of light from the front of the holder; the filter paper is held by tape on the face of the holder away from the light (see Fig. 9).

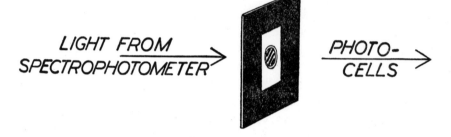

Figure 9. Method of measuring stains from a Gutzeit holder.

Arsine intoxication is occasionally met, usually as a result of an industrial accident. A renal shut-down is usual, and no urine can be collected. Using neutron activation techniques, high levels of arsenic in the root of the hair can be detected within a few days of exposure, and such tests provide valuable confirmation for the clinician. If a muscle biopsy is performed, elevated levels over normal may also be found (see Part II).

METHOD 2. (Fisher Scientific Company). Concentrated hydrochloric acid (2 ml), 2 ml of 15% potassium iodide solution and eight drops of a stannous chloride solution containing 40 g of stannous chloride in 100 ml concentrated hydrochloric acid are added to the solution containing the arsenic salt in 35 ml of water. Swirl the flasks and allow them to stand for fifteen minutes to ensure complete reduction to the trivalent stage; 3 g of granulated zinc are then added, and the liberated arsine is passed through a scrubber of lead acetate on glass wool, then through 3 ml of a 0.5% solution of silver diethyldithiocarbamate in pyridine. The scrubber and the reagent with which arsine forms a red complex are part of special Gutzeit-type of apparatus known as an arsine generator. The reaction is usually complete in thirty minutes after which the color is read at 560 nm. Standards are prepared in the range 0 to 15 μg. Stibine gives a red color as well and could therefore interfere, but this has maximum absorbance at 510 nm.

OTHER METHODS. Freeze-dried tissue can be irrdiated in a nuclear reactor which has a flux of about 10^{13} n/cm^2, and the resulting radioactive arsenic separated by the arsine/Gutzeit procedure. Clearly it is impossible to give full details here, but the toxicologist must remember that this is a recognized procedure, and in some areas may be available as a routine service. It is unrealistic, however, to consider it in every case of unnatural sudden death. Similarly, some laboratories may have the specially sensitive atomic absorption apparatus (normal flame atomic absorption is unsuitable), but descriptions are clearly inappropriate here. What needs to be emphasized is that arsenic must be sought at this stage of the analysis. For further details see Part II.

4. Test for Yellow Phosphorus and Phosphides

If a fatty, yellow liver is found at autopsy, four poisons must be considered immediately; these are arsenic, carbon tetrachloride, *Amanita phalloides* and yellow phosphorus. The writer has also seen a liver of this type in a young child following ingestion of ferrous sulphate. The circumstances of the death will undoubtedly be closely investigated in such cases, and enquiries will have been started at the instigation of the pathologist.

In children, there is a condition characterized clinically by repeated vomiting and increasing drowsiness preceding the onset of coma by intervals of a few hours to three days. Wild delirium may also be seen. The usual provisional diagnosis is encephalitis, but at autopsy the characteristic finding is a uniformly bright yellow or orange-yellow liver with fat distribution in small vacuoles within the parenchymal-cell cytoplasm. This condition is now known as *Reyes syndrome,* and hundreds of cases have been reported. At the time of writing, it is close to top of the popularity league in clinical medicine literature, and, thanks to alleged correlations with aflatoxin or influenza viruses, it seems unlikely that all these children have been deliberately poisoned.

The presence of an alkaloid in urine fluorescing blue under 254 nm light having an Rf = 0.45 in the butanol/citrate system (see Chap. 4) with λ max in 0.1N sulphuric acid = 255 and 330 nm and λ min = 280 nm, has been the only potentially significant finding for the toxicologist. The alkaloid has not been identified, but, on the basis of microbiological activity it has been tentatively classed as a pteridine (Curry, Guttman and Price, 1962).

Notwithstanding this special enquiry, the following test should be done routinely in areas where yellow phosphorus is available to the general public. Its most common form in the United Kingdom used to be as a sugar paste containing bran sold as a rodenticide. In the United States 3% phosphorus in a rat poison paste is available.

METHOD (SCHWARTZ *et al.*, 1955). From the center of the liver 50 g are cut into small pieces and covered with water in tube B of the apparatus shown in Figure 7. Tube A is used as a water bubbler to show the flow rate of nitrogen which is passed slowly through the apparatus. The Gutzeit holder shown in Figure 8 is placed at the exit with a filter paper which has been soaked in a saturated methanolic silver nitrate solution and dried. The head is filled with glass wool that has been soaked in lead acetate solution and dried. Nitrogen is passed through the apparatus for thirty minutes. A black stain on the filter paper indicates the presence of phosphine in the liver. Any stain is oxidised to phosphate by exposing it to chlorine vapor (made in a small generator by dropping concentrated hydrochloric acid onto solid potassium permanganate) for five minutes. The stain should be completely decolorized. A cold air stream, which is conveniently obtained from a hair dryer, is then blown over the paper for five minutes to remove excess chlorine.

The phosphate is converted to phosphomolybdaté by dropping on one drop of ammonium molybdate solution (5 g ammonium molybdate dissolved in 100 ml of water and mixed with 35 ml of concentrated nitric acid), and after standing at room temperature for three minutes is evaporated to dryness on a Petri dish or white tile over a boiling water bath. It is then removed and allowed to cool. When absolutely cold, one drop of benzidine solution (0.05 g benzidine in 10 ml glacial acetic acid is diluted to 100 ml with water) is dropped on the center of the paper which is then very carefully exposed to the fumes of ammonia. A positive result is shown as a blue color which is not stable and which in the lowest range of detection—about 0.1 μg phosphorus—is very transient.

The same procedure is repeated after adding 10 ml dilute sulphuric acid to the liver, and again after surrounding the tube B with a heating jacket and raising its temperature to 100 degrees C. The second passage of nitrogen liberates phosphine which may be present from any unchanged phosphide—the rodenticide zinc phosphide is the only one that need be considered—or from a yellow phosphorus metabolite which is as yet still uncharacterized. The third passage of nitrogen distils out any unchanged yellow phosphorus.

The oxidation and production of reduced phosphomolybdate blue is exactly the same in each case; the paper may have to be changed several times if large quantities of poison are present. Fatty livers and intestine walls not containing poison produce a yellow stain on the silver nitrate paper which is of no significance. A silvery sheen to a faint stain should also be regarded with suspicion; in all cases it is essential to confirm by the phosphomolybdate test.

INTERPRETATION OF RESULTS. The test is very sensitive and has detected phosphorus in a liver exhumed after thirteen months' burial. In other cases positive results have been obtained even though eight days elapsed between ingestion and death. Artefacts have not been reported.

No quantitative estimate of the ingested dose can be given from the result of this test on the liver. If no phosphorus can be detected in the intestinal tract, a positive test on the liver is the only available chemical evidence for poisoning and, even then only the metabolite may be present. In the writer's opinion, this is sufficient; it must be admitted, however, that in putrefied tissue there is the possibility of phosphine production from bacterial reduction of phosphate. This might cause difficulty in interpretation if it was suspected that zinc phosphide had been ingested because phosphine is the major metabolite of this rodenticide.

Levels of 49 $\mu g\%$ in liver, 9.5 $\mu g\%$ in kidney and 780 $\mu g\%$ in liver were found by Winek *et al.* in the three cases when tissue was steam distilled into silver nitrate, the precipitated silver phosphide was oxidised to phosphate which was then measured colorimetrically by the well known Fiske and Subbarow method (Fiske and Subbarow, 1925).

See also Bougeois *et al.,* 1971; Chang *et al.,* 1973; Curry *et al.,* 1962; Linnemann *et al.,* 1974; Reye and Morgan, 1963; Winek *et al.,* 1973.

B. THE SECOND STAGE
1. Metals
a. Thallium

In the forms of the soluble acetate and sulphate, thallium is a highly toxic rodenticide and is favored by criminal poisoners. Therapeutic accidents occur because the effective dose is too close to a toxic one. Dermatologists should be warned that 8.5 mg/kg is likely to cause death in children. The outstanding point of interest for the toxicologist is that symptoms are delayed for several days after ingestion, and death for much longer.

The outstanding symptoms are burning sensations over the lower extremities so that even the bedclothes become an intolerable burden, and the loss of hair occurs about fourteen days after ingestion. A microscopical examination of the hair root is most useful because the medulla becomes grossly enlarged, virtually filling the bulb. It is said that repeated doses lead to similar enlargements along the length of the hair, but this requires further substantiation. There is, similarly, no published evidence to show whether thallium is incorporated like arsenic into the growing hair. The loss of hair, presumably because of the toxic action of the metal, is apparent from small doses, so chronic criminal administration from low doses over a long period is probably less likely than with arsenic.

There is a danger that thallium could be missed if analysis is confined to the alimentary tract, and it is recommended that a portion of tissue be analysed routinely. Kidney is probably the best theoretical choice, but the limited amount, which may be required for other purposes, leaves liver or muscle with the second highest expected concentration. Such an analysis must therefore be done at this stage in a routine screen.

The choice of method depends on the instrumentation available; direct introduction of urine into a flame atomic absorption spectrophotometer is an easy, rapid screen. Alternatively, liver must be used if urine is not available, and, after atomic absorption, wet ashing followed by isolation and identification of thallous iodide is necessary.

METHOD (CURRY *et al.,* 1969). Blood or tissue (1-2 g) is heated in a Kjeldahl flask with 1 ml concentrated nitric acid and 1 ml concentrated sulphuric acid. More nitric acid is added as required until no further charring occurs on evolution of white fumes; cool; transfer with water washings to a boiling tube to a total volume of 10 to 15 ml. Add a few drops of thymol blue and adjust the pH with drops of concentrated ammonia with cooling until the solution turns yellow; 0.5 ml of 48% hydrobromic acid and one drop of liquid bromine are added, and the solution is boiled until it is colorless or a constant pale yellow color. Transfer to a 50-ml separating funnel and shake with 5 ml of water-saturated methyl-isobutyl ketone for one minute. Separate and shake the organic phase with 5 ml 1N hydrobromic acid. Separate and centrifuge the organic phase for five minutes in a capped vial and aspirate into the flame of a Perkin-Elmer 303 Atomic Absorption Spectrophotometer set at 2768 Å with a Boling three-slot burner (scale expansion $\times$ 3, noise $\times$ 2). Recovery is better than 98 percent. Standards of added thallium to tissue in the range 0.5 to 2.0 μg g are suitable.

Urine. Direct aspiration into the flame is suitable; aqueous standards are used. One percent absorption is found for 80 μg/ 100 ml. An alternative method is given by Berman (1967).

ALTERNATIVE METHOD. Liver, 50 g, is boiled with 200 ml of dilute hydrochloric acid and 100 volume hydrogen peroxide is added periodically in 5-ml aliquots until there is complete solution of the tissue. The cooled, aqueous solution is then extracted with three times an equal volume of ether which is separated and evaporated. This procedure extracts thallic chloride which is soluble in ether, and also any remaining fatty material. After evaporation the organic matter is destroyed by boiling with drops of mixed nitric and sulphuric acid. After dilution, reduction with sulphur dioxide and adjustment of the pH to approximately 5, thallous iodide is precipitated by the addition of potassium iodide solution. Let the solution stand for several hours for the yellow-green precipitate to form. Do *not* assume that the absence of an immediate precipitate is a negative case. It is important to keep the volume as small as possible. The precipitate can be assayed gravimetrically after collection and washing on a weighed Gooch crucible. Confirmation of identity is obtained by arc emission spectroscopy, the indicating line being at 3262.3 Å. An accurate microbalance is essential if the gravimetric method is used.

INTERPRETATION OF RESULTS. The minimum lethal dose for an adult is said to be about 0.8 g or 12 mg/kg. In fatal acute poisonings tissue levels can be expected in the range of 0.5 to 10 mg/100 g of tissue. The method described above whereby thallous iodide is precipitated is sufficiently sensitive provided 50 g of tissue at least are used.

Urinary excretion is said to vary considerably over even a twenty-four hour period and, therefore, estimates of dose from a single urine concentration are very difficult. In nonfatal poisonings, excretion has been shown to extend over a period of months. Concentrations vary from several milligrams per twenty-four hours to as low as 30 μg/litre. The analyst must, therefore, be able to demonstrate certain detection at the lower end of this range. Blood levels in nonfatal cases have also been reported as low as 10 μg/100 ml.

Levels in the normal population are known to be of the order of nanograms per gram, so no problems should exist in deciding cases in which death is thought to have occurred from acute thallium poisoning.

The toxicologist should take note that, repeatedly, clinicians do not recognize thallium poisoning, and only when the pathologist finds the hair of the deceased comes out easily or a detective meets a forensic toxicologist do such cases come to light. The same has been said in relation to arsenic; although Hausman and Wilson (1964) referred to thallium as a social menace, the criminal poisoner is one too, and therefore the tests described above must be performed.

See also Curry *et al.,* (1969) ; Domnitz (1960) ; Hubler, (1966); Loos and Timperman, (1959) ; Matthys, (1958) ; Prick, *et al.,* (1955) ; Sunderman, (1967) ; Weinig and Zink, (1967).

b. Other Metals

The metals which need to be seriously considered are lead, copper, iron, zinc, cadmium and mercury. As far as these are concerned it is likely they will be detected by tests on the alimentary tract, but specific details for each are given in Part II and the toxicologist must not forget them.

The following test has been included in the third edition of this book for two reasons. First, it is common sense to try and test for all metals, and secondly, if one does not have a spark source mass spectrometer it is difficult to know what else to recommend. One could run a battery of atomic absorption tests, but in a look for an unknown poison one has to balance initiative and subjective judgment against practicalities.

METHOD. Liver, 100 g, is heated on a boiling water bath with 100 ml of concentrated nitric acid in a Kjeldahl flask. After the reaction has subsided, 10 ml of concentrated sulphuric acid are added, and the mixture is gently boiled over a Bunsen flame. When the first signs of charring are seen, 5 ml of nitric acid are added and the heating repeated. This procedure is continued until all the organic matter is destroyed. If necessary, more sulphuric acid may be added during the digestion. The digest is then diluted with 20 ml of water, cooled and neutralized to pH 5 with ammonia. Any precipitate is removed by centrifuging. Hydrogen sulphide is passed, and, after allowing several hours for precipitation, any solid is removed. More hydrogen sulphide is passed after making the solution alkaline when a copious black precipitate is seen. This is also removed and washed. Ammonium phosphate is then added to the supernatant, and, after warming, any Group V precipitate is centrifuged off.

Examination of the precipitates is preferably done by arc spectroscopy, but paper chromatography is an acceptable and simpler method. Full details given on page 149. The paper chromatographic method enables any gross abnormality to be detected immediately by visual inspection.

It is rare for the toxicologist to perform, routinely, quantitative assays for the common metals, but if any suspicion of abnormality is detected, then obviously such analyses must be done.

2. Continuous Extraction with Alcohol

If the reader has already performed the previous analyses on liver it is doubtful if it is worthwhile to perform the following test. This is based on opinions of practicalities, not on perfection. This section of the book has been kept because in many countries tissues are submitted to the laboratory already preserved in alcohol. The apparatus described below is then cost-effective compared to the Stas-Otto procedure. For the perfectionist and the toxicologist who are required to use the technique there is no doubt that it is valuable.

METHOD (CURRY AND PHANG, 1960). Liver, 250 g, is macerated with 500 ml of 95% ethanol and 5 g of tartaric acid and placed in the left-hand flask (1 litre capacity) shown in the apparatus in Figure 10. This is known as the extraction flack. Additional ethanol is added to bring the level just to the point of overflowing into the conical flask which is filled with absolute ethanol. The 500-ml evaporation flask on the right of the figure is filled to approximately three-fourths full, also with absolute ethanol. This evaporation flask sits on a water bath held at 90 degrees C. Its upper surface is covered by cotton wool to reduce heat losses. When pressure is reduced in the apparatus by means of a water pump to 14 cm of mercury, the ethanol in the evaporation flask boils, aided by a fine air leak, is condensed by the triple surface condenser, and is returned to the extraction flask under the settled tissue. A clear circulating flow of liquid ethanol from left to right is thus established through the apparatus. The conical flask acts as an intermediate settling tank, and the plastic or rubber con-

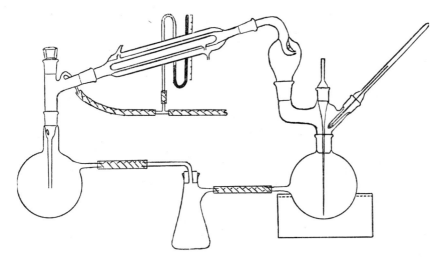

Figure 10. An apparatus for the continuous extraction under reduced pressure of tissue with ethanol.

nectors between the flasks allow for easy assembly. The small hole in the return from the condenser to the extraction flask equalises pressure to avoid disturbance of the tissue when slight unavoidable pressure changes occur.

There are many advantages to the use of this simple apparatus; the extraction is at room temperature, and, because of the reduced pressure, it is at no time higher than 30 degrees C to 35 degrees C. These conditions are so mild that glycosides and such labile alkaloids as atropine and cocaine are not destroyed. The volume of ethanol is kept to a minimum by the use of continuous extraction and, even if pressure is accidentally allowed to rise, all the extracts and tissue are safe and cannot be lost down the pump. The other outstanding advantage is the fact that this type of extraction, which used to take days, can now be completed in a matter of hours.

The only precautions that are necessary are to ensure that the pressure does not fall too low so that there is a gross loss of ethanol down the pump; the water flow through the condenser must be as cold and as fast as possible to ensure efficient cooling of the

ethanol vapor. Sufficient heat must be applied to the evaporation
flask to ensure a rapid boiling of the solvent.

When the extraction is finished, which can be seen by observing the clearance of color above the tissues, the fluid in the
evaporation flask is evaporated to dryness under reduced pressure.
It is then re-extracted with hot absolute ethanol which is filtered
and evaporated to dryness. The fatty solid is then shaken with
150 ml of cold 0.001N sulphuric acid for at least thirty minutes
in an effort to bring into solution, without loss, heat labile alkaloids and glycosides. After filtration the solid is again extracted
with 150 ml of 0.001N sulphuric acid, but this time by boiling.
After filtering, the filtrates are combined when cold and extracted
with ether, first from acid and then from ammoniacal solution.
Morphine, caffeine, antipyrine and the glycosides can then be extracted from the neutralized combined aqueous solutions by
chloroform + isopropanol $(4 + 1)$. In general, the volume of the
organic phase should at least equal that of the aqueous. Subsequent examination follows that detailed in Chapter 4.

If solanine poisoning is suspected, warm pentanol will extract
it from alkaline solution. Detection is by dipping a citrated chromatogram run as for other alkaloids in 1% paraformaldehyde in
concentrated phosphoric acid. A blue color at Rf 0.23 indicates
this poison. See Clarke (1958).

The most common glycoside in medicinal use is probably digoxin; it is commonly eaten accidentally by young children. The
obvious place to seek it is in the alimentary tract, but the liver
should not be neglected. It can be extracted in the apparatus described above and recovered from the chloroform phase. Some
measure of purification can be achieved by shaking a 70% ethanol
in water solution of the glycosides with carbon tetrachloride; fat
is removed and the poisons can be recovered after evaporation of
the ethanol phase by distillation under reduced pressure. Paper
chromatographic separation followed by color tests on the paper
or screening of eluates on the isolated frog heart are then indicated. In chloroform:methanol:water (10:2:5), organic layer,
it has an Rf of 0.71. Detection is by a spray of 5% m-dinitroben-
zene in benzene (beware fumes) followed by heating at 80 de-

grees C for fifteen minutes, and, finally, dipping in 20% sodium hydroxide when the blue colors are obtained.

For a separation using TLC plates the reader is referred to Part II, See Digitalis Glycosides.

A TLC separation of cardiac glycosides has also been reported by Johnston and Jacobs. Activated (120°C) plates of Silica-Gel G are used with a solvent of benzene:ethanol (7:3 v/v). Detection is achieved either by a spray of perchloric acid which produces spots fluorescing under 365 nm light, or by a spray of p-anisaldehyde which produces blue spots (oubain, yellow) after heating at 100 degrees C for a few minutes. Rf values are ouabain, 0.09; deslanoside, 0.27; lanatoside C, 0.36; digoxin, 0.62; digitoxin, 0.72; and acetyldigoxin, 0.82. Jelliffe has reported the detection of urinary digitoxin and digoxin in man in twenty-four-hour urine samples using a chloroform extraction and TLC (see Part II). Clearly, radioimmonoassay can also be used.

See also Brown *et al.*, (1956).

INTERPRETATION OF RESULTS. The main purpose of this extraction process is to extract sufficient poison to enable identification. When this has been done it is probable that another quantitative analysis on a smaller quantity of tissue will be done using a method of extraction and assay most suited to that particular poison.

As was indicated above and in Chapter 4, the main approach to the analyses consists of paper chromatographic examinations coupled with color tests, ultraviolet spectrophotometry and infrared spectroscopy. The importance of routine sublimation of an aliquot of the neutral ether and of the chloroform extraction fractions must be stressed because these usually consist of several milligrams of fatty material from which crystalline poison can often be obtained by this simple technique. The absence of crystals, however, should not indicate the absence of poison—in such cases the challenge to the toxicologist is even greater.

Full consideration of the interpretation of results cannot be given because each poison requires specific mention, and the number to be discussed would amount to many thousands. It is important to remember that an assumption that a poison is evenly distributed in the body tissues must not be made without experimental verification. In some cases a much higher concentration of poison can be found in the liver than in any other organ, for example in poisonings by orphenadrine, Nupercaine® and imipramine, but in others, notably salicylate in aspirin poisoning, the concentration is usually lower than in the blood. The ratios may also vary greatly with the time between ingestion and death.

Some poisons do not appear in the liver unchanged, but must be sought as metabolites; for example, 2,4-dichlorophenoxyacetic acid from its ethyl ester, and diethylacetyl urea in carbromal intoxication.

The difference in half-lives must also be considered—some are very short, measured in minutes, while those of drugs like quinine are so long that the drug can be detected for days after the ingestion of therapeutic quantities.

Generally, phenothiazines, orphenadrine, propoxyphene, amitriptyline, opipranol, pethidine, morphine, imipramine and desipramine have toxic blood levels well below 0.5 mg/100 ml, but, for the majority of these drugs, the liver should contain concentrations of milligrams/100 g. Choroquine, hydroxychloroquine, methaqualone, nicotine and tolazoline will probably appear in the blood with levels over 0.5 mg/100 ml, but even in these cases liver tissue will give higher levels. There is, in the writers view, in fatal cases, the strongest support for analysing liver tissue both by a tungstic acid and a strong hydrochloric acid digestion if a general search for alkaloid-type bases is required.

It should be noted that morphine is a most elusive poison to find, and before a negative report is presented, liver, kidney, bile and urine should have been analyzed. Methaqualone, whose highly toxic blood range is over 3 mg/100 ml, is a very weak base, and to extract from organic solvent at least 2N acid strength is required. It has a high ultraviolet absorption suitable for quantitative assay (see Table XIII and Part II).

3. Conclusion

It must have been obvious throughout this chapter that the analysis of liver is one of the most important series of analyses that must be done in a toxicological analysis in relation to the *general unknown*. It falls between rapid screening tests on blood and urine, the screening of the alimentary tract and the *special tests* on other fluids and tissues.

Without a complete understanding of this fact, the investigation of a possible poison case will almost inevitably fail.

REFERENCES

Algeri, E.J., Katsas, G.C., and McBay, A.J.: The toxicology of some new drugs; glutethimide, meprobamate and chlorpromazine. *J Forensic Sci, 4:* 111, 1959.

Algeri, E.J., and Walker, J.T.: Paper chromatography for identification of the common barbiturates. *Am J Clin Pathol, 22:*37, 1952.

Anders, M.W., and Mannering, G.J.: Gas chromatography of some pharmacologically active phenothiazines. *J Chromatogr, 7:*258, 1962.

Berman, E.: Determination of cadmium, thallium and mercury in biological material. *Perkin Elmer Atomic Absorption Newsletter, 6:*57, 1967.

Bladh, E., and Norden, A.: A method for determining 1-butyl-3 p-tolyl sulphonylurea (Tolbutamide) in human blood serum. *Acta Pharmacol Toxicol, 14:*188, 1958.

Bogan, J., Rentoul, E., and Smith, H.: Fatal poisoning by primidone. *J Forensic Sci Soc, 5:*97, 1965.

Bogan, J., and Smith, H.: Analytical investigations in barbiturate poisoning. *J Forensic Sci Soc, 7:*37, 1967.

Bougeois, C.H., Shank, R.C., Grossman, R.A., Johnson, D.O., Wooding, W.L., and Chandavimol, P.: Acute Aflatoxin B., toxicity in the Macaque and its similarity to Reye's Syndrome. *Lab Invest, 24:*206, 1971.

Bramlett, C.L.: Determination of phenothiazine and several of its derivatives by GLC. *JAOAC, 49:*857, 1966.

Brown, B.T., Shepheard, E.E., and Wright, S.E.: The distribution of digitalis glycosides and their metabolites within the body of the rat. *J Pharmacol, 118:*39, 1956.

Chang, L.W., Gilbert, E.F., Tanner, W., and Moffat, H.L.: Reye Syndrome: Light and electron microscopic studies. *Arch Pathol, 96:*127, 1973.

Clarke, E.G.C.: The identification of solanine. *Nature, 181:*1152, 1958.

Clarke, E.G.C., and Williams, M.: Microchemical tests for the identification of alkaloids. *J Pharm Pharmacol, 7:*255, 1955.

Comstock, E.G., Comstock, B.S., and Ellison, K.: A turbidimetric method for the determination of pentachlorophenol in urine. *Clin Chem, 13:*1050, 1967.

Curry, A.S.: The barbiturates. In Stewart, C.P. and Stolman, A. (Eds.):

Toxicology, Mechanisms and Analytical Methods. New York, Academic, 1961, pp. 153-158.

Curry, A.S.: The interference of β-methyl β-ethyl glutarimide in the determination of barbiturates. *J Pharm Pharmacol, 9:*102, 1957.

Curry, A.S., Grech, J.L., Spiteri, L., and Vassallo, L.: Death from thallium poisoning. *Eur J Toxicol, 2:*260, 1969.

Curry, A.S., Guttman, H.A.N., and Price, D.E.: A urinary pteridine in a case of liver failure. *Lancet, i:*885, 1962.

Curry, A.S., and Phang, S.E.: A continuous extractor for use in toxicological analysis. *J Pharm Pharmacol, 12:*437, 1960.

Curry, A.S., Read, J.F., Brown, C., and Jenkins, R.W.: Infrared of gas chromatographic fractions. *J Chromatogr, 38:*200, 1968.

Curry, A.S., Read, J.F., and Knott, A.R.: Determination of thallium in biological material by flame spectrophotometry and atomic absorption. *Analyst, 94:*744, 1969.

Curry, A.S., and Sunshine, I.: The liver/blood ratio in cases of barbiturate poisoning. *Toxicol Pharmacol, 2:*602, 1960.

Domnitz, J.: Thallium poisoning—a report of six cases. *South Med J, 53:*590, 1960.

Dubost, P., and Pascal, S.: Determination of chlorpromazine in biological material. *Ann Pharm Franc, 11:*615, 1953.

idem, ibid, *Ann Pharm Franc, 13:*56, 1955.

Fisher Scientific Company. Technical data: TD142. 633, Greenwich Street, New York.

Fiske, C.J., and Subbarow, Y.: *Biol Chem, 66:*375, 1925.

Forrest, I.S., and Forrest, F.M.: A colour test for all phenothiazines (F.P.N. reagent). *Clin Chem, 6:*11, 1960.

Hausman, R., and Wilson, W. J.: Thallotoxicosis, A social menace. *J Forensic Sci, 9:*72, 1964.

Haywood, P.E., Horner, M.W., and Rylance, H.J.: Thin layer chromatography of neutral drugs. *Analyst, 92:*711, 1967.

Hubler, W.R.: Hair loss as a symptom of chronic thallotoxicosis. *South Med J, 59:*436, 1966.

Jelliffe, R.W.: A chemical determination of urinary digitoxin and digoxin in man. *J Lab Clin Med, 67:*694, 1966.

Johnston, E.J., and Jacobs, A.L.: Thin layer chromatography of cardiac glycosides. *J Pharm Sci, 55:*531, 1966.

Kofoed, J., Fabierkiewicz, C., and Lucas, G.H.W.: A study of the conversion of phenothiazine derivatives to the corresponding sulphoxides on thin layer plates. *J Chromatogr, 23:*410, 1966.

idem, *Nature, 211:*147, 1966.

Linnemann, C.C., Shea, L., Kauffman, C.A., Schiff, G.M., Partin, J.C., and Schubert, W.K.: Association of Reye's syndrome with viral infection. *Lancet, ii:*179, 1974.

Loos, H., and Timperman, J.: A case of subacute thallium poisoning. *J Forensic Med, 6:*166, 1959.

Matthys, R., and Thomas, F.: Criminal thallium poisoning. *J Forensic Med, 5:*111, 1958.

Olsen, O.V.: A simplified method for extracting phenytoin from serum and a more sensitive staining reaction for quantitative determination by TLC. *Acta Pharmacol Toxicol, 25:*123, 1967.

Pilsbury, V.B., and Jackson, J.V.: The identification of the thiazide diuretic drugs. *J Pharm Pharmacol, 18:*713, 1966.

Plaa, G.L., Hall, F.B., and Hine, C.H.: Differentiation of barbiturates for clinical and medico-legal purposes. *J Forensic Sci, 3:*201, 1958.

Plaa, G.L., and Hine, C.H.: A method for the simultaneous determination of phenobarbital and diphenylhydantoin in blood. *J Lab Clin Med, 47:* 649, 1956.

Prick, J.G., Sillevio Smith, W.G., and Muller, L.: *Thallium Poisoning.* New York, Elsevier, 1955.

Rehling, C.J.: Poison residues in human tissues (report of 150 barbiturate and 90 barbiturate/alcohol combinations). In Stolman, A. (Ed.): *Progress in Chemical Toxicology.* New York, Academic, 1967, vol. 3.

Reye, R.D.K., and Morgan, G.: Encephalopathy and fatty degeneration of the viscera. *Lancet, 2:*1061, 1963.

Schreiner, G.E., Berman, L.B., Kovach, R., and Bloomer, H.A.: Acute glutethimide poisoning. *AMA Arch Intern Med, 101:*899, 1958.

Schwartz, H., Posnick, D., and Schenkel, S. Detection of yellow phosphorus in biological material. *Exp Med Surg, 13:*124, 1955, modified by Curry, A.S., Rutter, E. R., and Lim, C.H. *J Pharm Pharmacol, 10:*635, 1958.

Stevens, H.M., and Bunker, V.W.: The assessment of various protein precipitation methods for the extraction of basic drugs from tissue. *Forensic Science,* in press.

Stone, H.M., and Henwood, C.S.: The spectrophotometric determination of low levels of barbiturates in blood. *J Forensic Sci Soc, 7:*51, 1967.

Street, H.V.: The separation of barbiturates by reversed phase paper chromatography at elevated temperatures. *J Forensic Sci Soc, 2:*118, 1962.

Sunderman, F.W.: Diethyldithiocarbamate therapy of thallotoxicosis. *Am J Med Sci, 107/*209, February, 1967.

Turner, L.K.: Some applications of acceleration thin layer chromatography in toxicology. *J Forensic Sci Soc, 5:*94, 1965.

Turner, L.K.: Sulphoxides of the phenothiazine drugs. *J Forensic Sci Soc, 4:*39, 1963.

Weinig, E., and Zink, P.: Quantitative mass spectrometry of the thallium content of the human body. *Arch Toxicol, 22:*255, 1967.

Winek, C.L., Collom, W.D., and Fusia, E.P.: Yellow phosphorus ingestion—three fatal poisonings. *Clin Toxicol, 6:*541, 1973.

Chapter 7

ANALYSIS OF THE CONTENTS
OF THE ALIMENTARY TRACT

INTRODUCTION: DIVISION

AT THIS STAGE of the analysis the toxicologist usually pays close attention to the details of the case submitted on the form shown in Table I. Screening tests on blood and urine will have been completed, and the first simple tests on the liver for arsenic, zinc phosphide, phenothiazines and the many organic solvent-soluble poisons that can be isolated following the easy, quick tungstic acid protein precipitation such as the barbiturates, glutethimide and meprobamate, and some alkaloids including morphine (see Chap. 6), will have been done. He will therefore be approaching the alimentary tract either to confirm positive findings or to search for further poisons.

It is desirable to analyse the section of the alimentary tract which is likely to contain the highest concentration of poison. This is easy to say, but more difficult to do. If death has obviously been rapid, the stomach contents will be examined. If there is a good history, then clearly the relevant part of the intestines likely to contain the most poison should be taken. In the *found dead* case then *vide infra*. Fluoride is sometimes localized as the calcium salt in the wall of the stomach so the wall should also be analyzed. Barbiturate sometimes crystallizes under the stomach mucosa and can be seen macroscopically looking rather like a mould growth.

The stomach contents can be easily separated from the wall, and, after noting their weight, it is convenient to wash the wall and add this to the contents. The separation of the intestinal contents is sometimes a tedious procedure if the pathologist has not separated the intestines from adherent fat. This must be done so the contents can be squeezed into a previously weighed beaker. The wall then can be opened, inspected and washed. The washings are added to the beaker.

The contents and washings after weighing should be carefully inspected, smelt and their pH taken. If any abnormal degree of acidity or alkalinity is noted, this lead should be followed. Sodium barbiturates give an alkaline reaction and irritate the mucosa. Tablets generally resist disintegration better than capsules, and often can be picked out of the stomach contents in a relatively fresh condition; enteric-coated tablets are very stable and clinicians would be well-advised to consider performing stomach washes not only on the admission of the patient to hospital, but also if the clinical condition suddenly deteriorates several hours later. This often coincides with the solution of the enteric coating. The mucosa should be inspected for signs of corrosion or irritation or, in the intestines, for pathological changes associated with salmonella infection. Toxicologists who are not medically qualified should make sure of this facet of their training by instruction from a pathologist. Recognition of normal and abnormal conditions comes only from experience.

If an adequate time chart has been obtained, the chosen contents and washings are taken, their volume is measured and their weight taken. They are divided as described below. If a time chart is not available the stomach contents, the small intestine contents and the large intestine contents are separately isolated and measured. One third of each is bottled and put into reserve. The other aliquots are combined, diluted if necessary to give fractions that can be easily handled, and divided into the following fractions—one third of which is put into a flask ready for distillation, one ninth is put into the dialyser, and two ninths of the total is put into a beaker ready for isolation of organic poisons. With one-third in reserve, this accounts for the total. The following tests are then made.

A. TESTS ON ONE THIRD

1. Distillation from Acid Solution

This fraction is made to pH 2 with dilute hydrochloric acid and distilled; 25 ml of distillate are collected. If any test on the distillate is positive, the distillation is continued to completion.

The first test on the distillate is that of smell. Cyanide is one example that makes its presence obvious to those blessed with the hereditary ability to smell it, but there are many other poisons that can be detected in small amounts by this very simple and important test.

a. One ml of distillate is tested for volatile reducing substances by heating with 5 ml of dilute sulphuric acid and a few crystals of potassium dichromate. Any alcohols or aldehydes will turn the orange colour to green, and ethanol which is oxidized to acetaldehyde can be detected by smell and by heating the condensed products with pellet sodium hydroxide to give the characteristic colour and smell of aldehyde resin. Methanol, ethanol, isopropanol, ethylene glycol, acetaldehyde and paraldehyde are the common poisons found in this fraction, and their identification and assay must follow. Isopropanol is oxidized to acetone by acid dichromate; this can be detected by Rothera's reagent or by an Acetest® tablet.

If the test is positive, gas chromatography is the obvious choice for separating and identifying the members of this group, and even aqueous solutions can be put directly onto the column. The column and technique are described on page 94.

b. One ml of distillate is added to 2 ml of Schiff's reagent with which formaldehyde and acetaldehyde react to give a violet colour. Formaldehyde can be identified by the chromotropic acid test (see p. 282) and acetaldehyde by the aldehyde resin test described above.

c. One ml of distillate is heated in a test tube in a boiling water bath with 1 ml of pyridine and 2 ml of 20% sodium hydroxide for one minute. Colours in the pyridine layer are noted. Red indicates halogenated hydrocarbons while yellow results from p-nitrophenol, from the insecticide parathion or aldehyde resin from acetaldehyde or paraldehyde. This is a very sensitive test; 1 μg of chloroform can be detected. Parathion itself also distills in steam readily, and can be extracted from the distillate with benzene. The paper chromatographic identification of this very important insecticide is considered in Table XXII and Part II because it also appears in the neutral organic solvent-soluble poisons with other organophosphorus compounds. Parathion and p-nitrophenol have distinctive ultraviolet absorption spectra; blood cholinesterase levels should be depressed if an organo-phosphorus compound has been absorbed.

d. Ten ml of distillate are extracted with 10 ml of ether which are separated and carefully evaporated. The residue is examined and smelt. A large number of compounds can be detected by this simple test—camphor, methyl salicylate, cresols, chlorinated phenols, benzene and nitrobenzene are but a few. This method of concentrating the smell often enables the poison to be detected when the original distillate has such an objectionable odour that it overpowers the senses.

Pentachlorophenol is one of the compounds that will readily crystalise in the distillate; when this occurs identification is easy by comparison of melting points.

e. Several other simple tests should be done. These are as follows:

1. CYANIDE. This should be a routine test and the methods described in Chapter 5B1b are suitable. It should be remembered that postmortem production of small quantities (nanogram amounts) of cyanide can occur in the stomach and intestine contents. If a positive test is obtained, recheck the blood result (Chap. 5) and examine the undecomposed central area of the brain.

2. ACETONE. This can be detected in trace amounts by putting a drop of distillate on an Acetest tablet.

3. PHENOLS. If there is any suggestion of a smell of phenols in the ether extraction test described above, a drop of bromine water acts as a suitable chemical screening test. Brominated phenols are precipitated from solution. Salicylic acid will steam distil and give a faint positive in this test.

4. METHYLPENTYNOL. This hypnotic is detected by adding 1 ml of distillate to 1 ml of ammoniacal silver nitrate. A white precipitate of a silver acetylide is a positive result. Care must be taken to ensure that the precipitate is not silver chloride from distilled hydrochloric acid by making sure that the ammonia is in excess.

5. YELLOW PHOSPHORUS AND PHOSPHIDES. The distillation is done in the dark under nitrogen if yellow phosphorus is suspected. Distillation in the dark must be done if the screening test for phosphorus and phosphides that is always done beforehand on the liver (see Chap. 6) is positive. Phosphine and yellow phosphorus are distilled from the contents and collected

in silver nitrate solution from which they are oxidised to phosphate by boiling aqua regia and quantitatively determined.

ALTERNATIVE METHOD (Oliver and Funnel, 1961). The distillate (45 min) is cleaned from sulphide by a lead acetate trap, then collected on a plug of 0.3 g of powdered mercuric bromide. The plug is then washed with 4x2 ml portions of 0.003N iodide solution. 1 ml of ammonium molybdate solution (14 ml concentrated sulphuric acid are added to 60 ml of water with 1 g of ammonium molybdate added, the solution is then made up to 100 ml) is added to the washings together with 0.5 ml of freshly prepared 0.15% aqueous hydrazine sulphate solution. The mixture is then put in a boiling water bath for ten minutes. After cooling, the volume is made up to 10 ml and the optical density measured at 710 nm. Calibration measurements are made with standards from 0 to 50 μg of phosphorus.

6. ULTRAVIOLET SPECTROPHOTOMETRY. Normal aqueous distillates of intestinal contents usually show absorption peaks in the region 270 to 280 nm and the optical density reading is up to about 1.0 when the volume of distillate is 25 ml. Phenols and parathion increase the readings in this region. If additional peaks are found they should be investigated. Aromatic compounds such as benzene show fine structure bands about 240 to 270 nms and use of a recording spectrophotometer is advantageous.

INTERPRETATION OF RESULTS. The presence of ethanol in the gastrointestinal tract does not necessarily mean that it has been ingested. This particular alcohol is a fairly common artefact, usually in trace quantities. Positive tests have also been obtained for traces of isopropanol when none had been ingested. The presence of alcohols should always be fully investigated, however, as they are common constituents of many medicines, liniments and household commodities.

Chloroform is the most common halogenated hydrocarbon to be found as it is often present in medicines. As with the alcohols, gas chromatography is the best method of differentiating these halogenated hydrocarbons. Carbon tetrachloride used to be a common household cleansing agent of high toxicity with a fatal dose of the order of 5 ml; cases of death from the inhalation of the vapours of halogenated hydrocarbons are known, and even in the absence of a positive test in the gastrointestinal tract the brain should always be examined.

Ethyl salicylate with a smell reminiscent of methyl salicylate can be found as a result of esterification of ethanol and salicylic acid in the postmortem stomach contents. Camphor is difficult to detect in trace quantities other than by smell; a common liniment contains aconite, belladonna and camphor, and the importance of smelling a carefully evaporated ethereal extract of the distillate cannot be overemphasized. A fatal dose of camphor for a one-year-old child is probably about 1 g.

Cyanide is extremely toxic with a fatal dose of about 60 mg of the acid. Alkali cyanides are rarely pure, but are generally toxic in doses of this magnitude.

Methylpentynol and similar alcohols either free or their carbamates are generally of relatively low toxicity with therapeutic doses in the order of about 100 mg or slightly higher.

In the case of yellow phosphorus poisoning, on many occasions no unchanged poison can be detected in the alimentary tract. It is rare for more than 1 or 2 mg to be found in any case. Phosphorus has, however, been found in a body exhumed after thirteen months, and generalisations are difficult. A negative result in the alimentary tract does not exclude phosphorus as the causative agent in a case of acute fatty degeneration of the liver.

Note that distillation from alkaline solution can also be performed on the residue, but usually this is very difficult because of frothing, and volatile alkaloids can usually be found from tests described elsewhere. However, if amphetamine or nicotine are suspected, this alkaline distillation is useful. If collection in hydrochloric acid is practiced it should be remembered that nicotine hydrochloride is very volatile, and evaporation of the aqueous hydrochloride is best avoided. Careful evaporation of an alkaline ether extract is better.

2. Tests for Metals

After distillation, the volume of the residue in the flask is measured and a division is made into four equal parts.

The Reinsch test (boiling a small copper foil in dilute hydrochloric acid on which metallic arsenic, antimony, bismuth or mercury is deposited) is a worthwhile test because it is so quick to perform. It is therefore done on the quarter aliquot remaining after distillation which is boiled for five minutes with an equal volume of dilute hydrochloric acid and a piece of acid-cleaned copper about 0.5 cm by 0.5 cm in area. If no stain is seen on the copper in this time the flask is put on a boiling water bath for a further period of one hour when, if the foil is still bright, the test is considered negative. Black stains indicate arsenic, antimony or bismuth. Arsenic can be sublimed off and recognized as crystals of arsenic trioxide. Mercury also is obvious and the shiny deposit can be sublimed off the foil by heating.

Another quarter of the residue remaining after distillation is examined comprehensively for metals. This can be done in many ways and new techniques appear regularly. Destruction of organic matter by a nitric-sulphuric acid digestion can be followed by the classical metal group separation. After centrifuging off any insoluble chlorides or sulphates (Group I), this involves passing hydrogen sulphide gas through the solution first at pH 3 to 4 (Group II), then in ammoniacal solution (Group III and IV), and finally precipitating magnesium with warm ammonium phosphate solution (Group V). Twenty-four hours are recommended for sulphide precipitations; it must be remembered that although mercury will have been lost in the wet digestion, its detection should have been ensured by the Reinsch test which, because the interfering sulfides have been removed during the distillation, is usually very sensitive.

The group precipitates are centrifuged off and examined by arc emission spectroscopy, by paper chromatography or by specific spot tests. The first is a specialist technique requiring experience, but is most useful in detecting and identifying all the toxic metals. Paper chromatography is also valuable because it can separate those metallic ions which often mutually interfere in color tests. The sulphides and any magnesium salt from Group V are dissolved in a drop of hot dilute hydrochloric acid before application to the paper. Rf values, coupled with color tests on the purified ions, are criteria of identification. There are many papers published on this aspect of analysis, but a solvent consisting of the top layer of n-butanol: 3N hydrochloric acid (1:1) is suitable as demonstrating the method. To detect copper, lead, zinc, iron, bismuth, tin, mercury and many other metals, the paper is dipped in a solution of 0.005% dithizone in chloroform, then removed to allow the chloroform to evaporate when the multicolored dithizonates are visible. Prior inspection in 254 nm light detects lead as a brilliant green fluorescence and some other metals as absorbent spots (see Table XXI). If a particular metal is being sought, tests for it are applied directly on the paper and any spot can be examined by arc emission spectroscopy. Magnesium, which is commonly taken as the sulphate, must not be forgotten and is precipitated by warming with alkaline ammonium phosphate solution after the acid and alkaline sulphides. After solution in diluted hydrochloric acid is detected on paper by dipping in 0.01% solution of titan yellow in 1N sodium hydroxide; excess reagent is removed by washing in

TABLE XXI

PAPER CHROMATOGRAPHY OF METALS

Appearance in Daylight		Appearance in uv* Acid Conditions	Appearance in uv* (Ammonia Fumes)	Colour with Dithizone	Rf
Pb	Nil	Green	Fades to negative	Pink	0.29
Cu	Green	Strongly Absorbs	No change	Brown	0.19
Bi	Nil	Strongly Absorbs	No change	Pink	0.63
Hg	Nil	Weakly absorbs	No change	Orange	0.83
Fe	Yellow	Very strongly absorbs	No change	Brown	0.28
					0.42
Cr	Green	Strongly absorbs	No change	Slowly grey/blue	0.11
As	Nil	Nil	Nil	Nil	—
Sb	Nil	Absorbs	No change	Pink-orange	0.78
Sn	Nil	Orange-red	No change	Red	0.78
Ni	Green	Absorbs	Intensified	Weak red	0.12
Co	Blue-red	v.weak absorbs	Intensified	Red-magenta	0.20
Mn	Nil	Nil	Absorbs	Pink	0.19
Zn	Nil	Yellowish	No change	Scarlet	0.78
Cd	Nil	Yellowish	No change	Yellow-orange	0.78
Tl	Nil	Absorbs	No change	Weak red	0.00

*254 nm radiation.

System: n butanol 100: 3N hydrochloric acid 100 (top layer).

water when magnesium can be seen as a red spot on a yellow background. The very toxic metal, thallium, should be detected by precipitation as the insoluble thallous iodide. A portion of the original digest should be reduced by passage of sulphur dioxide and potassium iodide solution added. A green-yellow precipitate is obtained. For quantitation, see Part II.

In this writer's view, although examination of the alimentary tract contents for metals is most useful and obviously necessary, a negative result should not weigh too heavily. It is advisable to cross check by analyses of liver tissue for the main toxic metals such as arsenic, antimony, mercury, lead and thallium, and these are considered under the relevant sections.

3. Dialysis for Anions

The two remaining parts of the distillation residues are combined, made to pH 7 and, after concentration by evaporation to approximately 20 ml, are dialysed. It is usual for the dialysis of this extract, which is one sixth of the total stomach or intestine content, to *follow* the dialysis of the untreated one-ninth portion of the content described below. The only reason for this second dialysis is to check the dialysis of the untreated fraction. If the analyst is certain of his initial findings it can be ignored, but often it is extremely useful to have a separate fraction for confirmation.

In addition there will be the equivalent of one sixth of the contents in this fraction as opposed to only one-ninth in the direct dialysis.

Dialysis can be performed against about 300 ml of distilled water either through the conventional Visking or by stirring in a bag of cellophane. Two hours are usually sufficient for thin grade cellophane, but checks should be made routinely. The dialysate is concentrated by boiling to 2 ml to give a clear brown solution. The tests are described immediately below.

B. DIALYSIS

1. Dialysis of One Ninth Aliquot

This aliquot of the alimentary tract contents untreated in any way is dialysed through cellophane or Visking against 2 by 250 ml portions of distilled water: the dialysate is then exactly neutralized and concentrated to 2 ml, and the following spot tests are performed:

a. Nitrate, Chlorate and Bromate

One drop of dialysate is mixed with five drops of a 0.5% solution of diphenylamine in concentrated sulphuric acid. A blue color indicates the presence of one of these ions which is not present in normal extracts. They can be distinguished by the following additional tests. A solution of indigo carmine is made in dilute sulphuric acid and diluted to a very pale blue color. A few crystals of sodium sulphite are added, followed by one or two drops of dialysate. Microgram quantities of chlorate or bromate will completely decolorize the solution. Green colors indicate a negative reaction. Confirmation of chlorate and bromate can also be accomplished as follows: silver nitrate solution acidified with nitric acid is added to an aliquot of the dialysate until completion of the precipitation of silver chloride; the precipitate is removed by filtration and a weak solution of sodium nitrite added dropwise. Any silver chlorate or bromate in the filtrate (both are soluble) is thus reduced to chloride or bromide and can be seen as a further precipitate. Nitrate may be found after the ingestion of nitrite.

Thin layer chromatography separates oxidising anions. Use silica gel plates with a solvent of n butanol : glacial acetic acid : water (60:40:6). Spray with acetone : diphenylamine : Aniline (100:1:1 to which orthophosphoric acid has been added to just redissolve the precipitate, approx. 10) : heat at 110° for 5 minutes (Loveland, personal communication).

b. Hypophosphite

One g of granulated zinc and 10 ml of dilute hydrochloric acid are added to 0.5 ml of dialysate in a Gutzeit apparatus where phosphine is liberated. The paper in the Gutzeit holder is soaked in alcoholic silver nitrate or mercuric bromide. A black or yellow-brown stain depending on which paper is used can be converted to reduced phosphomolybdate blue (see p. 128).

Hypophosphite is not itself particularly toxic, but it is a metabolic product of the rat poison, zinc phosphide, and may be ingested as hypophosphite in the form of *tonics* containing strychnine or quinine.

c. Bromide

The simple fluorescein test described in Chapter 3B is most suitable; 1 μg can be detected. Bromide is found not only from the ingestion of bromide sedatives, but also as a metabolite of organobromo sedatives and of bromate which is used in *home perm* capsules. Large quantities of chloride interfere in this test, and when bromide is present in trace amounts this test may be negative because of interference by the hydrochloric acid added in the distillation stage when this test is done on the 1/6th aliquot obtained from the check dialysis described above. A similar test on the untreated one ninth dialysate may be positive.

d. Oxalate and Fluoride

Five-tenths ml of dialysate is acidified with dilute acetic acid, and calcium chloride solution is added dropwise. Any calcium oxalate is precipitated; this reaction can be assisted by heating slightly. The precipitate is removed by centrifuging and examined microscopically and by classical techniques. Calcium fluoride may also be precipitated and sulphate if present in large amounts. Fluoride may not have survived the distillation, but differentiation of the ions is possible by testing portions of the isolated precipitate in the alizarin-complexone diffusion test for fluoride (see p. 102) and by warming the washed precipitate with very weak acid permanganate to indicate oxalate. The crystal form of calcium oxalate is distinctive. Traces of fluoride can also be detected by Goldstone's hanging drop technique; 2 mg of powdered silica are added to the dried calcium salt before carrying out the test described below under silicofluoride. The fluoride electrode can also be used (see p. 153).

e. Thiocyanate and Thioglycollate

Thiocyanate may occasionally be ingested by laboratory workers and by schoolboys who mistake it for cyanide; thioglycollate is used in hair setting. Both can be detected by the formation of colors with a drop of ferric chloride solution on a drop of dialysate.

Often a violet color is noticed, and this usually results from salicylate following ingestion of aspirin.

f. Fluoracetate and Fluoroacetamide

This ion and compound are of great toxicological importance because of their availability as rat poisons. Rodenticides seem to be specially favored by criminal poisoners, and methods for their detection should be reliable. Fluoroacetamide, a volatile compound, may be hydrolysed to the ion *in vivo* or during the concentration of the dialysate, but indeed it is likely that the early preparations of fluoroacetate and fluoracetamide were contaminated by fluoride, thus leading the toxicologist to a false sense of security regarding the detection of these compounds. It is highly unlikely that clinicians or pathologists would suggest them to the toxicologist as a probable cause of death in a routine sudden death case. It is also equally unlikely that every toxicologist has the means to check for them in every case, but at this stage in the analysis they must be considered. If no cause of death has yet been found, then consider the analyses described in Part II.

g. Borate

This ion does not normally dialyse, even if present in stomach contents, presumably because of the formation of sugar complexes. This is why the determination of total boron in blood or tissue is advisable in any general search. If large excesses of borate are present a positive test may be obtained, but it should be remembered that evaporation of the dialysate in borosilicate glass can give a positive result in the test. A 1:10 dilution if still positive indicates a positive result from the content and not from the glass. The test consists of evaporating to dryness on a tile on a water bath a drop of dialysate with a turmeric paper wetted with dilute hydrochloric acid. A red color turning blue on wetting with dilute ammonia is a positive.

In borate deaths, which occur sometimes in young children accidentally given boric acid solutions, the blood is frequently a bright red color.

h. Silicofluoride

Five-tenths ml is made acid with hydrochloric acid and 0.5 ml of 10% barium chloride is added. Sulphate and silicofluoride are precipitated as barium salts. There is usually a faint positive result at this point from sulphate normally present from foods. This can be distinguished from silicofluoride by an examination of the centrifuged, washed crystals. Barium sulphate is usually amorphous while those from barium silicofluoride are boat-shaped. The well-known hanging drop test for silicofluoride can also be used in which fluorosilicic acid is liberated by concentrated sulphuric acid and captured in a hanging drop of sodium chloride solution to give characteristic crystals of sodium fluorosilicate. Goldstone has re-investigated this reaction and recommends the following procedure.

METHOD (Goldstone, 1955). Approximately 0.5 mg of powdered calcium carbonate are placed with the fluorosilicate in a 10-ml crucible and dried on a hot plate. After cooling, two small drops of concentrated sulphuric acid are added and the crucible is placed on a hot plate at 170 degrees C. A glass slide on the underside of which has been placed a small drop of sodium chloride solution is quickly placed over the crucible and a 50-ml beaker containing an ice cube is put on top of the slide to prevent evaporation of the drop during the twenty minutes required for the distillation. The sodium chloride solution is made by dissolving 1 g of sodium chloride with 3 g of glycerol in water and two drops of 40% formaldehyde and making the volume up to 100 ml. When the liberated fluorosilicic acid has all been collected by the sodium chloride the slide is removed, the top surface blotted and the drop is then dried out by placing the slide in a warm place for a few minutes. A microscopic examination shows the sodium fluorosilicate as faintly pink hexagonal or six-pointed stars at the peripherary of the drop among the well-known and easily recognizable sodium chloride crystals. 1 μg of fluorosilicate is easily detectable; the limit is about 0.2 μg.

i. Nitrite

A drop of dialysate is put on a powder made by mixing 6.2 g of α-naphthylamine, 1 g of sulphamic acid and 25 g of citric acid and drying the powder in a dessicator. Although this is a very sensitive test, controls should be done at the same time to show that deterioration of the stored powder has not occurred. In deaths from nitrites the blood is usually a chocolate color.

j. Iodide

A drop of dialysate is acidified with dilute sulphuric acid and a drop of copper sulphate solution is added. Free iodine is liberated if iodide is present which can be detected as a violet color in a chloroform extraction or by the blue of a starch iodide reaction.

Iodide is another ion which is bound in some way to protein, and if there is any suspicion of ingestion of iodide, blood or tissue should be ashed as described in Part II. Iodide does not appear in deproteinised filtrates of blood, and there is a grave doubt as to whether it will always dialyse from stomach contents.

k. Thiosulphate

A drop of dilute sulphuric acid and a weak solution of iodine in potassium iodide is added to a drop of dialysate. Decolorisation indicates thiosulphate which photographers and laboratory workers might ingest.

l. Ferrous and Ferric Ions

These ions will not dialyse if the contents were neutral or alkaline; if acid, they may be found. Spot tests with potassium ferrocyanide and ferricyanide acidified with dilute hydrochloric acid are suitable and sensitive tests.

m. Check Tests

Chloride and phosphate are normally present in the stomach and intestine contents, and serve as an internal control. Tests for their presence should always be done to check the efficiency of the dialysis.

2. Dialysis from Acid Solution

After the dialysis of the ninth part of the content, the contents of the cellophane or Visking are made acid with hydrochloric acid, and a second dialysis made again against 2 by 250-ml portions of distilled water. After evaporation, tests for ferrous, ferric, oxalate and fluoride ions are repeated. In deaths from ferrous sulphate in young children tests for ferrous ions are often obtainable before evaporation, and, in this way, any oxidation during evaporation does not complicate the interpretation. The dialysate should be neutralized before concentration to 2 ml by evaporation so that loss of hydrogen fluoride does not occur.

INTERPRETATION OF RESULTS. Nitrate and chlorate will cause serious symptoms of poisoning and sometimes death in doses of about 15 g of their sodium or potassium salts. Bromates are said to be slightly more toxic. Nitrates are found in fertilizers; chlorates, in weedkillers and also as an ingredient of mouthwashes and throat lozenges; and bromate is a very common ingredient of *home perm* kits. All may therefore be encountered. In the complete analysis for these ions it is likely that their presence will be detectable in the alimentary tract in only milligram amounts, and the inference that they were responsible for the poisoning must rest to some extent on the circumstantial evidence coupled with the clinical history and the findings at the postmortem examination.

The very high toxicity of the fluoroacetates, 50 to 100 mg being a lethal dose, means that the detection of microgram quantities in the alimentary tract is of great significance. Because of the ways in which interference with the tricarboxylic acid cycle manifests itself, death may be delayed for many hours or even days, and there is often an early quiescent period. Reported cases of poisoning by these compounds are to some extent complicated by the fact that inorganic fluoride was present in many early commercial samples.

Borates are found in most households either as boric acid or as borax. The interpretation of tissue levels of boron is discussed in Part II.

Nitrite and nitrate can be found in some water supplies, and can cause poisoning of children and animals. Methaemoglobinaemia is an outstanding clinical finding. Nitrite is used as a rust preventative and also in the chemical industry. Very small amounts are used to preserve the color in pickled or salted meats. Death has resulted in an adult from the ingestion of 2 g sodium nitrite, but the more usual fatal dose is about 10 g.

Ferrous sulphate is commonly taken by young children by accident because parents underestimate the climbing capabilities of the young child. Anaemia tablets hidden in a cupboard or drawer are attractive sweets to a youngster. In such cases the intestine contents are frequently blue in color from the formation of iron phosphates and tests for ferrous ion can often be obtained by a direct test on the faeces. The ingestion of five to ten tablets, each containing an adult therapeutic dose of ferrous sulphate, by a young child can be expected to lead to poisoning. Ferrous phosphate is also encountered in *tonics*. It is likely that ferrous ion intoxication will have been detected while the patient is still alive, and serum iron levels will be diagnostic. However, this is not always the case and haemolysed blood must *not* be used as a substitute for serum. Ferric salts cause irritation of the gastric mucosa, and, like ferrous sulphate, have been taken in attempts to procure an abortion. Traces of ferric ion are sometimes found in normal intestinal contents and faint positive tests on a drop of solution from a 2-ml sample of evaporated dialysate of one ninth of the alimentary tract contents should be ignored.

Silicofluoride is very toxic; a dose of 1 g of the sodium salt can be fatal. If more than a few milligrams of sulphate have been detected, the metal they have been derived from must be considered. Magnesium sulphate is one example, but ferrous and zinc sulphates are of more toxicological significance.

The detection of hypophosphite may lead to the discovery of the medicine whose other constituents are responsible for the illness or death of the patient.

If a positive bromide test is obtained, then blood and tissue levels must be determined (see Part II).

Both oxalate and fluoride are toxic ions, and ingestion in both cases leads to gastrointestinal disturbances. The fatal dose of oxalate is usually about 10 g while fluoride can kill in doses of about 5 g. In both cases death may be delayed for several hours, and the toxicologist must be prepared to detect milligram or even smaller quantities. Oxalate occurs in several plants, for example rhubarb, and a full history of what the patient has eaten in the forty-eight hours prior to the illness or death is therefore desirable coupled with a close examination of the vomit and the contents of the alimentary tract. See also Burden, 1961; Jackson, *et al.*, 1961; Polson and Tattersall, 1959; Sawyer *et al.*, 1967.

C. EXAMINATION OF THE TWO NINTHS ALIQUOT FOR ORGANIC SOLVENT SOLUBLE POISONS

1. Extraction

Which method should be used to extract these poisons? This is a difficult question to answer, but four methods are commonly used. They are as follows:

a. Direct extraction without prior treatment

b. Protein precipitation by ammonium sulphate

c. Continuous extraction by acid ethanol

d. Prior treatment of the content in 40% hydrochloric acid at 100 degrees C for five minutes.

In all the processes the extraction is made with an organic solvent, first from acid solution and then from alkaline solution. It is subsequently divided into the strong acid, weak acid, neutral, alkaloid and morphine fractions. Evaporation of the alkaline ether fraction must be done very carefully so that such volatile alkaloids as nicotine are not lost. If the presence of an unstable alkaloid such as atropine is suspected, very mild extraction procedures must be used; continuous extraction with alcohol under reduced pressure is suitable.

If screening tests on liver for phenothiazines have been positive, the toxicologist may consider it advisable to hydrolyse half of this aliquot by method (d) to free protein-bound drug. Apart from a few acid labile alkaloids the method does not result in the loss of many compounds, and, as usual, extraction from acid solution should precede that from alkaline solution. Filtration after the acid treatment gives a clear solution which does not usually emulsify when shaken with organic solvent.

Direct extraction of the content or diluted content, preferably with a large excess of solvent, may be the easiest method, but often emulsions occur, and protein precipitation is obviously necessary if the content is thick or bulky. Methods (b) or (c) may be used as experience indicates.

Stomach contents vary so much in their volume and consistency that it is difficult to give definitive advice on which method of extraction to use. However, direct extraction either using ether or chloroform should always be followed by a hydrochloric acid treatment. If the bulk is large, ammonium sulphate can be used, but its efficiency is low.

It should be noted that strychnine and phenazone are two bases that are very poorly extracted by ether, and after an alkaline-ether extraction, a second extraction with chloroform is worthwhile. Special mention must be made of methaqualone which will appear in the neutral fraction unless the first acid-ether extraction is made at least 2N with respect to sulphuric acid.

METHOD (b) (Nickolls, 1956). The contents are diluted to a gruel consistency and sufficient dilute hydrochloric or acetic acid is added to make the pH approximately 2 to 3. Solid ammonium sulphate is then added to make a saturated solution, and the digest is warmed without stirring in a boiling water bath for fifteen minutes. Filtration without suction through a paper pad on a sintered glass Buchner funnel gives a clear, protein-free filtrate that is suitable, after cooling, for extraction with an equal volume of ether. The solid on the paper pad is washed with warm acid water, then with ether, and all the extracts are combined.

The aim of these extraction procedures is to produce, first, an aqueous acidic phase and an organic solvent phase. If chloroform is used as the organic phase, then the aqueous acid should be sulphuric acid. This is because many base hydrochlorides are soluble in chloroform, and, in the subsequent division into strong acids, weak acids, neutrals and bases, they would be lost. The separation is as shown in schematic outline in Figure 6 with the additional extraction at pH 8 after the addition of a little sodium sulphite with chloroform:isopropanol (4:1) to isolate morphine.

The extracts will contain between them the possible presence of a very large number of poisons together with coextracted fat, cholesterol and other natural products.

A really comprehensive list of compounds to be sought in these fractions would contain many hundreds and possibly thousands of substances covering the whole range of chemicals in use in every branch of life. The toxicologist must consider the weed killer or insecticide in the same fraction as the medicament and household poisons. Several screening tests are necessary to detect any abnormal compound among those occurring in the normal stomach or intestines.

There are four stages in the approach to these analyses; these are considered in order below.

2. Analyses

a. Spot Tests

1. Strong acid and weak acid fraction. Test each for salicylates with ferric chloride solution; see page 66.

2. Neutral fraction. Test for carbamates with furfural-hydrochloric acid; see pages 65 and 69.

3. One percent of the neutral fraction is boiled over a microflame with two drops of 10% sodium hydroxide solution to dryness on a white tile. One drop of 50% saturated fluorescein solution, six drops of glacial acetic acid and six drops of 100 volume hydrogen peroxide are added and evaporated to dryness on a boiling water bath. A red color of eosin indicates the presence of an organobromo compound such as carbomal.

4. Test for DDT. A simple spot test is given below, but it is worthwhile in examining the circumstances of a series of unusual deaths to consider contamination by accident of food by organo-chloro and organo-phosphorus pesticides and herbicides. Even inorganic and organic metallo compounds (mercury and cadmium, for example) should be considered in this context. Clearly, gas chromatography with mass spectrometry will find answers quickly, and TLC separations using phenoxyethanol sprays (see Part II) are valuable for the organo-chloro compounds. O-P compounds and metallics are dealt with elsewhere in this book, but one is hesitant to exclude simple tests such as the one described below.

METHOD (Irudayasamy and Natarajan, 1961). An alcoholic aliquot of the neutral fraction is evaporated to dryness and treated with 10 ml of a chilled nitrating reagent consisting of 1:1 v/v nitric acid and sulphuric acids. It is then transferred to an eight by $\frac{3}{4}$ test tube and heated in a boiling water bath for one hour. If any carbonaceous material remains, heating is continued for another half an hour. After cooling, dilute with 50 to 100 ml of ice cold water, and extract with 20 ml, then 10 ml of chloroform. Wash the combined chloroform extracts with 50 ml of 1% potassium hydroxide solution, then with 3×50 ml portions of water. Dry the separated chloroform with anhydrous sodium sulphate and evaporate to dryness. Transfer the residue in chloroform to two separate spots on a white tile and evaporate off the solvent. To one spot add one drop of a 20% alcoholic potassium hydroxide solution (made by dissolving 5 g potassium hydroxide in 2.5 ml of water and diluting with 22.6 ml of ethanol). A positive reaction of colors going from rose to bright blue to green to yellow is obtained if DDT, DDE, DDA, DDD, DFDT or methoxychlor in even 1-μg quantity is present. To the other spot, addition of one drop of the alcoholic potassium hydroxide solution is followed by addition of one to two drops of acetone. A positive result is a bright blue color changing to bright purple to grey to yellow.

5. Test for α-naphthyl thiourea (Dybing, 1947). An aliquot, 1 percent, of the neutral fraction is dissolved in chloroform and shaken for thirty seconds with a few drops of bromine water. Excess sodium hydroxide solution is then added, and the whole shaken again. A positive result sensitive to 1μg or 50 μg/ml is obtained if a blue color is seen in the chloroform layer which is unchanged by shaking with 60% sulphuric acid.

Again, it is questionable whether such tests as this for unusual substances should be excluded from this book. Not many cases of poisoning from this rodenticide are known, but if the test is not done the poisoner will get away with his crime.

6. An aliquot, 1 percent, of the neutral fraction in alcohol is *carefully* evaporated. One ml of 20% sodium hydroxide solution and 1 ml of pyridine are added, and the reaction test tube is immersed in a boiling water bath for one minute. A red color in the pyridine layer indicates the presence of chloral hydrate or chlorbutol in the neutral fraction. This is a very sensitive reaction and chloroform must be absent from the environment. Positive tests should also be obtained in the volatile fraction.

7. One percent of the neutral fraction is treated with alkaline Folin-Ciocalteau reagent; a blue color indicates methyprylone.

8. One percent (10% if a 1% fraction gives a negative reaction) of the alkaloid fraction in ethanol is spotted on a filter paper and a drop of potassium bismuth iodide solution (Dragendorff's reagent,

p. 80) allowed to run into it. An orange color indicates the presence of an alkaloid. Three positive reacting aliquots are examined by paper or TLC chromatography.

This follows the procedure outlined in Chapters 4 and 6. A positive reaction is most unusual except in cases where putrefaction has occurred (see p. 27).

9. One percent of the alkaloid fraction is spotted on a filter paper and a drop of FPN reagent is allowed to flow onto it. This reagent is made as follows: five parts 5% ferric chloride, forty-five parts 20% perchloric acid, fifty parts 50% nitric acid. It gives a variety of colors with different phenothiazines. If the test is positive it is necessary to differentiate the many drugs that have the phenothiazine nucleus. Chlorpromazine is the most commonly found, but several of the others are very popular in medicine. For their separation, see Tables XIX and XX. This test is included as it gives such beautiful colors that are so distinctive that the toxicologist knows he has a lead to follow.

10. The procedure followed for the detection of an unknown alkaloid in the alkaloid fraction is followed with the morphine fraction. Detection of any morphine is accomplished either by spraying with Dragendorff's reagent or by dipping the dried chromatogram in a 2% solution of 40% formaldehyde in concentrated sulphuric acid (Marquis reagent). Full identification follows the ine suggested above. See also p. 90.

b. Ultraviolet Spectrophotometry

The second stage consists of measuring the ultraviolet absorption spectra for every fraction between 220 and 320 nm. It is usual to take 10 percent aliquots and use the following solvents:

1. Strong acid fraction—0.45N sodium hydroxide
2. Weak acid fraction—this fraction is read at three pH's; 0.45N sodium hydroxide is followed by 0.45N sodium hydroxide + 16% ammonium chloride (3 ml + 0.5 ml; pH = 10) then after adding 50% sulphuric acid to the pH 10 solution to change it to a pH of 2
3. Neutral fraction—alcohol
4. Basic fraction—0.1N sulphuric acid.

Normally, 5 to 10 ml is a suitable volume to dissolve each aliquot for taking the readings. In the absence of poison there are normally no inflexions in the curves whose optical density decreases slowly as the wavelength increases. If poison is present considerable dilution may be necessary.

Barbiturates in the weak acid fraction form the most common group of poisons, and their spectral changes with pH are illustrated in Figure 4. Normally the presence of barbiturate, glutethimide, and paracetamol will have been established by the first stage of the liver analysis which precedes that described here. In the neutral fraction, phenacetin, with an absorption maximum at 245 nm, is common; most of the carbamates do not show inflexions although mephenesin peaks at 270 nm. Caffeine may be found in both the neutral and the alkaloid fraction and has a peak at 273 nm. It does not react with Dragendorff's reagent. In the case of the alkaloids, a routine examination by ultraviolet spectrophotometry, and, if possible, infrared spectroscopy is worthwhile because such common drugs as benzocaine and theobromine also do not react with the common general alkaloid reagents, and spectroscopy is the only method for their easy detection.

The alkaloids show a great variety of absorption spectra with $E_{1cm}^{1\%}$ values ranging from over 1,000 to less than 5 with wavelength maxima from below 220 nm to above 360 nm. Comparison of the observed spectrum with known spectra enables identification to be easily and rapidly achieved if the curves are sufficiently characteristic. Often a chromophoric group is common to a series of drugs; for example, the phenothiazines show similar spectra with a maximum at 255 nm, and in the writer's opinion, a chromatographic separation using paper, thin layer or gas chromatography is a valuable and, in many cases, an essential additional tool for identification. If infrared is available only a few micrograms are necessary for absolute identification to be achieved, but purity is, again, most important, and prior chromatography is of the greatest value. Details of the absorption peaks to be commonly found in each extract are given in Tables V, X, XV and XVI.

It is obvious that the toxicologist must characterize for himself the poisons and drugs that are common in his area, and study such collections of data that are published. Any abnormal curve or chromatographic spot must be tracked to its source. A visit to the scene of the poisoning may be a great help.

c. Sublimation

Many compounds will sublime provided a sufficiently low pressure is used, 10^{-2}mm is essential, preferably lower. A temperature of 100 degrees C is used. Crystals are characterized by melting points (see Table XVII) or by any of the other available methods, x-ray diffraction, infrared and mass spectroscopy, for example. If any of the tests described above have given a positive result, sublimation is worthwhile trying. Even in negative cases its use is recommended.

TABLE XXII
SOLVENT SYSTEMS FOR ELEMENT PAPER CHROMATOGRAPHY

Element	Refs.	Solvent	Paper Treated with	Compounds Detected
Chlorine	[1,2]	Pyridine + water (3 + 2)	Soya bean oil at 2 mg per square inch	Aldrin, Dieldrin BHC
Phosphorus	[3]	Light petroleum + 10% aqueous solution of acetonitrile (3 + 1)	Saturate paper and chamber with vapour	p-nitro phenol Paraoxon, Parathion
Phosphorus	[4]	Chloroform Carbon tetrachloride	Nil	try for organo phosphorous compounds
Nitrogen	[5]	Glacial acetic acid + water (1 + 1)	20% olive oil in acetone and dried	Carbromal Bromvaletone Sedormid
Nitrogen	[5]	Methanol + water (18 + 2)	20% olive oil in acetone and dried	Methyprylone Glutethimide Thalidomide Bemegride Sedulon Persedon all carbamates

[1]Mitchell, L. C., and Patterson, W. I.: *J Assoc Agric Chem, 36:*553, 1953.
[2]Mitchell, L. C.: *ibid,* 1183.
[3]Karlog, O.: *Acta Pharmacol Toxicol, 14:*92, 1957.
[4]Otter, I. K. H.: *Nature, 176:*1078, 1955.
[5]Jackson, J. V., and Moss, M. S.: In Smith, I. (Ed.): *Chromatographic and Electrophoretic Techniques,* 2nd ed. New York, Interscience, 1960, vol. 1, p. 404.

Cantharidin and the halogenated insecticidal compounds form examples which are detected most simply by the isolation of crysalline material.

d. Determination of Elements

Four elements, bromine, chlorine, phosphorus and nitrogen, are usually sought in the various fractions. Bromine has been considered in test 3 above and will not be discussed further here. Paper chromatography is a useful step prior to the tests because they can all be carried out on the paper for the detection of microgram quantities of the organically combined elements. The solvents and sprays for use are detailed in Tables XXII and XXIII.

TABLE XXIII
SPRAY REAGENTS FOR ELEMENTS

Element	Ref.*	Spray for Chromatography
Chlorine	1,2	0.5 silver nitrate in ethanol; air dry for thirty minutes. Spray with 37% formaldehyde; air dry thirty minutes. Spray 2N potassium hydroxide in methanol. Heat at 130 degrees C for thirty minutes; cool; spray concentrated nitric acid + 30% hydrogen peroxide (1+1); air dry overnight; expose to sun. Alternatively — Spray with 0.5% ethanolic silver nitrate containing 1% phenoxyethanol. Expose to ultraviolet radiation.
Phosphorus	3	1.0N ethanolic sodium hydroxide
Phosphorus	4	1% N-bromosuccinimide in acetone; dry; then spray with molydate reagent and dry in the oven at 70°C. for 8 minutes. Remove and expose to ultra-violet light for ten to twenty minutes. Molybdate reagent is made by mixing 15 ml 72% perchloric acid, 25 ml 5% ammonium molybdate reagent and dry in the oven at 70°C. for 8 water.
Nitrogen	5	Expose paper to chlorine vapour for ten minutes; suspend in a current of air. Spray with 2% starch + 1% potassium iodide when paper itself does not give a deep stain. An alternative to exposure to chlorine is to dip the paper in sodium hypochlorite solution with 2.5% available chlorine.

*Refs. as in Table XXII.

Details for the further investigation of organo-chloro, organo-phosphorus and nitrogen-containing compounds are given in Part II. The continued use of a paper chromatographic examination at this stage instead of going direct to TLC systems is justified on the grounds that the neutral extract, in which the bulk of the toxicologically significant compounds of these groups occur, often contains a lot of fat. In the writer's opinion, paper is a far better medium than TLC in these particular circumstances.

If a positive result is obtained and the amount of drug responsible for it is present in only trace quantities, this is another occasion when a visit to the scene will probably produce more worthwhile results than days of semi-inspired guessing in the laboratory.

e. Interpretation of Results

These can be divided into three main categories as follows:

1. When a toxic dose of a particular poison can be isolated from the alimentary tract, the interpretation is straightforward.

2. When the presence of a highly toxic material is established, even in trace amounts, the inference that poisoning is the cause of death is also usually wholly justified.

3. When a small quantity of drug is found in the alimentary tract and the question arises as to whether it is the residue of a toxic or a therapeutic dose.

The question of the time interval that has elapsed between ingestion and death may also be posed.

In all cases the amount remaining in the stomach at death is what remains of that ingested after vomiting and absorption have occurred. If both of these two unknowns can be established by other analyses, the total ingested can be determined; if not, the calculation is, at best, a guess. The experience of the toxicologist is then the overriding factor, and it would be foolish here to indulge in generalizations. It is sufficient to say that 50 mg of barbiturate can be found in the stomach of a person who died less than an hour after the ingestion of a large overdose, and in another case the same quantity may be found after a period of forty-eight hours spent in coma. Simultaneous ingestion of alcohol can increase the absorption rate very considerably because of the dilation of the stomach's vascular system. Although it is frequently believed that the small intestine is the main site for the absorption of many poisons, in the writer's opinion, as far as large overdoses are concerned, this is not so— it is, in fact, the stomach. On many occasions it is possible to show by analysis that the poison has not reached the small intestine, yet the concentration of drug in the tissues is at a fatal level.

General principles hold relating the position of maximum concentration of drug in the alimentary tract to the time of ingestion although there are two complications. Firstly, diffusion of toxin after death and during the postmortem examination, and, secondly, secretion of some drugs by the bile. Unless the content is highly fluid the first is usually unimportant, but the second is of some significance—drugs which have been injected may be only demonstrable in the intestines; for example, nalorphine. On such occasions the interpretation becomes very much a guess based on experience.

REFERENCES

Burden, E.H.W.J.: The toxicology of nitrites with particular reference to the potability of water supplies, *Analyst, 86:*429, 1961.

Dybing, F.: Detection of α-naphthylthiourea (ANTU) in forensic chemistry. *Acta Pharmacol, 3:*184, 1947.

Goldstone, N.J.: Microchemical detection of fluorides—sodium fluosilicate crystal test. *Anal Chem, 27:*464, 1955.

Irudayasamy, A., and Natarajan, A.R.: Spot test micro determination of DDT and its related compounds in biological material. *Anal Chem, 33:*630, 1961.

Jackson, R.C., Elder, W.J., and McDonnell, H.: Sodium chlorate poisoning complicated by acute renal failure. *Lancet, ii:*1381, 1961.

Nickolls, L.C.: *The Scientific Investigation of Crime.* London, Butterworth, 1956, p. 382.

Oliver, W.T., and Funnel, H.S.: Determination of phosphorus in biological material. *Anal Chem, 33:*434, 1961.

Polson, C.J., and Tattersall, R.N.: *Clinical Toxicology.* London, English Universities Press, 1959, p. 140-Fluorides.

idem ibid, Clincal Toxicology. London, English Universities Press, 1959, p. 274-Boracic acid (Boron®).

Sawyer, R., Grisley, L.M., and Cox, B.G.: Separation and determination of fluoroacetamide residues in water, biological materials and soils. *J Sci Fd Agri, 18:*283, 1967.

Chapter 8

BRAIN AND KIDNEY

A. VOLATILE POISONS

Inhalation of many volatile poisons can cause death, and the tests on the gastrointestinal tract which were described above will not reveal their presence. It is essential, therefore, that they be sought in a blood-containing organ.

In theory, tests on the lungs would be desirable, and, indeed, many toxicologists do perform these. However, it is unusual for the lungs always to be submitted for analysis, and, because it is said that the brain retains chloroform exceptionally well in putrefied bodies, it seems logical to analyse this organ on a routine basis. At the same time other volatile compounds can be sought, such as the anaesthetics, fluothane and ether and the cleaning agents, carbon tetrachloride, trichloroethylene and perchlorethylene as well as other toxic solvents such as benzene. All of these are highly volatile, and special care must be taken to ensure an efficient cold trap. All the joints of the apparatus must be Teflon®-sleeved because gross loss of poison will occur by its solution into any grease. The best method of identification and assay is undoubtedly gas chromatography.

METHOD. Brain, 100 g, is macerated and diluted to approximately 500 ml with water, 25 ml of dilute sulphuric acid are added, and distillation is commenced. The precautions outlined above must be observed. Three ml of distillate are collected, and this is divided into 3×1 ml aliquots. One aliquot is mixed with 1 ml of pyridine and 2 ml of 20% sodium hydroxide in a test tube. The time is taken T_0. The test tube is then immersed in a boiling water bath for exactly one minute when it is removed and cooled in icewater; four ml of water are added and, at exactly thirty minutes from T_0, the optical density is read at 520 nm against a reagent blank. For 1-cm cells the calibration graph is made from 0 to 250 μg of chloral hydrate per millilitre of solution. This gives optical density readings in the range 0 to 1.0. For interpretation of results see Chapter 5B1(c).

The other two aliquots are examined by gas chromatography (see Chap. 5B1(a)). If gas chromatography is not available, apart from ultraviolet spectrophotometry, there is no alternative but to distil at least 500 g of brain tissue and attempt to isolate the few milligrams of volatile poison in a pure state. Fractional redistillation and the use of dry ice traps are essential and rewarding techniques. Identification can be by measurement of microboiling points although infrared examination is a more sensitive and more specific choice.

B. CHOLINESTERASE

In some cases the quantity of blood that the pathologist can obtain from a body is severely limited, and there is not enough for the toxicologist to perform all the tests that normally would be done. Tissue must then be used, and, for the assay of cholinesterase activity, brain is recommended. Poisoning by organo-phosphorus compounds manifests itself in a gross reduction of this normal body enzyme, and even when the blood level is depressed in cases of poisoning, a reduction in brain activity should also be sought.

C. METALLIC POISONS

In a routine search the kidney should be analysed for mercury, manganese and cadmium. The details for these metals are given in Part II.

D. TOXIC ANIONS

Because death may not follow for several days after the ingestion of such toxic anions as chlorate or oxalate their concentration in the alimentary tract may be too low for certain detection, and a search in the kidney may be considered desirable. This is often the case if methaemoglobinaemia has been noticed and chlorate poisoning is suspected. The tissue should be well macerated before dialysis, and the tests descibed in Chapter 7B1 carried out. Negative results are usually obtained even in strongly suspicious circumstances, but the efficiency of the extraction and tests can be easily demonstrated. Even though there is little hope for successful detection, the possibility cannot be ignored.

E. OTHER TESTS

At this stage of the analysis the toxicologist will no doubt be relieved to know that he has nearly finished! However, there still remain poisons which may have escaped detection so far. The quaternary ammonium compounds such as succinylcholine and tubocurarine are obvious examples, the former of which figured in a famous murder case in the United States. Details for their analyses are given in Part II (p. 297). Insulin may have escaped detection, and at the present time, if the pathologist has not excised a portion of tissue from around the injection site, there is little the toxicologist can do. If tissue is available, the tests described in Part II can be done. Finally, the heart drug, digoxin, and similar glycosides can be sought by radioimmunoassay. The introduction of this test in the United Kingdom in the last few years has dramatically increased the number of analytical requests. In 1973, twenty-seven cases were encountered in which it was thought digoxin might be involved. Obviously, in a screen for an unknown poison such a test must be included. Finally, cannabis and LSD abusers occasionally get themselves in situations where death results, albeit they have driven off the road or jumped out of a window, and a toxicological examination is required. These tests are also discussed in Part II.

PART II

ALPHABETICAL LIST
OF POISONS

ABORTION ENQUIRIES

If oral ingestion of an abortifacient is suspected, the death usually occurs many days afterwards, and, unless quinine is involved, very little can usually be done analytically. Often herbal brews figure where chemistry and pharmacology can only be a matter of conjecture. Even herbal pills and tablets are a great problem, and without a control collection of local manufacturers' products, the analysis becomes more a matter for the pharmacognisist.

Pennyroyal can be readily detected by smell and GLC. Extraction from aqueous acidic solution with ether followed by a TLC separation of the concentrated extract enables aloes, rhubarb and cascara to be differentiated. Benzene:chloroform (30:70) is used as the developing solvent on Silica-Gel G plates, and the spots are inspected in visible 254 and 365 nm light before and after exposure to ammonia vapor. Spot tests for ferrous and ferric ions should also be routine. The problems of the analyst can be exemplified by one case in which the dose was a teaspoonful of a mixture of an ounce of pennyroyal plant, an ounce of Canadian ginger and an ounce of thyme simmered for two hours and decanted into a bottle of stout. The mixture was not successful!

Where death follows suddenly after the introduction of disinfectant or soap solution by enema syringe into the vagina, then analysis can often help. Vaginal swabs should be examined first by GLC, using the head space method (Chap. 5B1(a)). Isopropanol is a common constituent of disinfectants. The smell of the swab or drainings can often give a valuable lead. Its pH should be measured. Local irritation may be associated with alum, borax or permanganate. To detect soap, a portion of the swab and separate 2 ml blood samples from the heart, peripheral veins and uterine contents are heated with 10 ml ethanol at 80 degrees C for five minutes. The filtrates are evaporated, redissolved in hot ethanol, refiltered and evaporated. The resulting solids are dissolved in water, 5 ml, acidified with O.1N H_2SO_4 and extracted with ether, 20 ml. The separated ether fractions are evaporated to dryness, redissolved in 10 μl of ethanol and examined by paper chromatography or GLC. For paper, a Whatman No. 1 paper is dipped in 10% liquid paraffin in benzene, drained and dried. After applying control spots of soap fatty acids in ethanol and the extracts, the paper is run in glacial acetic acid. The spots can be detected as follows: (a) dip in 1% lead acetate solution; wash thoroughly in running distilled water and then immerse in water saturated with H_2S; or (b) dip in 5% mercuric oxide in 20% sulphuric acid, wash thoroughly in running distilled water, drain, and dip in 0.1% diphenylcarbazone in ethanol. The fatty acids show up as a series of spots between Rf 0.5 and Rf 0.8.

Gas chromatographic separations after esterification of the fatty acids can also be achieved.

For ergometrine see Curry, 1959.

AMANITA PHALLOIDES

A general screening test for detecting toxins in the amanita mushrooms has been described, and it may prove useful in confirming a fresh botanical specimen.

METHOD (Block, Stephens, Barreto, and Murrill, 1955.)

The plant tissue is extracted with ethanol, and after evaporation is examined by paper chromatography. A solvent consisting of methyl-ethyl ketone:acetone:water:butanol (20:6:5:1) is used, and development takes forty minutes. The spray is 1% cinnamaldehyde in methanol after which the paper is exposed to fumes of hydrochloric acid. Violet or blue colors indicate amanita toxin, and the test is sensitive to 0.1 g of fresh tissue. Thin layer chromatography can also be used.

METHOD (Palyza, 1972. See also Palyza and Kulhanek, 1970.) The best TLC system was found to be Butyl-Cellosolve—25% aqueous ammonia (7:3) with 0.2% cinnamaldehyde incorporated in the plate. After running and drying, the plate is exposed to HCl fumes for thirty minutes Rf values of 0.36 for α-amatin, 0.32 for β-amanatin, 0.51 for γ-amanatin and 0.59 for amatin were obtained. (= 1 mg fresh mushroom.) This paper is in German; and Czecholovakian silica gel thin layer plates were used—Silufol®.

In the examination of intestinal contents for this toxin, which is a peptide, the alcohol extraction procedure is recommended. Obviously, some of it must be used to test for other poisons, but the proportion used to test for phalloidin must be decided with regard to the circumstances of the case. Acetone is also a suitable solvent for this poison which can be purified on cellulose powder columns eluting with a methanol, acetone, water mixture. Paper chromatography is, however, simple, and because of the very high toxicity of phalloidin—50 μg will kill a mouse—is a convenient purification procedure for crude extracts. The following solvents have been suggested: ethyl formate:acetone:water (100:145:40), and methyl-ethyl ketone:acetone:water (20:2:5) .

In each case the spray reagent is 1% cinnamaldehyde in methanol followed by exposure to hydrochloric acid fumes. Phalloidin gives blue colors. Extracts from similar positions on other chromatograms should be eluted and injected into mice after solution in saline. It is also desirable to show that extracts from other positions on the chromatogram are nontoxic and that other color tests for peptides such as the chlorine-starch iodide reaction (Table XXIII are also positive. Phalloidin shows an absorption maximum about 290 nm in water.

Many workers have suggested that the spores of *Amanita Phalloides* should be sought in the intestinal tract. These are said to be 8 to 11 μ by 7 to 9 μ white subgloboid bodies, each with a central oil drop. Expert mycological advice informs us that this approach is unsatisfactory on specimens isolated from the large intestines, although several workers have found such bodies, and, in any such cases, the isolation of the peptide followed by its examination chemically and biologically is obviously desirable. If negative, an examination for spores is still necessary.

A fatal case with fourteen references was reported by Abul-Haj, *et al.* (1963) in which a methanol extract of 400 g of liver, after purification, gave the expected ultraviolet and paper chromatographic results. See also Wieland and Schmidt (1952) .

AMITRIPTYLINE AND NORTRIPTYLINE

Special mention must be made of the fact that amitriptyline base is unstable (Henwood, 1967) , and strong acid or alkaline hydrolysis is necessary before attempting to isolate the drug by solvent extraction from tissues. A method which will detect these tricyclic antidepressants from urine five days after a single dose has been described by Wallace and Dahl (1967).

The following general methods may be used. The ultraviolet methods will give values that may reflect the presence of metabolites, depending on which solvent has been used for extraction. For isolation of the unchanged drug, ether is the preferred solvent. For some unknown reason chloroform is unsuitable.

Blood and Urine

a. Blood (Based on Sunshine and Baumler, 1965)

Stir 10 ml blood with 2 ml water and 8 ml concentrated hydrochloric acid; heat in a boiling water bath for five minutes. Remove and place in an ice bath. When cool, add 12 ml 60% w/v potassium hydroxide which has previously been washed with ether. Keep cool and check the pH for alkalinity. If acid, add more alkali. Shake with 150 ml ether, breaking any emulsion by centrifuging. Separate and shake the aqueous phase with a 50-ml portion of ether. Combine the ether fractions and wash in sequence with 10 ml 2.5% sodium hydroxide, 10 ml water and 5 ml water. Extract the ether with 5 ml 0.1N H_2SO_4 which is separated and read from 230 to 280 nm. Amitriptyline peaks at 240 nm with an $E_{1cm}^{1\%}$ value of 470. Nortriptyline has a very similar curve.

b. Urine

METHOD 1. Extract 10 ml of urine after alkalinisation to pH 14 with 25 ml ether. Wash the separated ether with 10 ml water which is rejected. Extract the ether layer with 5 ml 0.5N sulphuric acid and read from 230 to 280 nm.

THIN LAYER CHROMATOGRAPHY. After ultraviolet spectrophotometry, the acid solutions can be made alkaline and extracted with 5 ml ether and examined by TLC. Methanol:acetone:triethanolamine (10:10:0.3), and isopropanol:water 80:12 (one-third saturated with sodium chloride) have been used. On Kieselgel G a solvent of benzene:acetone: 25% aqueous ammonia (8:4:1) gives good separations of nortriptyline and amitryptline.

METHOD 2. (Gard, Knapp, Walle and Gaffney, 1973).

Ten ml of urine or bile are incubated at 37.5 degrees C with 3 ml of β-glucuronidase (Warner-Chilcott Ketodase) and 6 ml pH 5 acetate buffer (0.4M), then adjusted to pH 2 with hydrochloric acid. Add a measured amount of protriptyline as an internal standard. Extraction of amitriptyline and its metabolites, nortriptyline, and 10-hydroxyamitriptyline is done with an equal volume of 5% isobutanol in benzene (beware toxicity hazard) after alkalinisation to pH 14 with 50% w/v sodium hydroxide. Extract the organic layer with 1 ml of 1N sulphuric acid and back extract the acid layer after alkalinisation to pH 14 with 5 ml of 5% isobutanol in hexane. Separate and concentrate the organic layer to a small volume by warming under a stream of nitrogen. Inject 1 μl onto an 2% OV17 on Chromosorb W column at 220 to 230 degrees C, using nitrogen as the carrier gas and a flame ionisation detector.

RAPID METHOD 3. (Munksgaard, 1969 [modified]). Extract three ml blood, urine or liver homogenate with 10 ml 1 M sodium carbonate and 25 ml ether. Evaporate 15 ml of the ether layer to dryness and do TLC on Silica Gel PF254 plates previously activated at 110 degrees for thirty minutes. Clean the plate by developing first in chloroform: ether (80:15). Run in chloroform, acetone, diethylamine (50:40:10). Spray with iodoplatinate. Experience obviously has to be gained in recognizing the patterns of the drug and up to four of its metabolites.

INTERPRETATION OF RESULTS. Massive differences (8-78 ng/ml) have been found in blood of patients who took the same eight-day dose of 0.2 mg/Kilo three times daily (Asberg *et al.* 1970), and Swedish workers (Kragh-Sorensen *et al;* 1973) found that in endogenous depression the best therapeutic effect was obtained with a plasma level below 175 ng/ml. However, some patients went up as high as 238 ng/ml. Sjoqvist (1968) has reported therapeutic (150 mg/day nortriptyline) plasma levels of 3μg/ml after two weeks.

Braithwaite and Widdop (1971) found up to 303 ng/ml for amitriptyline and 246 ng/ml for nortriptyline in the plasma of volunteers and patients taking the drug over a period of time.

Blood levels in fatal overdose cases are very low; only 400 ng/ml has been found in a twenty-five-year old male who took between 1.25-2.5 g and died within three hours. Liver levels are much higher and can be expected to be over 1 mg/100 g. Urinary excretion is normally small; Forbes *et al.,* (1965) found only 50μg/100 ml in urine after consumption of 50 mg and 1 mg in a twenty-four-hour sample after 100 mg intake. See also Sunshine and Yaffe (1963). Thus, there is an overlap between overdose and high therapeutic dose blood levels.

Most workers think that liver concentrations are more useful in postmortem cases. Bonnichsen (1970) thinks 5 mg/100 g in liver is necessary to account for death where amitriptyline is the sole cause, but it is obviously impossible to be dogmatic.

However, in the writer's opinion, values over 1 μg/ml in the blood and/or 1 mg% in the liver would be worthy of toxicological consideration.

One of the great problems is the differing recovery of the drug and its metabolites, depending on the solvent used and its method of measurement. Ultraviolet measurement measures more than a G-C determination because metabolites contribute to the spectrum; Stevens found the hydrochloric acid recovery to be 32 percent while other workers have used a perchloric acid precipitation which Stevens found gave only an 8 percent yield. See Table XVIII.

As far as urinary excretion is concerned, recoveries ranging from 1.3 percent to 58 percent of the ingested dose in a twenty-four-hour sample of urine have been noted. Difficulties in interpretation are to be expected.

See also: Amundsen and Mathey, (1966) ; Balazar, *et al.,* (1973); Barnes, *et al.,* (1968); Betts, *et al.,* (1968) ; Blackwell, (1968) ; Blazek and Hronikova, (1967) ; Bonnichsen, *et al.,* (1970) ; Bruno and Lambiase, (1969) ; Burston, (1968) ; Charalampons and Johnson, (1967) ; Drabner, *et al.,* (1966) ; Eschenhof and Rieder, (1969); Hannsson and Cassano, (1966) ; Hucker and Miller, (1968) ; Milner, (1967); Milner, (1968); Nobel and Matthew, (1969); Norheim, (1974) ; Orepoulous and Lal, (1968) ; Sisenwine, *et al.,* (1969); Stinnelt, *et al.,* (1968) ; Winek, *et al.,* (1968) ; Worm, (1969) .

AMPHETAMINE AND OTHER STIMULANTS

Amphetamine and a host of similar amines are frequently abused, and a request for a rapid test is not unusual. Experienced workers all have their favorite methods; the following methods have been selected from the writer's personal preference. The TLC screen takes only a few minutes.

METHOD 1 (ULTRAVIOLET) (Stevens, 1973). Ten ml of urine is made alkaline to pH 12 by the addition of approximately 2.0 ml of 1.0N sodium hydroxide and shaken with 50 ml ether. The ether layer is separated and washed with three successive 15-ml portions of saturated sodium chloride solution, care being taken to drain out the last few drops of wash liquid each time. The ether extract is then shaken with 4 ml 0.03N sulphuric acid; this layer is then separated. Two ml are warmed and a current of air blown through it for five to ten seconds to expel ether. It is then carefully neutralized to pH 6 or 7 using 1.0N and 0.25N sodium hydroxide using universal indicator paper. 0.1 ml of 1% w/v sodium tetraborate ($Na_2B_4O_7$ 10 H_2O) and 0.4 ml of freshly prepared 10% w/v carbon disulpide in ethanol are then added.

Heat in a waterbath at 60 degrees C for seven minutes. Scan in a recording spectrophotometer from 240 to 300 nm against a reference blank containing tetraborate and CS_2. The amphetamine dithiocarbamate derivative has peaks at 254 and 284 nm with a trough at 272 nm. The peaks are about equal in size but the size of the 284 nm maximum is very susceptible to small changes in pH. Many amines behave in this way so the remaining 2 ml of the sulphuric acid extract is examined by TLC.

METHOD 2 (THIN LAYER CHROMATOGRAPHY). The other 2 ml acid extract obtained above are made alkaline to pH 12 and extracted with 10 ml ether. The ether is separated and carefully evaporated to about 100 μl (never let the solvent completely evaporate). This is then transferred to a silica-gel plate onto two separate spots and run in chloroform:methanol (90:10). (see Table IX.) After running, the part of the dried plate containing one spot is exposed in a tank of carbon disulphide vapour for five minutes. The plate is then examined in 254 nm light when even 1 μg of amphetamine can be seen as a dark-absorbing spot. A subsequent spray with 1% silver nitrate in 1N nitric acid brings up a dark brown spot.

Control spots of amphetamine and other amines such as methylamphetamine, ephedrine and phenmetrazine should also be run. The other spot after inspection in 254 nm light is sprayed with iodoplatinate solution (p. 81) when tertiary amines will reveal themselves (again, see Table VIII) as dark purple spots.

METHOD 3 (GAS CHROMATOGRAPHY) (Beckett, Tucker and Moffatt, 1967).

EXTRACTION FOR AMPHETAMINES AND EPHEDRINES. Urine (1 to 5 ml) is pipetted into a glass-stoppered centrifuge tube together with 0.5 ml 20% sodium hydroxide. The urine is then extracted with 2x2.5 ml freshly distilled ether using a mechanical test shaker; it is centrifuged, and the ether extracts transferred to a 15-ml Quickfit® test tube with a finely-tapered base. The extract is then concentrated to approximately 50 μl on a water bath at 40 degrees C.

EXTRACTION FOR PHENOLIC TYPE AMPHETAMINES. Urine (10 ml) is made alkaline to pH 9 to 10 with solid sodium carbonate and extracted, the extracts concentrated as described above except that 3x5-ml portions of ether are used.

One to 5-μl portions of the ether extracts are examined. Beckett and his co-workers give four columns for general use. For screening, the following is recommended: An acid-washed silanized support medium, i.e. Anakrom ABS or Chromosorb G (AW-DMCS) (80 to 100 mesh) is coated with 5% potassium hydroxide in ethanol which is evaporated off; it is then coated with 5% Apiezon L in ethylene dichloride and evaporated in a rotary evaporator below 40 degrees C. A 6-foot column is used at 160 degrees C. Table XXIV shows the retention time for a number of compounds.

IDENTIFICATION (FORMATION OF DERIVATIVES DETECTED BY GLC). a. Five tenths ml of acetone is added to 50 μl of the concentrated ethereal extract; it is then evaporated to 50 μl on a water bath at 60 degrees C. The Schiff's base formed with primary amines has a different retention time to the unchanged drug; 90 percent conversion is usually achieved.

b. Five tenths ml carbon disulphide is used instead of acetone in test a. This converts primary and secondary amines to give dithiocarbamates, but only primary amines are converted to the isothiocyanate which gives a peak on GLC.

c. Acetyl derivatives can be formed from primary and secondary amines by adding 5 μl acetic anhydride to the concentrated ethereal extract and injecting 5 μl of the mixture on the GLC.

TABLE XXIV
RETENTION TIMES FOR AMPHETAMINES

Base	Mean Retention Time in Minutes
Cyclopentamine	2.75
Amphetamine	3.5
Methylamphetamine	4.0
Pargyline	4.4
Nicotine	9.1
Phenylpropanolamine (dl-Norephedrine)	10.0
Ephedrine	11.9
Chlorphentermine	12.2
Methylephedrine	13.1
Phenmetrazine	15.0
*Diethylpropion	17.3
Nikethamide	22.7
Benzphetamine	100.0

*Diethylpropion; Major peak at 17.3 min. Smaller peak at approximately 19 min.
Instrument: Perkin-Elmer F11, with F.I.D.
Column: 5% Apiezon L + 5% KOH on A. S. Anakrom:-
Oven Temp. 160°C; Carrier Gas; N_2 at 60 ml/min. Inj. Port. Temp '4' (approximately 200°C)

This method is very suitable for the detection and identification of amphetamine and methylamphetamine in very small volumes of urine. Naturally, control results must be obtained first, and the toxicologist will soon build up his own table of retention times for the common drugs found in this fraction.

Direct injection of urine (10 μl) onto this column will also reveal amphetamine, providing the amplifier settings of the chromatograph can be set high enough. If control experiments show that less than a nanogram of amphetamine can be detected easily, then preliminary extraction is superfluous. This is the most rapid, convenient method of screening for amphetamine. Confirmation by acetone derivatives is achieved by warming the urine with an equal volume of acetone and injecting 10 μl again onto the column.

INTERPRETATION OF RESULTS. Abuse of amphetamine and methamphetamine usually results in very large concentrations in the urine, but therapeutic levels can be up as high as 10 to 20 μg/ml. (Clearly these figures have to be borne in mind when applying the TLC spots.) Deliberate taking of bicarbonate to make the urine alkaline and to so reduce the concentration of drug in the urine is well-known and clearly adds to the biochemical hazard for the abuser.

Methamphetamine is partially metabolized to amphetamine (up to about 10%). Urinary excretion depends tremendously on the pH of the urine; a change from pH 5 to pH 8 can alter the amount excreted from 3 to 63 percent.

ANTABUSE
(Tetraethyldithiuram Disulphide)

This drug inhibits acetaldehyde oxidation, and therefore gives rise to toxic and occasionally fatal results when ethanol is ingested, even as long as a week after cessation of drug therapy. Because acetaldehyde disappears rapidly from the blood, it may be worth attempting to show the presence of antabuse and alcohol, and therefore by inference, that acetaldehyde intoxication has taken place. However, antabuse itself is rapidly metabolized *in vitro,* the blood level is not proportional to the dose, it is not excreted in the urine and it is not extractable from tissues.

Heparin and sodium fluoride can cause interference, and sodium oxalate is the recommended anticoagulant.

METHODS (Divatia, Hine and Burbridge, 1952).

To 1 ml of whole blood or plasma add 1 ml of 0.002M copper sulphate solution. Add 1 ml of phosphate buffer at pH 7.4 and 10 ml of redistilled ethylene dichloride. Shake for thirty minutes, then centrifuge. Read the dichloride at 270 nm and at 320 nm. The optical density difference at these two wavelengths is proportional to the concentration of antabuse. Ethylene dichloride is used in the compensatory cell; standards are prepared in the range 5 to 200 μg/ml of blood.

ARSENIC

The methods described on page 125 will be suitable for normal analyses. As they form part of the general screen and were described earlier in this book, they will not be repeated here.

It cannot be too often emphasised that arsenical poisonings do escape a diagnosis. In the Stoneleigh Abbey case (Barrowcliffe, 1971) the victim was seen by twenty doctors on a teaching discussion round, and the possibility of arsenical poisoning was not raised.

OTHER METHODS. Neutron activation analysis is the preferred method for analyses of arsenic in hair, indeed for the analysis of only a few hairs it is the only method. After irradiation, in parallel with standards, the reduction to arsine and its trapping and counting provide the required results.

The older methods for atomic absorption determinations of arsenic are not sensitive, but new machines and devices are already on the market which can be used; for example, Hoover *et al.* (1974) report a sensitivity of 0.1 μg/As per gram. Flameless atomic absorption of liberated arsine has also been described (Chu *et al.*, 1972).

INTERPRETATION OF RESULTS. In general, the figures of Hansen and Moller (1949) show accepted levels and their interpretation. These are shown in Table XXV; all concentrations are in mg/100 g.

The clinical chemist must remember that the blood concen-

TABLE XXV
ARSENIC CONCENTRATIONS IN TISSUE

	Liver	*Kidney*	*Blood*	*Brain*
Normal healthy adults	0.001-0.01	0.001-0.01	0-0.002	—
Treated with inorganic arsenicals	—	—	0.01-0.025	—
Treated with organic arsenicals	ca 0.1	ca 0.02	ca 01	—
Acute arsenical poisoning	1 - 50	0.5-15	0.1 -1.5	0.05-2.0

trations are much lower than the liver or kidney figures. The writer's experience indicates that if the patient survives for a period of about four days then the blood figure can be even lower than that suggested by Hansen and Moller. Twenty μg/100 g was the figure in one fatal case following ingestion of arsenious oxide. In a case of death following the insertion of thirty pessaries of Stovarsol into the vagina over a period of three days, the concentration of arsenic (as trioxide) in the liver was 1.6 mg/100 g (Bowen *et al.*, 1961).

Smith (1967), using neutron-activation analysis on freeze-dried tissue, found values of 0.5 to 24.6 μg/100 g in *normal* liver, 0.2 to 36.3 in kidney and 0.1 to 92 in blood. This last figure seems extremely high, and Smith (personal communication) reports later work in which his highest dried blood value is 20 μg/100 g. Smith (1967) gives the following most useful table (Table XXVI) for results on freeze-dried tissues. These must be divided by 6 to get corresponding wet figures. See also: Smith, (1959).

Smith (1967) has also published most useful information on the distribution and measurement, using activation analysis, of arsenic in hair. There seems little doubt that exposure results in the deposition of arsenic in the root, and as the hair grows, repeated administration causes concentration peaks along the hair length. It is, therefore, possible by sectional analysis to deduce when arsenic was ingested and on how many occasions.

Pearson and Pounds (1971) record hair arsenic levels measured in centimetre lengths following long-term administration of Fowler's solution, and levels up to 88 ppm were found. Their results confirm the fact that arsenic is incorporated into the growing root, then grows out with the hair so that a good analytical picture can be obtained of administration against time of ingestion months later. This subject has been reviewed at length in *Advances in Forensic and Clinical Toxicology*, (Curry, A.S. 1972) especially in relation to murder enquiries.

Clinicians very often underestimate the quantity of hair the analyst requires for these analyses. If the Gutzeit procedure is used, about 3,000 hairs (1 g) are necessary. This will enable analysis on about half-inch lengths to be done. If an atomic reactor is

TABLE XXVI
NORMAL ARSENIC CONCENTRATIONS IN TISSUE SAMPLES
(Smith, 1967)

Tissue	No. of Samples	Maximum	Minimum	Median	Mean
Adrenal	22	0.293	0.002	0.029	0.061
Aorta	29	0.570	0.003	0.031	0.063
Blood (whole)	12	0.920	0.001	0.038	0.147
Bone	20	0.240	0.010	0.057	0.080
Brain	19	0.036	0.001	0.013	0.016
Breast	3	0.221	0.030	——	0.095
Hair	1250	8.17	0.030	0.510	0.650
Heart	23	0.078	0.002	0.024	0.027
Kidney	25	0.363	0.002	0.033	0.050
Liver	27	0.246	0.005	0.028	0.057
Lung	56	0.514	0.006	0.082	0.113
Muscle (pectoral)	24	0.431	0.012	0.063	0.091
Nail	124	2.90	0.020	0.300	0.362
Ovary	13	0.260	0.013	0.037	0.071
Pancreas	30	0.410	0.005	0.045	0.088
Prostate	10	0.090	0.010	0.046	0.045
Skin	76	0.590	0.009	0.090	0.124
Spleen	23	0.132	0.001	0.020	0.032
Stomach	21	0.104	0.003	0.037	0.037
Teeth	75	0.635	0.003	0.050	0.070
Thymus	11	0.332	0.003	0.015	0.047
Thyroid	22	0.314	0.001	0.042	0.079
Uterus	23	0.188	0.010	0.031	0.058

*Results are given as ppm in freeze-dried tissue. (Courtesy of the Editor of *J Forensic Sci Soc*).

available, the quantity need only be about 50 hairs. The hair should be cut as close to the head as possible, tied immediately in locks, and the cut end clearly indicated.

It is most important that, if the hair has been pulled from the scalp by the pathologist (which is the recommended procedure), before analysis *each hair* be aligned by the roots. This is a tedious procedure taking several hours work, but it is essential. The act of pulling the hairs from the scalp causes slipping of a few roots into the body of the lock. In a case of acute arsenical poisoning the concentration in the roots can be very high—several milligrams per 100 g, and it requires only a few hairs to slip to give a misleading impression that the concentration of arsenic along the length is uneven and that levels are above normal, i.e. a case of chronic poisoning being superimposed on an acute case. Alignment is therefore essential to overcome this artefact. Smith says categorically that the hair should *not* be washed before analysis.

In the United Kingdom in people not exposed to arsenic, the overall concentration median values of arsenic in hair are 0.62 and 0.67 $\mu g/g$ for males and females respectively. Smith says that values over $2\mu g/g$ merit further investigation, *but* this advice must include the caveat that, in acute poisoning, the roots must be separately analysed. He quotes a case with a whole hair value of 0.86 $\mu g/g$ with 90 $\mu g/g$ in the first millimeter from the root.

The rate of hair growth varies over a fairly wide range. The average rate is said to be about 13 mm a month, although Stewart and Stolman, in a review of the literature, give a range of 9.3 to 10.2 mm per thirty days.

Teichmann and his co-workers reported at the first International Meeting in Forensic Toxicology, London, 1963, the range of *normal values* for urinary arsenic excretion. It is clear from the literature quoted in this paper, involving over 500 persons and eight surveys, that the majority of workers found mean values of the order of 1 $\mu g/100$ ml, although amounts varied considerably, presumably due to diet and industrial exposure. Levels can rise up to 200 $\mu g/100$ ml in arsenic workers. In acute arsenic poisoning values higher than this are normally found, but if several days have elapsed between ingestion and the taking of the sample, the interpretation of levels in the range 1 to 200 $\mu g/100$ ml may be necessary and will be difficult.

Kingsley and Schaffert (1951) showed that *therapeutic* arsenic solutions (Fowler's solution) gave urinary excretions up to 30 $\mu g/100$ ml which dropped to 2 $\mu g/100$ ml in ten days.

See also Taylor, (1956).

BARBITURATES

The extraction and rough quantitation of the common 5:5 disubstituted barbiturates as a group has been described on page 47. For accurate quantitation, using ultraviolet spectrophotometry. Table XXVII shows the $E_{1cm}^{1\%}$ values for several barbiturates.

TABLE XXVII

$E_{1cm}^{1\%}$ VALUES OF COMMON BARBITURATES

$E_{1cm}^{1\%}$ values at 240 nm in 0.05 M borax buffer*			
Phenobarbitone	431	Quinalbarbitone Secobarbital	374
Barbitone	538	Hexethal	400
Methylphenobarbitone	458	Sigmodal	271
Dial	442	Butallyonal	280
Vinbarbitone	446	Allyl, sec-butyl barbiturate	401
Cyclobarbitone	423	Sandoptal	415
Cycloheptenyl, ethyl, barbiturate	400	Nostal	301
Amylobarbitone	424	Aprobarbital	438
Butobarbitone	453	Probarbital	452
Butabarbitone	439	Allyl, phenyl, barbiturate	401
Pentobarbitone	411		

*Stevenson, G. W.: *Anal Chem, 33*:1376, 1961.

An alternative approach is to use gas chromatography.

METHOD (Berry, 1973).

Berry had a critical look at gas chromatographic columns and methods of extraction. He recommends tetraphenylene ethylene as the internal standard. For toxic levels 1.0 ml of plasma is extracted with 15 ml of chloroform by gentle shaking for ten minutes. After centrifuging and pouring the chloroform layer through a glass wool plug, the barbiturate is back extracted into 5 ml of 0.5N sodium hydroxide. After acidification it is re-extracted into 5 ml of chloroform and evaporated. He favors 4% CDMS on Chromosorb W, HP at 220 degrees. Retention times are given in Table XXVIII. Leach and Toseland (1968) and Blackmore and Jenkins (1968) have also described reliable methods. The latter workers' results (Table XXIX) are similar to those of Berry.

It is essential to identify the barbiturates involved before attempting to interpret the quantitative result into probable clinical effect. GC-mass spectrometry is an ideal solution, but most workers will probably have to stick to paper or thin layer chromatography for some time yet.

Chromatographic Methods for Identification. After the ultra-

TABLE XXVIII

Compound	4% CDMS
Allybarbituric acid	4.0
Amylobarbitone	4.1
Barbitone	2.5
Butobarbitone	3.8
n-Butylallylbarbitone	4.7
Cyclobarbitone	14.3
Glutethimide	4.2
Heptabarbitone	19.4
Hexobarbitone	4.1
Methaqualone	8.6
Methohexitone	1.8
Nealbarbitone	4.5
Pentobarbitone	23.4
Phenobarbitone	4.5
Quinalbarbitone	5.6
Tetraphenylethylene	7.8
Thiopentone	6.2

violet curves have been read, the acidified solution from the cuvette is re-extracted into 5 ml of ether which is separated, dried with a little anhydrous sodium sulphate, decanted and evaporated. If barbiturate has been found by ultraviolet spectrophotometry an estimate of its total weight in the extract can be made. The amount necessary for good results in the chromatographic identification depends on the particular technique that is to be used. For paper 10 μg should be put on one spot; for TLC, about 5 μg; for Eastman® Chromatogram sheet, 0.5 μg; for GLC, about 10 ng. The most common other drugs to be sought are glutethimide and phenytoin. Recommended systems for paper, TLC and Eastman sheet follow.

Paper. Systems are as follows:

1. Whatman No. 4 paper: solvent, n-butanol:880 ammonia: water (100:33:66). Use the top layer.

2. (Fox, personal communication.) Whatman No. 1 paper is pretreated by dipping in 10% w/v trisodium phosphate, blotted and dried. Before use, dip in acetone:water (75:25), blot, and in the two to three minutes during which time the acetone evaporates at room temperature, apply the spots. Run

TABLE XXIX
RETENTION TIMES OF BARBITURATES

Compound	Mean Retention Time Column 1	Relative R.T. c.f. Buto- barbitone Column 1	Mean Retention Time Column 2	Relative R.T. c.f. Buto- barbitone Column 2
Barbitone	4.05	0.67	7.5	0.60
Butobarbitone	6.30	1.00	12.55	1.00
Amylobarbitone	6.8	1.08	14.60	1.16
Hydroxyamylobarbitone	26.8	4.25	64.0	5.1
Hexobarbitone	6.70	1.06	13.85	1.10
Pentobarbitone	7.60	1.21	15.15	1.21
Cyclobarbitone	22.30	3.55	48.80	3.90
Methylphenylbarbitone	9.65	1.53	19.3	1.54
Quinalbarbitone	9.60	1.52	18.8	1.50
Phenobarbitone	33.50	5.33	75.2	6.05
Secbutobarbiturate	6.25	0.98	12.55	1.00
Glutethimide	6.40	1.02	12.60	1.01

Column 1
Column Neopentyl Glycol adipate and trimer acid on A.W.—DMSC Chromosorb
W. 80-100 mesh. 3: ¾: 96¼
Temperature: 220°C. Carrier gas: N_2 at 60 ml/min.
Inj. Temp. '5'
Gas Chromatograph: Perkin-Elmer F-11. with F.I.D.
Column 2
Temperature 200°C. Other conditions as above. All times in minutes.

either for a four-inch run ascending in a beaker, or for a ten-inch descending run in a tank using ethylene dichloride as the developing solvent with water in the bottom of the tank.

3. (Abernethy and Hensel, personal communication.) Whatman No. 1 paper pretreated by dipping in 5% sodium silicate, blotted and dried. The paper is run in the bottom layer of chloroform:880 ammonia (100:50) after equilibrating the paper for forty-five minutes in the vapour of the top layer. The developing solvent must be introduced without disturbing the atmosphere; a symmetrical paper arrangement is best.

Systems 2 and 3 are recommended but system 1 is useful for the beginner. Rf's are given in Table XXX, but the values are not absolute ones, and control spots should be run on all occasions.

TABLE XXX
RF VALUES OF BARBITURATES ON PAPER CHROMATOGRAMS

System 1	System 2	System 3	Compound	Melting Point
.43	.02	.05	Barbitone	188 — 190
.50	.05	.05	Phenobarbitone	193 — 195
.58	.20	.22	Cyclobarbitone	171 — 174
.69	.30	.36	Butobarbitone	127 — 130
.73	.65	.66	Amylobarbitone	152 — 156
.73	.75	.66	Pentobarbitone	122 — 130
.77	.85	.77	Quinalbarbitone (Secobarbital)	96 — 100
.75	.45	.44	Nealbarbitone	155 — 157
.60	.65	.65	Phenytoin	295 — 298
.75	.90	.90	Glutethimide	87

Practice is needed during which the reader will obtain his own values.

If there is any yellow color in the ether extract in this fraction, system 1 should be used. Control spots of DNOC and p-nitrophenol should be run as well. Sometimes decomposing blood and tissue contains a yellow chalcone which is separated in this system from these poisons.

Detection is achieved by one of the following methods: (a) Inspect the paper under 254 nm light; alkaline papers used in solvents 2 and 3 enable the barbiturate spots to be seen without prior treatment. In the case of solvent 1 the paper is inspected before and after exposing it to ammonia fumes. Phenobarbitone and cyclobarbitone can be seen before exposure to ammonia because they exhibit slight absorption at this wavelength in neutral conditions. Glutethimide is decomposed if solvents 2 or 3 are used and is not detected by this method. (b) Dip the paper in 5% mercuric oxide dissolved in 20% sulphuric acid; wash well with three rinses of distilled water and then dip in 0.1% diphenylcarbazone in ethanol. The spots are colored various shades of purple. (c) Spray with saturated aqueous mercurous nitrate solution. The spots are black. Not suitable for system 1. (d) Spray with 0.1% aqueous potassium permanganate solution. Those compounds with allyl groups in the molecule (nealbarbitone, quinalbarbitone) give immediate yellow colors. Cyclobarbitone gives a yellow color in about thirty seconds. (e) Expose the paper to chlorine or bromine fumes for five minutes. Aerate for fifteen minutes; spray with 1% w/v potassium iodide containing freshly boiled starch solution to reveal blue-black spots.

Thin Layer Chromatography. Solvent systems are as follows:

1. Chloroform:acetone (9:1) on Silica-Gel G plates.

2. (Richardson, 1964.) Chloroform:isopropanol (8:2) on Silica-Gel G plates in an atmosphere of ammonia.

3. (A.S. Curry and R.H. Fox, 1968). Merck cellulose-coated plates (with fluorescent indicator) GF254 pretreated by dipping in 10% w/v trisodium phosphate aqueous solution, blotting and drying for twenty minutes at 80 degrees C. Before applying the spots dip in acetone:water (75:25) and aerate for two to three minutes for the acetone to evaporate. Run in methyl n-amyl ketone.

4. (R.H. Fox, personal communication.) Treat Eastman Chromatogram Sheet Cellulose No. 6065 and run in the same way as the Merck plates in system 3 in the Eastman Chamber No. 104 or the 20 by 20 cm size.

As for the paper systems, the reader should obtain his own Rf values running controls on every occasion. Systems 3 and 4 are recommended but require practice. See Table XXXI for typical values.

TABLE XXXI

RF VALUES OF BARBITURATES ON THIN LAYER CHROMATOGRAMS

System 1	System 2	System 3	System 4	Compound
.20	.47	.20	.20	Barbitone
.24	.33	.30	.30	Phenobarbitone
.24	.62	.38	.38	Cyclobarbitone
.33	.67	.70	.70	Butobarbitone
.33	.74	.82	.82	Amylobarbitone
.33	.74	.85	.85	Pentobarbitone
.44	.77	.90	.90	Quinalbarbitone
.38	.68	.75	.75	Nealbarbitone
.00	.62	.00	.00	Phenytoin
.75	.97	.99	.99	Glutethimide

For detection, use the methods as for paper except that the mercury/diphenylcarbazone treatment is modified as follows: Spray with 5 g mercuric oxide in 100 ml of 20% sulphuric acid diluted to 250 ml. Barbiturates are seen as white spots. Overspray with .01% diphenylcarbazone in chloroform to reveal blue spots. To see spots on Silica-Gel G plates in 254 nm light, spray with .04% fluorescein in 4% w/v aqueous sodium hydroxide.

An alternative method for the chlorine/starch iodide method is to spray with commercial sodium hypochlorite, 1:20 dilution; after five minutes spray with ethanol, and after one minute with a solution of 0.5% amidon in 0.5% potassium iodide. Two tenths μg of barbiturates can be detected on the Eastman sheet with the mercurous nitrate spray.

Another useful test for differentiating barbiturates is to heat them with concentrated sulphuric acid. This will probably not be of much use to the clinical biochemist unless he has no chromatographic facilities, but, done on an aliquot of the liver extract in fatal cases, it can be useful. The test is usually done in a test tube, and 1 ml of concentrated sulphuric acid is added to an evaporated ethereal aliquot. A cotton wool plug is placed in position at the mouth of the tube which is then immersed in a boiling water bath for exactly one hour. The acid is then poured into 25 ml of water, cooled, and extracted with 20 ml of ether. The ether is separated, evaporated and dissolved in 0.5N ammonia solution. The volume should equal that used for the reading taken at pH = 10 (see p. 54). The ultraviolet absorption spectrum is measured between 220 and 320 nm. 5,5 disubstituted barbiturates substituted in the alpha position to the ring undergo attack and Table XXXII shows typical results of the acid treatment.

INTERPRETATION OF RESULTS

1. *The Living Subject.* There is a great deal of confusion in the literature concerning the interpretation of analytical results in cases involving barbiturates. In this writer's view, this is because doctors and toxicologists have tried to compare or contrast cases involving different barbiturates, patients with differing degrees of habituation, and blood samples taken at differing times since ingestion, then analysed by differing methods. On many

TABLE XXXII

EFFECT OF CONCENTRATED SULPHURIC ACID ON BARBITURATES

Barbiturate	Wavelength Maximum of Product at pH 10
Barbitone	240 nm
Amylobarbitone	240 nm
Butobarbitone	240 nm
Pentobarbitone	268 nm
Cyclobarbitone	268 nm
Quinalbarbitone	weak peaks at
(Secobarbital)	240, 266 and 315 nm
Phenobarbitone	completely destroyed
Nealbarbitone	240 nm major peak and 315 nm as minor peak

occasions the possible simultaneous ingestion of alcohol and other drugs has been ignored or no analyses for these have been performed. It is not surprising that some clinicians have given up trying to relate level to clinical effect, while others do not even bother to ask for an identification. In order to try and rationalize this confusion it is necessary to make some general remarks.

a. There is good evidence that barbiturates do not concentrate massively in any one organ, although liver levels are elevated. Consequently, the more one takes, the higher is the expected blood level. (Serum and blood are virtually synonymous for barbiturate.)

b. Barbiturates accumulate in the body when taken over long periods of time in therapeutic doses. A barbiturate addict will be taking massive doses, often many grams a day, and, hence, he or she will be walking around reasonably fit and well with blood levels perhaps ten times those that will account for death in a person not used to barbiturates.

c. It is easier to interpret blood levels than urine concentrations.

d. In cases of patients undergoing normal therapy with short acting barbiturates, i.e. one sleeping capsule at night, one would not expect blood levels over 0.5 mg/100 ml. The following general remarks apply: levels below 1 mg/100 ml in the blood can account for coma in the case of secobarbitone (quinalbarbitone: Seconal®) and pentobarbitone (Nembutal®). For butobarbitone (Soneryl®) and amylobarbitone (Amytal®), levels of about 3 mg/100 ml are usually required to account for a deep coma. Patients on phenobarbitone and barbitone may still be conscious at 10 mg/100 ml if they have been having one or two tablets three times a day or long-term, heavy night-time sedation.

f. If the patient has never had barbiturate before or takes alcohol as well, the effects are generally greater.

If the patient is addicted, then all the blood level will do is tell the clinician that the patient has taken a large dose of barbiturate, and indeed, as can be seen from the above rationale, this is all that can be determined in the laboratory. A very rough estimate of the total barbiturate in the body (excluding the stomach) can be made from the statement that a one-gm dose of barbiturate can be expected to lead to a *maximum* blood level of about 2 mg/100 ml in a 150-pound person. It is also usual to find that a blood level will drop by about 2 mg/100 ml in each twenty-four-hour period.

2. *The Dead Victim.* Many workers have correlated death cases with blood levels, but apart from showing that people who have taken overdoses occasionally die, there is little to be said. Gee and his co-workers in 1974, can still write, "the diagnosis of barbiturate poisoning even nowadays, is not foolproof as far as the pathologist is concerned."

As with cases involving alcohol, the source of the blood for barbiturate determination is important. Heart blood values are usually about twice the peripheral blood values with little difference between left and right heart. Portal vein blood should be avoided. The values in brain are normally about the same as in heart blood.

Gee *et al.,* (1974) presents convincing figures to show that the toxicologist agrees with the anatomist that, of the blood entering the inferior vena cava, roughly half is derived from the liver! The liver always has a higher concentration of barbiturate than the blood, usually at least twice, and sometimes twenty times as much. It is still speculative as to whether the high liver/peripheral blood ratios prove recent intake, i.e. within five hours, but the results from all sources are highly suggestive. (High means a ratio greater than 4.)

A liver left in a jar experiences depletion of fluid due to drainage, then a significant increase in the liver concentration occurs because the drained fluid is relatively free of barbiturate.

The computer at the Home Office Central Research Establishment has 347 references post 1966 on its barbiturate file not counting the many books on the subject. It would be invidious to single out a few. Surely each country has its *barbiturate expert* by now, and, in any case, entry to the literature is available via a library.

BENZENE

This is an extremely toxic solvent and a method for its colorimetric determination is described below. A gas chromatographic examination is also an obvious method of enquiry (see p. 94) .

METHOD (Gerarde and Skiba, 1960) .

Added to 5 ml of blood are 35 ml 0.1N hydrochloric acid in a two-ounce wide-mouthed bottle and mixed by inversion; 5 ml of carbon tetrachloride are added, and the whole is shaken for three to five minutes. The water layer is removed and the centrifuged, separated, carbon tetrachloride layer transferred to a test tube. Five ml of reagent (1 ml of 40% formaldehyde and 100 ml concentrated sulphuric acid) are added, and, after stoppering, the mixture is shaken for two minutes. After centrifuging at 2,000 rpm for five minutes the color is read at 490 nm. Standards are prepared in the range 1 to 10 mg/100 ml of benzene in blood.

INTERPRETATION OF RESULTS. Because of the leukaemia-inducing properties of benzene, the writer believes any measurable blood level must be regarded extremely seriously. It is most important that rubber-capped vials should not be used for the submission of blood samples in cases of suspected benzene intoxication. For a gas chromatographic method for benzene and toluene see also Szadkowski *et al.,* 1971.

BERYLLIUM

Industrial poisoning as a result of inhalation of dust containing beryllium compounds occasionally occurs. In such cases the metal can be detected in the lungs and in mediastinal lymph for periods up to at least ten years after exposure.

METHOD (Peterson, Welford and Harley, 1950) . Lung tissue,

100 g, is wet ashed with nitric and sulphuric acid in a Kjeldahl flask keeping the volume of sulphuric acid as low as possible. The total volume used should not exceed 5 ml of concentrated acid. The final destruction of organic material is effected by the addition of 0.5 ml of 60% perchloric acid, heating being continued to the production of white fumes. Decant and wash into a centrifuge tube with water and ethanol, then evaporate on a water bath. Make up to about 20 ml with water and add ammonia dropwise to appearance of a precipitate. Cool, and add 2 ml glacial acetic acid and dilute hydrochloric acid dropwise until the precipitate just redissolves. Now add 5 ml of 12% oxine in glacial acetic acid and adjust the pH to 6 with ammonia. Centrifuge and decant through a loose filter paper into a 125-ml separating funnel. Wash the filter paper with water and combine the washings and the filtrate. Extract filtrate with 10 ml of chloroform to remove the excess oxine and repeat the washing if the aqueous phase is not colorless. The aqueous phase is then transferred to a 50-ml centrifuge tube and the pH adjusted to 7; 1 ml of aluminum salt solution containing 2.5 mg of aluminium per millilitre is then added. The precipitate is centrifuged and washed, and the supernatant discarded. Forty mg of sodium chloride are added, and, after evaporating to dryness, arc spectroscopy is performed. Lines at 2348.6, 2650.8, 3130 and 3131 Å are examined. Suitable standards are in the range of 0.1 to 5 μg.

A gas chromatographic analysis, capable of detecting 0.01 microgram/ml of blood is also available (Foreman *et al.*, 1970; Taylor and Arnold, 1971). In this technique beryllium trifluoroacetylacetonate is obtained by heating samples with a benzene solution of trifluoroacetylacetone.

INTERPRETATION OF RESULTS. There is usually no difficulty in the interpretation of the results in a case of berylliosis, but the toxicologist must be aware that the amounts for which he is searching are usually very much less than with normal *poisons*. Lung tissue and lymph in such cases can contain less than 1 μg of beryllium per 100 g of tissue. In one case in which the writer was involved the analysis showed the levels were 20 μg per 100 g of formalin-treated lung tissue and 10 μg per 100 g of mediastinal lymph. Death occurred seven years after exposure to dust. See also: McCallum, *et al.*, (1961); Smythe and Whittem (1961).

BORON

This is usually encountered as borax or boric acid, especially in the accidental poisoning of young children by these medicaments. Because the borate ion will not dialyse, presumably because of the formation of sugar complexes in biological media, it is essential that a sample of blood or tissue be separately analysed for its total boron content.

METHOD (Smith, Goudie and Sivertson, 1955).

One tenth of a gram (0.1 g) of lithium carbonate and 2 ml of blood or tissue slurry are evaporated to dryness on a steam bath in a platinum crucible. The crucible is then transferred to a muffle furnace when the temperature is slowly raised to 650 degrees C where it is held for one and one-half hours or until the sample is free of carbon. After cooling, 2 ml of 6N hydrochloric acid are added, and after mixing well they are centrifuged. One ml of the supernatant is mixed in a boron-free test tube with 5 ml of concentrated sulphuric acid containing 250 mg of carminic acid per litre. The violet color from the reaction with boron develops at a rate dependent on the quality of carminic acid reagent. Some batches produce a stable color within a few minutes, but in others several hours are necessary. The zero blank reagent is put in the compensatory cell, and when the reading at 575 nm reaches a stable value, the optical density is measured. A calibration graph for 0 to 25 μg boron standards gives optical readings in the range 0 to 0.5 at this wavelength.

INTERPRETATION OF RESULTS. McBay, in a paper to the Toxicology Section of the American Academy of Forensic Sciences in 1961, reviewed the literature on boron poisoning in young children, and reached the conclusion that blood levels over 4 mg/100 ml total boron were suggestive of poisoning.

Cases of poisoning analyzed before the era of accurate colorimetry gave tissue values of over 25 mg/100 ml and sometimes over 100 mg/100 ml but these are much higher than the average case nowadays. Blood boron levels in normal healthy infants are in the range 0 to .08 mg/100 ml.

BROMIDE

This can be encountered either as a result of ingestion of inorganic bromide or as a metabolite of organo-bromo compounds such as carbromal or bromvaletone. Nonprescription medication is frequently involved.

METHOD 1. (Hall, 1943).

Mixed in the ratio 1:1 are 20% trichloracetic acid and 0.25% auric chloride solutions. One drop of serum is spread over the area of 1 cm², and one drop of reagent dropped into the center. The circular ring of precipitated proteins has a yellow color at bromide levels of about 25 mg/100 ml, and is red-brown at levels in excess of 50 mg/100 ml.

METHOD 2. (Street, 1960).

Two millilitres of blood diluted 1:1 with water are deproteinised with 10 ml of 20% trichloracetic acid. Nine ml of filtrate are extracted with 5 ml of ether. Seven ml of the aqueous phase are then mixed with 2 ml of 6N sulphuric acid and a knife blade point of potassium permanganate. It is then shaken with 3 ml of cyclohexane and the brown solution of bromine in the organic solvent read against exact standards at 405 nm.

A procedure for measuring bromide in serum filtrates has been described by Goodwin (1971). This involves tungstate/hydrochloric acid deproteinisation, oxidation to bromate with hypochlorite, and reaction with added bromide to give bromine which is reacted with rosaniline. In twenty-eight men, the maximum bromide level was 3.05 mg/100 ml. A flame photometric method may also be used (Gutsche and Herrmann, 1970) for bromide in urine.

INTERPRETATION OF RESULTS. After ingestion of a single overdose of an organo-bromo compound, blood levels do not rise above what may be present in normal blood, that is up to 5 mg/100 ml. In these cases the concentration of total bromide in the liver may be as high as 15 to 25 mg/100 g, and therefore provides a lead to the probable ingested poison. An alkaline fusion of the blood is necessary to destroy the organic compound in these cases, although continued therapy with these drugs will lead to blood levels of over 100 mg/100 ml of inorganic bromide at which level psychiatric disturbances manifest themselves.

Accumulation with inorganic bromide therapy also occurs, and mental disturbances and skin rashes at blood levels over 200 mg/100 ml are common. Its use as a sedative in the treatment of mentally ill patients should include routine blood determinations because of this probability.

BUTAZOLIDIN® (PHENYLBUTAZONE)

Because this drug has been noted as causing agranulocytosis, clinicians often ask for routine determinations of its concentration in blood. In the writer's experience it has not appeared in the usual deproteinised extracts, and the following method can be used.

METHODS (Stevens, 1970 Courtesy *Clin. Chem.*).

PLASMA. To 3 ml plasma, add 7 ml of water, followed by 1 ml of formic acid (98 to 99%). Shake this mixture vigorously with 30 ml of *n*-hexane. Separate the hexane layer and add to it a little anhydrous sodium sulfate to destroy any traces of emulsified liquids. Wash the hexane extract by shaking it with about one fourth of its volume of water and discard the wash liquid.

Add 5 ml of 0.5N sodium hydroxide to the hexane and shake the mixture vigorously in a separatory funnel. After the phases have separated, withdraw the aqueous alkaline layer from the funnel. It may be slightly opalescent at this stage; it can be cleared by keeping it at its boiling point over a small flame for fifteen to thirty seconds with gentle agitation. The slight turbidity will not be detrimental to the subsequent spectrophotometric assay in 1-cm cells at 263 nm versus 0.5N sodium hydroxide.

BLOOD. Mix 5.0 ml of blood with 10 ml of water, then add 15 ml of 0.5N sodium hydroxide. To the dark brown, clear solution add 1 ml of formic acid to render the mixture acid. Add 30 ml of hexane and shake the mixture vigorously. When the phases separate, remove and discard the excess of aqueous (lower) phase. Pour the emulsified hexane layer into a small flask and break the hexane emulsion by continually adding anhydrous sodium sulphate during brisk agitation. Separate the hexane extract, wash it with water, and extract with 0.5N alkali as described for plasma.

LIVER. Pulp a weighed quantity of liver (2-5 g) with 10 ml of water, add 15 ml of 0.5N sodium hydroxide, and continue maceration for about one minute. Add 1 ml of formic acid to make the mixture acid. Shake the mixture with 30 ml of hexane and complete the procedure as described for blood. *Blank* samples of plasma, blood or liver should be processed, and the corresponding alkali extracts used as reference solutions on the spectrophotometry.

Standards should be prepared using butazolidin added to plasma, blood or urine as relevant. The range should be 5 to 15 mg/100 ml. Recovery from plasma is 95 percent, and from blood, 65 to 70 percent.

The majority (about 90%) of phenylbutazone is bound to protein. Its main metabolite is p-hydroxyphenylbutazone (oxyphenbutazone) which appears in both the strong and weak acid fractions in routine extractions. In sodium hydroxide solution the unchanged drug has an absorption maximum at 265 nm $E_{1cm}^{1\%} = 820$, whereas the corresponding metabolite figures are 253 nm $E_{1cm}^{1\%}$ 630. In a fatal case of accidental poisoning in a child the writer found the drug could not be detected after a tungstic acid isolation method.

For a TLC separation of phenylbutazone and oxyphenbutazone silica gel plates are used in chloroform:acetone (9:1). Spray with 1% ammonium vanadate, dry and overspray with concentrated sulphuric acid. Phenylbutazone gives a purple spot; oxyphenbutazone, a yellow one.

Oxyphenbutazone is not very soluble in hexane. If a chloroform extraction is used, subsequent separation of phenylbutazone from oxyphenbutazone can be achieved by the use of hexane/chloroform partition coefficients.

INTERPRETATION OF RESULTS. Normal blood levels for patients under routine therapy are about 10 mg/100 ml. See also Whittaker and Price Evans (1970).

CADMIUM

Cadmium salts are highly toxic; most recorded cases of poisoning refer either to inhalation of fumes in industrial processes or to accidental ingestion from solutions of citrus fruits made in cadmium-plated containers, but Sachs and Calker (1959) noted an unusual case from the plating in a coffee percolator in which the clinical diagnosis was extremely difficult. This type of metallic poisoning usually manifests itself in an outbreak involving several persons with copper as the most usual impurity; Sachs and Calker's case, therefore, emphasises again the need for extensive toxicological investigations in unusual or unexpected deaths, and cadmium must not be forgotten. Atomic absorption spectrophotometry is the most suitable method for cadmium. The limit of sensitivity for cadmium in blood was found to be 23 x 10^{-12} g Cd by Cernik (1973) using a microtechnique in a nickel crucible. Hauser *et al.* (1972) used a tantalum boat technique.

Great care has to be taken when dealing with such low amounts to avoid contamination and loss by adsorption. Struempler (1973) recommends polyethylene containers for aqueous cadmium solutions.

METHOD 1 (Saltzman, 1953).

Tissue, 5 g, is heated in a Kjeldahl flask with 1 ml of concentrated sulphuric acid and 2 ml of concentrated nitric acid. When digestion is complete the clear solution is neutralized to just yellow to thymol blue with 40% sodium hydroxide. The volume is adjusted to 25 ml, and the following solutions are added in order: 1 ml of 25% sodium potassium tartrate, 5 ml of a solution containing 40 g of sodium hydroxide and 1 g potassium cyanide per 100 ml, 1 ml of 20% hydroxylamine hydrochloride and 15 ml of 0.008% dithizone in chloroform. After shaking, the chloroform layer is run into a second separating funnel containing 25 ml of 2% tartaric acid which should be ice-cold. Add 10 ml of chloroform to the first separator, shake and run it into the second separator. Shake the second funnel for two minutes and discard the chloroform. Add 5 ml chloroform, shake again and discard. Add 0.25 ml hydroxylamine hydrochloride solution (20%) and 15 ml of a 0.008% solution of dithizone in chloroform and 5 ml of a solution containing 40 g of sodium hydroxide and 0.05 g of potassium cyanide per 100 ml. Shake for one minute and run the chloroform through a cotton wool plug into the measuring cell. Read at 518 nm. The calibration curve is prepared with standards in the range of 0 to 10 μg of cadmium.

METHOD 2 (Berman, 1967).

Oxalated blood, 5 ml, and 10 ml 5% trichloroacetic acid are mixed in a centrifuge tube. After one hour the contents are centrifuged and the supernatant decanted into a 60-ml cylindrical separating funnel. The precipitate is washed with another 10 ml of 5% TCA and centrifuged. The washings are added to the separating funnel. Adjust the pH to 6 to 7.5 by addition of 2N sodium hydroxide; add 1 ml 1% aqueous sodium diethyldithiocarbamate and 2.5 ml of water saturated methyl-isobutyl ketone. Shake for two minutes; separate the organic phase and feed into the Perkin-Elmer 303 Atomic Absorption Spectrophotometer (at 2288 Å). For urine make 10 ml to pH 6 to 7.5 and proceed with the complexing extraction as described above. Tissue (1 g) is destroyed by a concentrated nitric and sulphuric acid digestion, diluted to 25 ml, made to pH 6-7.5 and analyzed as above.

METHOD 3 (Curry and Knott, Courtesy *Clin. Chim. Acta* 1970). APPARATUS. Perkin-Elmer Model 303 Atomic Absorption Spectrophotometer equipped with scale expansion accessory and an Hitachi Perkin-Elmer Model 165 recorder: Kjeldahl digestion apparatus

REAGENTS. Digestion mixture 1:1 *Foodstuffs* grade nitric acid: *Foodstuffs* grade sulphuric acid

Nitric acid, *Foodstuffs* grade

Concentrated ammonia solution, *Foodstuffs* grade

Bromo-thymol blue

Demineralized water

1000 p.p.m. standard cadmium solution made by dissolving 2.282 g 3 $CdSO_4$ 8 H_2O in demineralized water and making up to 1 litre.

For each determination about 2 g of sample are cut from the respective organ using stainless steel scissors; the samples are accurately weighed and placed in a 100-ml Kjeldahl flask. The tissue is digested by adding 2 ml of the digestion mixture, a couple of antibumping beads and electrically heating. One-ml aliquots of the nitric acid are added as required until no further charring occurs. Blanks are prepared in a similar manner. On completion, the digest is allowed to cool, then neutralized to about pH 3, using the ammonia solution and bromo-thymol blue indicator. The acidity adjustment is made in order to protect the burner of the spectrophotometer. The resulting solution is transferred quantitatively into a 25-ml volumetric flask and made up to the mark with demineralized water. Cadmium standards of 0.1, 0.2, 0.5 and 1.0 p.p.m. are made by dilution of the 1000 p.p.m. stock standard. The standards and samples are then compared on the atomic absorption spectrophotometer using the following instrumental settings:

Source	Cadmium hollow cathode lamp
Current	6 mA
Wavelength	228.8 nm
Slit	4 (bandpass 7 Å)
Burner	Boling 3-slot
Flame	air/acetylene
Scale expansion	$\times 1$, $\times 3$ as required
Noise suppression	$\times 2$

INTERPRETATION OF RESULTS. Cadmium is a normal constituent of tissues, and Stitch, using arc emission spectroscopy, said that *ashed* kidney can contain up to 10 mg/100 g. Because cadmium salts are toxic in doses of 50 mg it is clear that, as in the case of mercury, the analyses alone cannot in many cases provide unequivocal proof of poisoning, although its detection in kidney in amounts over 2 mg/100 g and the finding of a similar level in the liver would warrant a full investigation into the circumstances of the death. Normal urinary excretion is said to be 0 to 20 μg/litre, but in workers in the cadmium industry it can rise as high as 580 μg/litre.

In nonfatal cases reported by Berman the blood level was only 5 μg/100 ml with 710 μg/litre in the urine. The sources were silver polish and shoe whitener.

Curry and Knott (1970), in twenty cases in the United Kingdom not involving cadmium, found a mean liver concentration of 2 μg/g, and a mean kidney concentration of 11.7 μg/g.

In three cases involving long-term industrial intake values of 5, 180 and 200 μg/g in liver were found with corresponding kidney levels of 70, 170 and 300 μg/g.

Lewis *et al.* (1972) found means of about 4 mg per kidney 2.28 mg in the liver and 0.36 mg in lungs in thirty-four nonsmokers. Comparable values for 138 male smokers were 10.28 mg for kidneys, 3.06 mg for liver, and 0.81 mg in lungs (whole organ values).

See also: Manley and Dalley, (1957); Smith, *et al.*, (1955).

CANNABIS

The material either as plant or resin has a characteristic appearance. Tests for the presence of tetrahydrocannabinol, cannabidiol and cannabinol can then be done.

METHOD (Patterson and Stevens, 1970 Courtesy *J Pharm. Pharmacol.*)

An extract is prepared by shaking the cannabis or cannabis resin vigorously for one minute with sufficient stock solution of dibenzylphthalate (10 mg/ml) in light petroleum (40-60°) to produce a mixture containing approximately 20% w/v cannabis or 10% w/v of cannabis resin. The supernatant solution is used without further purification for chromatography.

In these experiments a Pye 104 Gas Chromatograph equipped with a flame ionization detector and a Kelvin Electronics servoscribe recorder was used. The column is glass, 5 feet by 4-mm internal diameter, packed with 80-100 mesh acid-washed, siliconized Diatomite C which is coated with 1% cyclohexanedimethanol succinate (CDMS). A hydrogen pressure of 18 lb/in²; air, 7 lb/in²; and a nitrogen flow rate of 50 ml/min was used throughout. The operating temperature is 220 degrees. One μl of the extract was injected onto the column at an appropriate attenuation, and the retention times of cannabidiol (CBD), Δ^1-3,4-*trans*-tetrahydrocannabinol (THC), and cannabinol (CBN) were calculated relative to dibenzylphthalate (DBT), the internal standard. The total analysis time was approximately fifteen minutes. Retention times of the cannabinols relative to dibenzylphthalate are cannabidiol, 0.26; THC, 0.39; cannabinol, 0.64.

For paper chromatography, Whatman SG81 paper (7 × 25 cm) is immersed in a 15% w/v solution of silver nitrate in distilled water, the excess solution is allowed to drain off, and the paper is then air-dried. After applying spots of the extract of suspected cannabis or cannabis resin, and of Δ^1-3,4-*trans*-tetrahydrocannabinol, the paper is developed in chloroform using the ascending technique. Location of the cannabinols is by spraying successively with a 1% solution of Fast Blue Salt B in water, then 2N sodium hydroxide. Development time is ten minutes for a 5-cm run. Rf values are cannabidiol, 0.3; THC, 0.6; and cannabinol, 0.8.

A method for the detection of cannabinols in the mouth and on the fingers of smokers has been described.

METHOD (Stone and Stevens, 1969).

EXPERIMENTAL MATERIALS.

1. Alumina column. Prepared from Hopkin and Williams® alumina, pH 10, mesh 100-200; $1\frac{1}{4}$ inch in a Pasteur pipette.

2. Gas chromatography. The instrument used was a Pye® 104, with FID detection, glass column, 5 ft x 4 mm internal diameter, filled with neopentyl glycol adipate, plus trimer acid, on silanized Chromosorb® W 80-100 mesh $(3 : \frac{3}{4} : 96\frac{1}{4})$.

3. Thin layer plates. Merck Kieselgel® F_{254}, and Merck Aluminium Oxide® F_{254}, ready prepared.

4. Tetrazotised tolidine.

Solution 1. Five g o-tolidine were dissolved in 25 ml 25% hydrochloric acid and diluted with water to 1 litre.

Solution 2. Aqueous 10% w/v sodium nitrite solution. Equal volumes of the two solutions were mixed just prior to use. This mixture could be kept for at least two to three hours.

EXPERIMENTAL METHOD.

1. The thumb and first two fingers of each hand were dipped into approximately 50 ml chloroform for a few seconds. This chloroform finger wash was stable overnight in the dark.

The chloroform was evaporated just to dryness on a water bath, and the residue dissolved in approximately 1 ml of a 1 : 1 mixture of benzene and petroleum ether (40°-60°).

The benzene/petrol ether solution was placed on an alumina column and washed through with a further 10 ml of the same benzene/petroleum ether mixture. This washing removed most of the fat. The cannabinols were then eluted from the column with 5 ml of a 1 : 1 mixture of chloroform and benzene. The chloroform/benzene solution was then evaporated to a few microlitres.

A portion of a Merck Silica gel F_{254} plate, cut to 7.5 cm by 7.5 cm, was pre-extracted with acetone by placing it in a small tank and allowing acetone to ascend to the top. In these investigations an Eastman® Chromagram jar, which takes plates up to 7.5 cm square, was found to be satisfactory. The acetone was allowed to evaporate and the top 5 mm of absorbent scraped off.

The concentrated chloroform/benzene solution was placed on the plate in two approximately equal compact spots along with but well-separated from control cannabinol or cannabis extract spots and the plate developed in chloroform/petroleum ether (80°-100°C) 80 : 20 v/v.

After evaporation of the solvent, the plate was observed under 254 nm UV light for the detection of any nonphenolic substances. The plate was then cut to separate the portion containing half of the finger dip extract which was put aside for further tests. The remainder of the plate was sprayed in a fume cupboard with tetrazotised tolidine. This reagent is sensitive to 25 ng of cannibinol.

The presence of cannabinol, as revealed by the presence of a red-brown spot of Rf 0.7 can be interpreted as evidence that cannabis has been smoked or handled. In these investigations, the handling of resin resulted in very strong positive reactions for cannabinol and also cannabidiol, but tetrahydrocannabinol (THC) could not be differentiated from the cannabinol (CBN) present by the TLC system.

2. Confirmation of the positive test for CBN could be obtained from the unsprayed portion of the plate as follows: A circle of the absorbent, in a position corresponding to the CBN found in the other portion, was scraped off and placed onto cotton wool in the base of a Pasteur pipette and the CBN extracted by pouring 5 to 10 ml of hot redistilled benzene through the pipette.

The benzene extract was evaporated in a conical centrifuge tube to a few microlitres for injection onto a gas chromatograph at 220 degrees. A peak corresponding to cannabinol was a further confirmation.

3. As a less satisfactory alternative to the GC confirmation, the benzene concentrate from the silica gel plate was spotted onto an alumina TLC plate. A suitable development solvent for Merck Alumina plates was CCl_4 : acetone : acetic anhydride, 92:4:4. The alumina plates were activated before use by heating at 110 degrees C for half an hour. The Rf of CBN is about 0.5.

It was considered advisable to precede the testing of a finger dip extract on the GC by (a) a 10 μl solvent injection to check the syringe for traces of CBN from previous injections, and (b) an injection of a 5 μl concentrate of the benzene solvent. The laboratory reagent-grade benzene, evaporated from 10 ml to 5 μl, produced a peak at a retention time close to that of CBN. Redistillation eliminated this impurity.

It was not possible to show the presence of CBN known to be present in the chloroform-benzene eluate from the alumina column by concentration and direct GC injection. Even CBN added to the concentrate just prior to injection failed to separate. This failure was interpreted as on-column reaction with concomitant extracted substances. It was for this reason the TLC separation on silica gel was necessary. Pink and blue-colored substances were clearly seen on the silica gel TLC plates before spraying at Rf values differing from those of cannabinols. These substances did not react with the spray solution.

After the emergence of the CBN peak on the GC, an intense peak at a retention time of 1.8 x RT of CBN appeared in all injections of finger dip extracts treated as described above. The technique described has been used successfully to differentiate between samples from (a) cannabis and tobacco smokers, (b) two hands where the reefer has been smoked while held in only one hand, (c) two hands where the resin has been handled by one hand.

DETECTION OF CANNABINOLS IN MOUTH WASHES. A method has been developed by which the presence of CBN can be shown in a mouthwash taken from a cannabis smoker thirty minutes, and in some circumstaces, one hour after smoking. The test is less assured of success than the finger dip method, but of many trials carried out in the laboratory, in only one or two instances have negative or very faint tests been obtained. The technique employed by the smoker, e.g. depth of inhalation, had an effect on the amount absorbed in the mouth. A description of the technique is as follows: The mouth is washed with four successive lots of 15 ml of aqueous 10% ethanol containing 1 percent w/v sodium chloride. An equal volume of 2% w/v sodium hydroxide is added to the wash and mixed. Forty ml of benzene (redistilled) is added, and the cannabinols extracted in a separating funnel by vigorous shaking. After standing, the lower aqueous layer is discarded, and any emulsion in the benzene layer is broken by the addition of anhydrous sodium sulphate.

The benzene extract is washed once with N hydrochloric acid and once with water, and evaporated just to dryness. The process is continued as described for finger dip with removal of fats on alumina, and elution of CBN.

Mouthwash containing cannabinol was stable overnight at room temperature and, when analyzed next day, still gave positive results.

Analyses on successive mouthwashes have shown that even in the third mouthwash cannabinol was still being extracted.

One percent aqueous sodium chloride as a mouthwash was found not to be very effective, and it appears that the presence of ethanol is essential. Sodium chloride was added principally as a deterrent to the swallowing of the alcohol. No cannabidiol could be detected in any of the washes.

There have been techniques published for the detection of cannabinols and their metabolites in blood and urine but they are complex procedures and the reader is referred to the references.

See also Agurell *et al.*, (1973) ; Fenimore *et al.*, (1973) ; Paton and Crown, (1972) ; Garrett and Hunt, (1973).

CARBON MONOXIDE

A few preliminary remarks must be made in relation to carbon monoxide. First, spectroscopic methods are unreliable in decomposing blood. This is most important as toxicologists have been known to come into head-on collision on differences in results when one has been using spectroscopy, and the other, a gas chromatographic procedure.

Methods for a general screen have been given on pages 59-61. In the living subject and the dead one who has been autopsied soon after death the CO-Oximeter is a most useful instrument. This measures HbO_2, $HbCO$ and Hb digitally with direct read out in a few seconds. The methods for carbon monoxide are so numerous that it is impossible to even review them here, and every toxicologist will have a favored one. Maehly's review (1962) is still an excellent starting place, and, in the writer's opinion, Blackmore's paper (1970) is *essential* reading. Also a chapter is devoted to the subject in *Advances in Forensic and Clinical Toxicology* Curry, A.S., (1972).

The definition of carboxyhaemoglobin levels needs to be studied closely. Spectroscopic methods can measure the relative amount of carboxyhaemoglobin to oxyhaemoglobin or carboxyhaemoglobin to total haemoglobin. When carbon monoxide is liberated from the blood, the volume, measured either gasometrically, by gas chromatography, or perhaps by infrared spectroscopy, has to be related back to the original blood. This may be done by measuring haemoglobin or perhaps total iron content.

In discussing the interpretation of results it is necessary to remember that these many analytical variables may be significant. The patient dies because of interference in the cytochrome C cycle due to carbon monoxide toxicity or because there is insufficient oxygen-carrying capacity remaining in the blood to maintain life. It may be very difficult to measure the latter accurately because, if the blood has clotted postmortem, a reliable percentage of haemoglobin in the antemortem blood may be difficult to extrapolate.

A passing word is necessary on the making up of 100% carboxyhaemoglobin and its dilution for the making of standard curves. The blood should be saturated with a nitrogen/carbon monoxide mixture (e.g. 90:10) or, after saturating with 100% carbon monoxide, it should be flushed with nitrogen to remove dissolved carbon monoxide if gasometric methods are to be used. Fully oxygenated blood (kept in 100% oxygen up to the mixing) is used to dilute the fully carboxylated blood. Many workers think that the avidity of blood for carbon monoxide is so great that a few minutes is all that is required for saturation. This is not so; old blood requires long periods. Blackmore (1970) showed that eleven-day-old blood stored at 37 degrees C could not be fully carboxylated until it had been diluted and treated with dithionite. Even then thirty minutes bubbling with carbon monoxide was necessary.

Method 1. The palladium chloride diffusion method can also be used as a quantitative procedure, either by measuring the quantity of palladium chloride used up in the reaction or by titrating the liberated hydrochloric acid. Both techniques require skill and should not be undertaken without much practice. A simpler method which gives a result in about one minute is described below.

METHOD 2. The apparatus devised by E. R. Rutter and shown in Figure 11 is set up. The principle of the method rests on the liberation of carbon monoxide from a measured volume of blood whose haemoglobin content has been found on a separate aliquot.

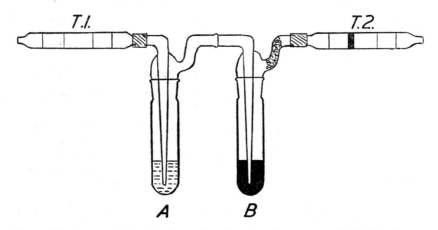

Figure 11. Apparatus for the determination of carbon monoxide in blood.

The gas reacts in a commercially available carbon monoxide detector tube, T2, to give a visible black stain whose length is proportional to the volume of gas. In this way, the volume of carbon monoxide per 14 g of haemoglobin can be calculated. In practice, 0.5 ml of blood is put in Tube B, diluted with 3 ml of water, and a mixture of lactic acid-potassium ferricyanide is quickly added; air is sucked through the apparatus from left to right at a rate of approximately 60 ml/min. The tube, T1, acts as a purifier of the air and Tube A contains water to act as a flow meter; in the neck of Tube B is a pack of cotton wool impregnated with lead acetate to remove any sulphide impurities. The length of stain for blood 100 percent saturated with carbon monoxide should also be obtained. The apparatus is equally suitable for measuring low concentrations

—that is, of the order of 5 percent saturation—by increasing the volume of blood used to 5 ml.

A haemoglobin determination should be done on an exactly similar aliquot of blood.

METHOD 3 (van Kampen and Klouwen, 1954).

This depends on reducing blood, diluted with 0.5N ammonia, with a small spatula end of solid sodium hydrosulphite to give a mixture of reduced haemoglobin (from the oxyhaemoglobin and any methaemoglobin in the sample) and carboxyhaemoglobin. The optical densities at the point of maximum difference of density, 540 nm (D_m), and the point of equal optical density, 579 nm (D_1) are measured. It can be shown that if a = the fraction of total haemoglobin present as carboxyhaemoglobin, then

$$\frac{D_m}{D_1} = a \left(\frac{1}{x} - \frac{1}{y} \right) + \frac{1}{y}$$

where $x = \dfrac{D_1}{D_m}$ for 100% COHb and $y = \dfrac{D_1}{D_m}$ for 0% COHb.

A calibration curve is prepared by plotting $\dfrac{D_m}{D_1}$, i.e. $\dfrac{\text{(reading at 540 nm)}}{\text{(reading at 579 nm)}}$

for 0%, i.e. reduced haemoglobin, and for 100% COHb. The dilution is relatively unimportant—one or two drops of blood are added to 5 ml of 0.5N ammonia—the ratio being independent of concentration. The readings should, however, be arranged to be in the most sensitive part of the scale of the spectrophotometer which is usually about 0.3 to 0.4. The ratio for 0% should be 1:10 and for 100%, 1:50. As the equation shows, the calibration is linear for intermediate samples.

The method is an excellent one, very sensitive, works well with postmortem blood and does not need a separate haemoglobin determination. It is not to be recommended to the beginner without full comparative controls. One precaution must be observed; the reading at 579 nm is taken on a very steep slope and the wavelength is critical. The spectrophotometer must be not only routinely aligned for wavelength calibration, but minor variations must be minimized by the following procedure: Set the wavelength first at 540 nm and take the reading of a control sample of 0% reduced blood against the compensatory ammonia. Knowing the ratio for

0% blood (1.10) the reading at 579 nm can then be calculated. The wavelength giving this reading (it may be 578 or 580 nm on the dial) is used for subsequent determinations.

The reduction of oxyhaemoglobin with sodium hydrosulphite has been the subject of a study by Dalziel and O'Brien, (1957) who have shown that it is a complex reaction fraught with the possibility of complications for spectrophotometry. Their paper indicates that 0.5N ammonia is too alkaline for rapid and full reduction, but, in contrast to ones at a lower pH, this strength gives clear solutions, and in practice does not lead to error. Theoretically more weakly alkaline buffer solutions are preferable, a pH of 8.5 and the taking of reading between ten and thirty minutes after adding the hydrosulphite are indicated.

METHOD 4 (D. J. Blackmore, 1970).

Three millilitres of reagent (20 g sodium hydrogen carbonate AR, 20 g sodium carbonate AR, 15 g potassium ferricyanide AR, 10 ml Triton-X 100 diluted to 600 ml with distilled water) are mixed with 1 ml of blood and 1 ml air for not less than ten minutes in one of two 5-ml plastic disposable syringes joined together with a short length of plastic tubing. After this time the 1 ml of air is withdrawn into the second syringe, and all of it is injected into a 5-ml gas loop on a gas chromatograph. It is essential that the whole of the syringe air space be injected if maximum sensitivity and linearity of recorder response to air/carbon monoxide volume are to be achieved. The column consists of a six-foot length of Linde molecular sieve 5A at 100 degrees C with helium carrier gas flowing at 45 ml/min. A Katharometer detector is used at ambient temperature with a detector current of 225 milliamps (Pye® 104 apparatus). Peak height measurements give excellent quantitation. Comparison to results from 100 percent saturated blood and to blood iron provide assay.

INTERPRETATION OF RESULTS. Problems do occur in interpreting results, but usually only when the circumstances of the case indicate poisoning and the blood levels are low, or when a high value is found and the circumstances seem to exclude carbon monoxide.

Blackmore (1970) found that, for no discoverable reason, values varied between blood samples taken from different sites on the same body. The differences were significant—for example, in one case, from 18 percent in the right ventricle to 33 percent in the femoral vein; in another case, 38 percent in the left ventricle, 56 percent in the right ventricle, and 60 percent in the femoral vein. In the light of this finding only generalities can be stated, rather than precise correlations between levels and probable clinical effects. It was stated above that the remaining oxygen-carrying capacity of the blood was important. This manifests itself particularly in persons with a low haemoglobin; the anaemic elderly person may show only a 25 percent saturation. However, if the blood is assumed to contain its normal 14 g/100 ml of haemoglobin, this leaves 10.5 g of oxyhaemoglobin to sustain life. If, however, the anaemia is so intense that in every 100 ml only 7 g of haemoglobin is present after deducting 25 percent, only 5.25 g of oxyghaemoglobin is available to maintain life—a very different picture.

A word must also be said of postmortem changes in apparent carboxyhaemoglobin. Several toxicologists have reported dramatic changes in stored blood—upward and equally dramatically downward. At this time no one has found out why, or if they have the writer is not aware of it. Crystal ball gazing then assumes its proper role.

To return to the problems noted at the beginning of this section it must be noted that in fires people do die with low carbon monoxide levels, and this can sometimes cause problems in deciding if a fire victim was breathing before the fire started. Clearly, it cannot be assumed that they were. Finally, the murder cases must be remembered in which a husband has put a gas pipe through the window of his wife's bedroom or a parent has held a child over a gas stove, and then, after putting the dead child back to bed, has rung the police to report a sudden death of unknown aetiology. Carbon monoxide is a killer which can be missed at autopsy. Toxicologists would do well to perform a screening test in all *sudden deaths.*

See also: Ainsworth, *et al.,* (1967) ; Betke and Kleihauer, (1967); Collinson, *et al.,* (1968) ; Cooper, (1966) ; de Bruin, (1967) ; Dominguez, *et al.,* (1964) ; Dominguez, *et al.,* (1959) ; Dubowski and Luke, (1970) ; Feldstein, (1967) ; Feldstein and Klendshoj, (1954);

Feldstein and Klendshoj, (1957); Freireich and Landau, (1971); Goralski and Januszko, (1968); Gramer and Ruof, (1968); Hessel and Modglin, (1967); Maas, *et al.*, (1970); Mant, (1960); Markiewicz, (1967); McCredie and Jose, (1967); Obersteg and Delay, (1966); Paulet and Chevrier, (1968); Porter and Volman, (1962); Roberts, *et al.*; Roche, *et al.*, (1960); Simpson (1955); Srch, (1967).

CHLORDIAZEPOXIDE (Librium®), DIAZEPAM (Valium®), NITRAZEPAM (Mogadon®) AND OTHER BENZODIAZEPINES

Although many cases of overdosage with these tranquillizers have been reported, the mortality is obviously extremely low.

METHOD 1 (Based on Smyth and Pennington, 1963).

Blood, 5 ml, is made alkaline by the addition of 0.5 g potassium carbonate and extracted with 3 x 20 ml chloroform. The combined chloroform extracts are washed with water and extracted with 3 ml 2N hydrochloric acid. The separated acid is centrifuged, then read in an ultraviolet spectrophotometer in a 1-cm cell from 230 to 320 nm.

Chlordiazepoxide shows a major peak at 245 nm with a minor peak at 310 nm. Diazepam peaks at 240 nm with a minor peak at 285 nm. Nitrazepam shows a peak at 278 nm. Standards should be prepared from the pure drugs at concentrations in 2N HCl of approximately 0.5 mg/100 ml.

It is probable that for diazepam and nitrazepam the background absorption will be too high for the necessary sensitivity to be achieved. If this is so and it is desired to confirm suspected intake, the best, quick approach is to re-extract the tranquillizers from the hydrochloric acid solution into chloroform after making it alkaline with ammonia. The evaporated chloroform extract should then be examined by TLC using methanol on Silica-Gel G plates sprayed with iodoplatinate (see below).

METHOD 2 (Jatlow, 1972 Courtesy *Clin. Chem.*).

Three ml plasma, 2.0 ml of 0.5 mole per litre phosphate buffer at pH 7.4, and 30 ml of chloroform are placed in a 50-ml round-bottomed, stoppered centrifuge tubes, shaken for about five minutes, and centrifuged ($1500 \times g$, 5 min). Twenty-five milliliters of the chloroform is collected, after filtration through Whatman No. 1

filter paper, in a second centrifuge tube containing 5 ml of NaOH (0.45 mol/liter). The contents are shaken for about five minutes and centrifuged. The NaOH (upper) layer is completely removed and either discarded or saved for barbiturate analysis. Five milliliters of HCl (0.5 mol/liter) is added to the remaining chloroform, and the tubes are again shaken and centrifuged. The aqueous layer is removed and divided into two 2-ml aliquots, A and B. One-half milliliter of HCl (0.5 mol/liter) is added to A, and 0.5 ml of NaOH (5 mol/liter) to B. A and B are each scanned separately, but on the same recording, against an identically processed aqueous blank. They are identified from the characteristic configuration of the ultraviolet absorption spectra at the two pH's. Absorbance at the major acid peak (245-250 nm) is used for quantification of chlordiazepoxide. Calculations are based upon absorbance values obtained from identically-processed plasma standards.

STANDARD CURVE. A standard curve was obtained by analysis of plasma containing various amounts of added chlordiazepoxide. Absorbance values at 247 nm were linear with concentration to an absorbance of at least 0.8, which is equivalent to a plasma concentration of 3.3 mg/100 ml.

Chlordiazepoxide is converted to 7-chloro-1:3 dihydro-5-phenyl 2H-1, 4-benzodiazepine-2-one 4 oxide by mild acid treatment. This is a weak acid, soluble in ether, and may be found in the weak acid fraction as it is a metabolite of the drug.

A strong acid hydrolysis results in the formation of 2 amino-5-chlorobenzophenone.

THIN LAYER CHROMATOGRAPHY (Stevens and Jenkins, 1971).

One system is a thin-layer system using Merck precoated aluminum oxide F254 plates (Type E) and a mobile phase containing chloroform/toluene/ethanol (40 : 60 : 2). In a 10cm run, which takes approximately 35 minutes, a separation between six of these drugs is achieved, Nitrazepam and Bromazepam running together (Fig. 12). Prior saturation of the chromatographic tank with solvent vapor is necessary for a good resolution, and it is advisable to run control spots of authentic samples alongside the mixtures on account of small fluctuations of the absolute Rf values.

The system complementary to the previous one employs

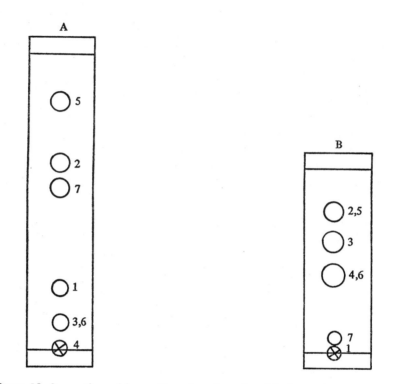

Figure 12. Separation of benzodiazepine drugs by thin layer chromatography (A) and the SG81 paper system B.

1 = chlordiazepoxide   2 = diazepam   3 = nitrazepam
4 = oxazepam   5 = medazepam   6 = bromazepam
7 = dibenzepine

silica gel loaded paper (Whatman S.G.81) and a mobile phase containing chloroform/ethanol 49 : 1. This is more rapid than the thin layer system, a 7-cm run taking about fifteen minutes. Satisfactory results were obtained, although not such a high degree of resolution as with the thin-layer method. In the paper system nitrazepam and bromazepam were resolved, but no resolution was obtained between diazepam and medazepam and between bromazepam and oxazepam.

The paper system has the added advantage that the prior equilibration of the chromatographic tank with solvent vapor is not such a critical factor for providing good resolution.

Spots containing about 5 to 10 μg of each drug were placed on the thin-layer plate or paper, and after elution, the compounds were located either by viewing under shortwave (254 nm) ultra-violet light, or by spraying with potassium iodoplatinate solution. The former method of location was more satisfactory for the thin-layer plate as the fluorescent background assisted in the detection of the absorbing spots.

S.G.81 paper has a considerable absorbance in ultraviolet light, giving a dark background against which it is more difficult to detect the spots, but all the spots develop well if the paper is sprayed with an acidified solution of potassium iodoplatinate (5 ml 2N hydro-chloric acid added to 100 ml of aqueous solution see p. 81), or with an aqueous solution of the reagent followed by blowing HCl fumes on the chromatogram. Iodoplatinate treatment of the alumina thin-layer plate also required the presence of acid for full development of the spots.

Further information to assist in identifying a particular benzo-diazepine can be obtained by spotting a solution of the compound on to Whatman No. 1 paper and examining it in ultraviolet light of both 254nm and 350nm wavelengths without treatment, and then after treatment with HCl fumes, and ammonia.

In Table XXXIII the properties of the seven benzodiazepine drugs examined are summarized.

Although ultraviolet measurements are suitable for the measurements of these drugs in blood, there are many alternatives. Spectro-fluorimetry and gas chromatography have been used, particularly.

Nitrazepam has also been measured in plasma by electron capture gas chromatography (Beharrell *et al.*, 1972) as has oxazepam (Knowles and Rueluus, 1972).

See also: Beyer and Sadee, (1969) ; Foster and Frings, (1970); Gjerris, (1966) ; Greaves, (1974) ; Koechlin and D'Arconte (1963); Weist, (1968).

URINE ANALYSIS

Chlordiazepoxide can be found unchanged in the urine as can nitrazepam, but the metabolic pathways are complex; for example,

TABLE XXXIII

Compound	Rf in TLC System	Rf in S.G.81 Paper System	Untreated Drug 254nm	350nm	Exposed to HCl Fumes 254nm	350nm	Exposed to Ammonia 254nm	350nm
CHLORDIAZEPOXIDE	0.20	0.02	absorbs	yellow	absorbs	yellow	absorbs	yellow
DIAZEPAM	0.67	0.84	absorbs	—	green*	green	absorbs	—
NITRAZEPAM	0.08	0.59	absorbs	absorbs	—	blue	absorbs	absorbs
OXAZEPAM	0.00	0.43	absorbs	—	green	green	absorbs	—
MEDAZEPAM	0.88	0.83	green	blue	orange	orange	blue	blue
BROMAZEPAM	0.05	0.42	absorbs	—	yellow	yellow	absorbs	—
DIBENZEPINE	0.50	0.07	greenish-blue	greenish-blue	greenish-blue	greenish-blue	greenish-blue	greenish-blue

*—Detection of 0.2 μg of this drug is possible using this reaction (Stevens, 1967).

medazepam is metabolised to oxazepam, desmethyl diazepam and 3 hydroxy diazepam, and the major urinary metabolite of diazepam is the oxazepam glucuronide (da Silva *et al.*, 1970). For the toxicologist it is probable that urinanalysis would be confined to demonstrating the presence of these drugs.

INTERPRETATION OF RESULTS

Chlordiazepoxide (Librium®). Cate and Jatlow (1973) showed that in the majority of cases most patients showing CNS depression (not coma) had serum levels below 1 mg/100 ml confirming the view expressed in the previous edition of this book. They say that if the patient cannot be aroused, other causes of coma should be investigated regardless of the serum concentration. Even at over 6.0 mg/100 ml two patients were discharged after minor routine therapy. Alcohol seems to be especially dangerous with this drug.

In their series 77 percent of ingestions of chlordiazepoxide involved other drugs, most often barbiturates and ethanol. Above 2.0 mg/100 ml, although drowsiness or stupor was observed, coma was not seen even at values of 6 mg/100 ml.

Zingales (1971) found plasma concentrations to range from 17 micrograms/100 ml after a single dose to 689 micrograms per 100 ml following administration of multiple 50-mg doses.

Diazepam (Valium®). Plasma levels following therapeutic doses of diazepam have been measured using gas chromatography by Berlin *et al.* (1972).

After a single dose of 100 mg, blood levels of about 25 micrograms per 100 ml can be expected, but on long-term therapy they may be about 100 μg/100 ml if very high doses (200 mg/day) (da Silva *et al.*, 1966) are given.

Garateini *et al.* (1969), however, found blood levels of patients on continuous treatment of diazepam to be in the region 0.1 to 0.24 microgram/ml. (10 − 24 μg/100 ml).

Nitrazepam (Mogadon®). Nitrazepam in therapeutic doses gives plasma levels of up to about ten micrograms per 100 ml (Rieder, 1973; Beharrell, 1972) Tompsett, (1968).

Medazepam (Nobrium®). da Silva (1970) noted a concentration of 0.98 microgram/ml in blood, one hour after a 50-mg dose.

After 50 mg per day for four days a blood level of 0.7 microgram/ml was reached. Oxazepam in the urine after medazepam dosage reached levels of less than 1 μg/ml.

CHLORPROMAZINE (Largactil®)
Chlorpromazine in Blood

METHOD. Blood, 10 ml, is stirred with 2 ml water and 8 ml concentrated hydrochloric acid and heated in a beaker in a boiling water bath for five minutes. Remove and place in an ice bath. When cool, add 12 ml 60% w/v potassium hydroxide which has been previously washed with ether. Keep cool and check the pH to ensure alkalinity. If acid, add more alkali. Shake with 150 ml ether breaking any emulsion by centrifuging. Separate and shake the aqueous phase with a further 50 ml portion of ether. Combine the ether fractions and wash in sequence with 10 ml 2.5% sodium hydroxide, 10 ml water and 5 ml water. Extract the ether with 5 ml 0.1N sulphuric acid which is separated and read from 230 to 280 nm. Chlorpromazine peaks at 255 nm and has $E_{1cm}^{1\%} = 960$.

Gas chromatography can also be used, e.g. Christoph *et al.* (1972).

Chlorpromazine in Urine

Chlorpromazine is very extensively metabolized, and in overdose cases a positive FPN reaction (p. 65) is to be expected.

INTERPRETATION OF RESULTS. Excretion of total chlorpromazine in the urine in patients receiving long-term therapy of 100 to 140 mg per day, varies from 21 to 70 percent of the ingested dose. The ratio of conjugated to unconjugated metabolites varies from 2.1 to 11.

The level to be expected in the blood after an acute toxic overdose of about 1 g or over is of the order of 100 μg/100 ml. Liver levels ar much higher (see Chap. 6A2).

See also: Bolt, *et al.*, (1966); (Curry, 1970); Curry and Marshall, (1968); Driscoll, *et al.*, (1964); Hammer and Holmstedt, (1968); Huang, (1967); Kaul, *et al.*, (1970); Korczak-Fabierkiewicz, *et al.*, (1967); Malik and Martin, (1970); Warren, *et al.*, (1967); Wechsler, *et al.*, (1967).

CHOLINESTERASE

This is an essential routine investigation because of the ready availability of organo-phosphorus insecticides in all parts of the world. Accidental contamination of foodstuffs leading to poisoning as well as their intentional ingestion for suicidal and homicidal purposes make a search for these compounds which depress the enzyme cholinesterase in the blood necessary. Fluoride does not inhibit this enzyme so the preserved sample of blood can be used. Refrigerated samples are stable for at least several weeks.

METHOD (Michel, 1949).

Buffer solution. 1.237 g of sodium barbitone, 0.136 g of potassium dihydrogen phosphate and 17.535 g of sodium chloride are dissolved in 900 ml of water, made up to nearly one litre with water, and the pH adjusted to 8 with 0.1 N hydrochloric acid. The volume is then accurately made up to 1 litre. A few drops of toluene are added as a preservative, and the solution keeps indefinitely in a refrigerator.

Substrate. 0.2 g acetylcholine bromide in 10 ml of water made fresh.

Take two stoppered test tubes and add 2.5 ml buffer and 2.5 ml substrate to each and 0.05 ml serum or whole blood to one. Take the pH immediately and again after incubation at 25 degrees C for one hour. The control should not have altered its pH by more than 0.05 units. The difference in pH between the control and the incubated blood gives the cholinesterase activity in pH units.

INTERPRETATION OF RESULTS. Normal whole blood gives values of 80 to 160 pH units; the average values are about 120, and the lowest value for a normal, fit human is probably seventy-five units. Normal plasma is in the range 50 to 100 units. Although depression of cholinesterase activity can rarely decrease to zero without the death of the patient, the ChE value gives a useful lead to the probability that the ingested poison is an inhibitor and, therefore, an organo-phosphorus compound. Accumulation of small quantities of poison can result in cumulative depression of ChE activity which returns to normal only slowly; as much as a month may be required after cessation of exposure. See Pickering and Martin, (1970) for modification of the method.

CLOMIPRAMINE (Anafranil®)

METHOD (Haqqani and Gutteridge, 1974 Courtesy *Forensic Science*).

Five or 10 ml of blood or urine (or 5 g of macerated tissue) were made alkaline by the addition of an equal volume of 0.1N sodium hydroxide, then extracted directly with 2.5 volumes of hexane. Suitable quantities of the hexane fraction were then used for identification and assay.

Half the hexane extract was evaporated on a boiling water bath and the residue dissolved in a known volume (1–5 ml) of 0.05 N hydrochloric acid. This solution was then scanned in a spectrophotometer. Clomipramine in 0.05N HCl shows an absorbance peak at 252 nm with a shoulder at 275 nm and minimum at 237 nm. Its $E_{1cm}^{1\%}$ was calculated to be 193.

Two thin layer chromatographic systems, both with silica gel G prepared with 0.1N sodium hydroxide were used—System A: running solvent, methanol; System B: running solvent, chloroform—methanol, 9:1.

Approximate R_f values for clomipramine were in System A, 0.4; and in System B, 0.65. The following location reactions were used: (1) ultraviolet inspection, weak purple fluorescence; (2) Dragendorff reagent, orange; (3) 50% nitric acid, transient deep blue; (4) 5% sodium nitrite in 20% aqueous methanol followed by heating at 100 degrees C for fifteen minutes, stable ochre.

Suitable aliquots of the hexane extract were run alongside clomipramine controls (0.5–10 μg) prepared by using a 0.1% w:v clomipramine solution as the hydrochloride in methanol. Visual assay after location by the nitrite oxidation procedure above enabled an estimate of the clomipramine present to be made.

The colorimetric assay used was the nitrite reaction described by Klinge and Beyer (1968) for determining imipramine and its derivatives. A suitable fraction of the hexane extract was evaporated to dryness and dissolved in 10 ml 80% acetic acid. Two drops of fresh 5% sodium nitrite were added to 5 ml of this solution which was then heated on the boiling water bath for fifteen minutes. The developed ochre color was read at 412 nm against the remaining 5 ml of solution without nitrite. Standard solutions equivalent to 0 to 20 μg/ml of clomipramine in the final assay solution were used to construct a calibration curve. An optical density of unity was given by a solution of 13 μg/ml using a 1-cm path length.

A glass column, five feet in length and of one fourth inch outside diameter, containing $2\frac{1}{2}\%$ SE30 on acid-washed celite (oven temperature, 225°C) was used for gas chromatography. A nitrogen flow of approximately 30 mls/min to the flame ionisation detector produced a well-shaped peak after 7.7 minutes for the free base of clomipramine in hexane.

INTERPRETATION OF RESULTS. The distribution as indicated by Haqqani and Gutteridge (1974) seems similar to imipramine. In their two cases, blood levels were 0.1 mg/100 ml and *trace,* but the livers contained 3 and 2.2 mg/100 g respectively. The brain in the second case contained 0.45 mg/100 g. These results included a metabolite, thought to be desmethylclomipramine.

CLONAZEPAM

METHOD (Naestoft and Larsen, 1974).

This gas chromatographic method uses an internal standard not readily available; it also requires an electron capture detector. Reference to the original work is required.

Plasma levels in twenty-five patients undergoing continuous treatment with 6 mg daily for fifteen to twenty-six days were found to be 29 to 75 ng/ml for clonazepam, 23 to 137 ng/ml for an amino metabolite, and 3 to 13 ng/ml for the acetamido metabolite.

CYANIDE

See Chapter 5B1b, but the following are alternative methods.
METHOD (Tompsett, 1959).

The following reagents are placed in an Öbrink diffusion vessel:

1. Sealing ring—6N sulphuric acid.
2. Outer ring—blood or tissue macerate—1 to 2 g; also 0.5 ml 6N sulphuric acid.
3. Inner ring—1.0 ml of 1N sodium hydroxide.

After mixing the blood and acid in the outer ring, diffusion is allowed to proceed at room temperature for two hours. To the sodium hydroxide in the inner ring add, in order, 0.1 ml of glacial acetic acid, 0.1 ml of bromine water, 0.1 ml of sodium arsenite solution, and, when the bromine has been decolorized, 0.5 ml of pyridine/benzidine reagent. The volume is then made to 3 ml by adding 1.2 ml of water. The mixture is transferred to a test tube and allowed to stand for fifteen minutes at room temperature then read against a reagent blank together with exact controls from 2.5 to 10 μg cyanide at 520 nm. The sodium arsenite solution is made by dissolving 1 g arsenious oxide in as little 2N sodium hydroxide as possible, and making up to 50 ml with water. The pyridine/benzidine reagent is made as follows: (a) 0.36 g benzidine is dissolved in 10 ml 0.5N hydrochloric acid; and (b) 12 ml of pyridine is made up to 20 ml with water; 2 ml concentrated hydrochloric acid is added. The reagent is made by adding 5 ml of (a) to 20 ml of (b). It does not keep.

For interpretation of results see page 98.

METHOD (Valentour, Aggarwal and Sunshine, 1974).

After diffusion (see above) 1.0 ml of the sodium hydroxide trapping reagent is added to 2.0 ml hexane, 2.0 ml of 1M sodium dihydrogen phosphate, and 1.0 ml of chloramine T reagent (0.25% w/v in water). After shaking, the solution is placed in an ice bath, and five minutes later the tube is thoroughly shaken, replaced in the ice bath, and 1 μl of the hexane layer is injected into the gas chromatograph (6' Halcomid M-18 on Anachrom ABS—90-100 at 55°C; 5% methane in argon as flow gas with a [63]Ni pulsed linearised detector to detect the cyanogen chloride).

See also: Ballantyne, (1974); Bonnichsen and Maehly, (1966); Curry, (1963); Curry, *et al.*, (1967); Gettler and Baine, (1938); Gettler and Goldbaum, (1947): Halstrom and Moller, (1945); Patty, (1921); Pettigrew and Fell, (1973); Sunshine and Finkle, (1964).

DDT, DIELDRIN, AND OTHER ORGANO-CHLORO COMPOUNDS

These compounds can be demonstrated in normal tissue provided sufficiently sensitive methods of detection are employed. Normal levels in tissues in mg/100 g are as follows:

	Fat	Urine	Blood	Liver	Kidney	Brain
DDT and DDE	0.3—1.3	.001—.004	.0012—.0046	.01—.1	.001—.003	.001—.02
HEOD	0.02—	.00005—	0.00014	—	—	—
	0.026	.00019				

Reported toxic levels are as follows:

	Blood	Urine	Liver	Kidney	Brain
Aldrin	4.0				
Dieldrin	over .02 (0.5—0.7)				
Endrin	.0053	.0004			
Toxaphene			.78	.67	1.4

METHOD (based on de Faubert Maunder, Egan, Godly, Hammond, Roburn and Thomson, 1964).

Tissue, 10 g, is ground in a glass mortar with an approximately equal weight of sharp sand and sufficient anhydrous sodium sulphate to a uniform dry powder. Transfer the ground material to a 150-ml beaker and simmer for about two minutes with 50, 20, 20 and 20-ml successive portions of hexane, stirring carefully. Allow each solution to cool for a few minutes before decanting them separately into 100-ml calibrated flasks. Dilute the solutions to the mark and take a 25-ml portion of each. Shake with 10 ml of dimethylformamide saturated with hexane and run the clear DMF phase into a 100-ml separating funnel, centrifuging if necessary. Repeat with two further portions of 10 ml of DMF and combine the extracts. Wash them with 10 ml of hexane saturated with DMF. Separate the hexane, wash this with a further 10 ml of DMF which is added to the original 30 ml of DMF. The DMF extract is shaken briskly for two minutes with 200 ml of 2% aqueous sodium sulphate solution and, after twenty minutes, the hexane previously held in solution separates and is collected. The stem of the separating funnel is washed with hexane, and the combined extracts are passed down the following, previously-prepared column; 10 g of activated alumina (heat aluminium oxide at 800°C for 4 hrs., cool, add carefully 5 % v/w water and mix thoroughly in a closed vessel; use within 10 days) in hexane is poured into a chromatographic column and kept covered in hexane; the alumina is covered with a 5-cm layer of anhydrous sodium sulphate, and the hexane level is allowed to fall to its upper level.

Run the solution prepared above, concentrated to 2 ml onto the column; wash with three successive 2-ml portions of hexane and elute with 90 ml of hexane. Collect a similar volume. Evaporate the eluate to 0.5 ml. This extract can be concentrated and half of it examined by a thin-layer system using a silica-gel plate with hexane or carbon tetrachloride as the solvent. Rf values for hexane are as follows:

Aldrin	0.7	op′ DDT	0.50	Heptachlor	0.58
α BHC	0.34	pp′ DDT	0.42	Heptachlor epoxide	0.17
γ BHC	0.21	Dieldrin	0.12	pp′ TDE	0.25
pp′ DDE	0.65	Endrin	0.13		

The spots are made visible by spraying with a solution of 0.5% ethanolic silver nitrate solution containing 1% phenoxyethanol and exposing to 254 nm ultraviolet light. Black spots appear in a short time. Alternatively, a GLC separation can be achieved on a 10 μl extract. A five-foot column of SE30 at 175 degrees C, using an electron capture detector, will demonstrate normal levels if the above procedure is followed and, hence, detection of poisoning is ensured. It should be noted that TDE and little DDT will be found in livers analysed more than a few days after autopsy.

A six-foot column of 2% OV-1 and 3% QF-1 on gas chrom. Q 80/100 at 180 degrees C is said to give excellent resolution.

See also Adamoric, (1966) ; Benyon and Elgar (1966) ; Brown, Hunter and Richardson (1964); Coble, *et al.,* (1967); Cueto and Biros, (1967); Fishbein, (1972); Hodge, *et al.,* (1967); Hunter, *et al.,* (1963); Kovacs, (1966); Maybury and Cochrane, (1973); Palmer and Kolmodin-Hedman, (1972); Robinson and Hunter, (1966); Schafer and Campbell, (1966), Richardson, *et al.,* (1965); Richardson, *et al.,* (1967) . For Toxaphene see Haun, (1967) .

DIGITALIS GLYCOSIDES

The accidental ingestion of these compounds by young children sometimes occurs and the toxicologist is asked to confirm by analysis the circumstantial suspicions of intake. The stomach contents, and any vomit, are probably the best sources, but

Doherty *et al.,* (1967) and Jelliffe (1966) have given certain basic information which is of assistance in this field. Doherty's work using tritium-labelled digoxin on human subjects indicates that the drug will be found in the highest concentrations in the heart muscle, liver and kidney. Recovery from tissue using continuous alcohol extraction has been discussed in Chapter 6B2.

METHOD (Jelliffe, 1966).

As much urine as can be obtained is used—If possible, a twenty-four-hour sample. It is stored under 50 ml heptane in a refrigerator and analysis performed within three days. The urine is diluted to 2 litres with water and extracted at 25 to 29 degrees C with 1,500 ml chloroform after making the solution to pH 4 with sulphuric acid. The separated chloroform is shaken three times with 50-ml portions of 1N NaOH. It is then washed with 50 ml water and, after separating again, evaporated to dryness at 30 degrees C in a rotary flask evaporator. The residue is dissolved in six washes of 2.5 ml chloroform:methanol (1:1) and the solvent evaporated to dryness under a stream of nitrogen. The urine extract is spread as a band on a TLC plate with controls. The plates (20 × 20 cm) are prepared by shaking 30 g Silica-Gel G with 60 ml 0.05N NaOH for one minute and spreading to 250 μ in the usual way. They are dried at 120 degrees C for one hour and cooled in a desiccator.

The solvent used is methylene chloride:methanol:formamide (90:9:1) with a filter paper liner to facilitate equilibration. Plates are run to 10 cm at 25 to 29 degrees C. They are then removed and allowed to dry for about five minutes. They are then slowly and gradually sprayed with water which reveals digoxin and digitoxin as frosty white spots just separated on the semitransparent background at Rf's of about 0.35. The positive reacting areas are scraped off into stoppered centrifuge tubes, 5 ml of xanthydrol reagent (30 mg in 100 ml redistilled glacial acetic acid plus 1 ml concentrated hydrochloric acid) is added, vigorously shaken for exactly two minutes, and placed in a boiling water bath for three minutes. It is then cooled in ice water for five minutes and centrifuged. The supernatant rose-wine color is read within twenty minutes at 550 nm and 580 nm. The optical density difference at these two wavelengths is proportional to the digitoxose in the sample. Reference standards in the range 5 to 30 μg of digitoxin and 30 to 50 μg digoxin should be used. Traces of nonspecific material may be found to the equivalent of 12.5 μg digoxin per day, but, in acute poisoning, the expected urinary concentration at its maximum should be considerably above this background. On a maintenance dose of 1 mg per day, digoxin patients excrete about 200 μg per day; on 300 μg digitoxin a day, excretion is about 45 μg per day.

There has been a considerable increase in interest in the toxicology of digitalis glycosides in recent years mainly because of the introduction of commercial radioimmunoassay kits.

Notwithstanding this, the above chemical method has been left in this edition for those toxicologists who do not possess β or γ counters. As far as the radiochemical method is concerned one follows the instructions on the kit, remembering that the erythrocyte/plasma ratio for digitoxin and digoxin are 0.09 and 0.90 respectively. Thus, for digoxin, whole blood values are similar to plasma and serum, but, for digitoxin, serum levels are higher than whole blood.

INTERPRETATION OF RESULTS. The interpretation of plasma levels of digoxin in patients undergoing routine therapy is outside the scope of this book except to say that these are usually in the region of 1 to 2 ng/ml. In patients who have taken or who have been given large overdoses, values are usually over 10 ng/ml, but may be over 100 ng/ml.

Karjalainen, Ojala and Reissell (1974) have reported on tissue concentrations of digoxin in autopsy material in thirteen cases where the persons had been on digoxin maintenance therapy. Blood levels were higher than normal, ranging from 1.3 to 8.2 ng/ml, but it must be noted that in the muscles, liver and renal cortex, values can be over 100 ng/ml. Thus, the lesson is learned that the blood sample must be a good one taken away from the main organs if a reliable interpretation is to be achieved. It is probably best if at least two samples are taken, and not be too surprised if these assay at slightly different values.

See also: Lukkari and Alha, (1967); Somogi, *et al.,* (1972); Wilson, *et al.,* (1967); Zeegers, *et al.,* (1973); Holt and Benstead, (1975).

Digitoxin. Serum levels for patients on therapy are usually about 20 ng/ml; Mercier (personal communication) had a case of a death fourteen hours after taking 15 mg of digitoxin where the plasma level was 320 ng/ml.

Lanatoside C. Plasma levels after 0.5 mg are a few ng/ml, and Moffat (personal communication) analysed an overdose case where death occurred after forty-eight hours where the serum level was 47 ng/ml.

Deslanoside. Normal levels are up to about 4 ng/ml. Iisalo and Nuutila (1973) reported a case of a man who died after taking one hundred tablets and had a serum level of 24.0 ng/ml. The myocardial concentration was 624 ng/ml.

See also Grade, Forter and Schulzeck (1967).

DINITRO-O-CRESOL

The toxicologist is occasionally asked to determine the concentration of this agricultural compound in blood because from it can be determined the exposure severity and the time that the worker must remain away from further spraying.

METHOD (Fenwick and Parker, 1955).

Blood, 1 ml, is shaken for thirty seconds with 5 ml of methylethyl ketone and 1 g of a 9:1 solid mixture of sodium chloride + sodium carbonate. The ketone layer is then filtered into the cell of a spectrophotometer and read at 430 nm. One drop of concentrated hydrochloric acid is added, any cloudiness is removed by centrifuging, and the optical density is again read. The difference in reading is plotted against the amount of DNOC. To prepare a standard curve; 0 to 40 μg give readings of 0 to 0.625 in a 1-cm cell in our hands.

INTERPRETATION OF RESULTS. Toxic effects in man appear at levels of about 3 to 4 mg/100 ml. Levels of 6.5 mg/100 ml are extremely serious, and above 7.5 mg/100 ml will probably be fatal. After cessation of exposure the blood level falls by about 0.1 mg/100 ml per day. See also Edson (1955).

DIPHENYLHYDANTOIN
PHENYTOIN (Dilantin®)

This drug should have been detected in a routine screen by a peak at about 230 nm in the weak acid fraction (p. 36), and by inspection of a paper or thin layer chromatogram (p. 190). However, serum levels are often requested by clinicians to monitor treatment, and the method used will depend on the available equipment. The following methods may be useful.

METHOD 1 (Dill *et al.,* 1971 Courtesy *Clin. Chem.*).

Using 16 by 150-mm glass-stoppered test tubes, take 1 to 2 ml of heparinized plasma (or of serum), 0.2 ml of phosphate buffer (1 mol/liter, pH 6.8), and 10 ml of 1:2 dichloroethane (EDC) (purified grade). Shake mechanically for fifteen minutes and centrifuge.

Transfer 8 ml of the EDC to a second glass-stoppered tube containing 3 ml of 1N sodium hydroxide. Shake for five minutes and centrifuge.

Transfer 2 ml of the NaOH extract to a third glass-stoppered tube, add 1.5 ml of NaOH solution (50 g/100 g), 4 ml of iso-octane* (2,2,4-trimethylpentane, pure grade) and 0.5 ml of saturated aqueous potassium permanganate. The tubes are inserted into a test tube rack in a steam bath through a close-fitting gasket (aluminum foil) so arranged that only the portion of the tube containing the aqueous phase is exposed to the steam, while the upper portion of the tube including the iso-octane layer is air-cooled.†

Heat for thirty minutes with stoppers loosely fitted, then cool the tubes to room temperature and shake them mechanically for five minutes to ensure completeness of extraction. (There is no appreciable loss of iso-octane by evaporation.)

Separate the iso-octane layer and measure the absorbance of

---

*The iso-octane is purified before use by percolation through a column containing layers of equal parts of acidic and basic alumina.

†A heating block could presumably be used if the tube is inserted only to the depth of the aqueous organic interface, and some heat shielding is provided at the level of the interface. Also, one would have to adjust the heating time and temperature for the particular conditions used to achieve complete oxidation.

the solution at 247 nm against a reagent blank in a spectrophotometer.

A similar method has been described by Thürkow *et al.* (1972). TLC has been used Simon et al. (1971) and Olsen, (1967).

Not surprisingly gas chromatography has been extensively used (Cooper *et al.*, 1972; Berlin *et al.*, 1972; Chin *et al.*, 1972; Flanagan and Withers, 1972; Larsen *et al.*, 1972; Meijer, 1971).

A method for phenobarbitone, carbamazepine and phenytoin in 3.0 ml of serum has been reported by Larsen *et al.* (1972). A column of 3% SE52 on Celite JJ CQ 100/120 mesh at 235/290 degrees was used, and Papadopoulous, *et al.* (1973) have described an elegant technique for separating and quantitating phenobarbitone, phenytoin, primidone and pheneturide in 0.2 ml of plasma using gas chromatography. Reference to the original paper is necessary for full working details.

INTERPRETATION OF RESULTS. Therapy as an antiepileptic usually aims at blood levels of about 1 mg/100 ml; toxic reactions tend to occur above this figure, and in fatal acute poisonings it is to be expected that the blood value will be 3 mg/100 ml or above.

DOXEPIN

METHOD (Randolph, Walkenstein, Joseph and Intoccia, 1974).

Five ml urine are pipetted into a 40-ml centrifuge tube followed by 1.5 ml of saturated aqueous potassium permanganate solution. Shake and stand for five minutes. The resulting doxepin ketone is extracted by shaking for ten minutes with 10 ml n-hexane. Centrifuge, separate and read the hexane layer absorption maximum at 266 nm. For quantitation use 266 to 295 nm readings. For standards use 1 to 3 mg/100 ml doxepin in urine. After 50-mg doses, urinary excretion in forty-eight hours varied from 4 to 18 mg. Amitriptyline gives an identical UV spectrum, and diazepam and chlordiazepoxide also interfere.

ETHANOL

Gas Chromatography

METHOD (Curry, Walker and Simpson, 1966).

A Pye® 104 gas chromatograph is used with five feet of 10%

PEG400 on 100-120 Celite with a flame ionisation detector at 85 degrees C. The temperature of the injection port is the same as that of the column. An integrator is fitted in parallel with the recorder. A Griffin and George "Type 221" Diluspence® or similar automatic device is used to dilute 10 μl blood with 100 μl of an aqueous n-propanol solution (approximately 20 mg/100 ml). (The diluspence gives accurately measured dilutions; the absolute dilution ratio is not important provided it is constant for standards and samples. A better than 1% accuracy is normally achieved over several months.) If a Diluspence or an equivalent device is not available, manual dilution (0.1 ml blood + 1 ml aqueous n-propanol) can be used, but operator fatigue introduces significant errors (up to 5%) late in the day if large numbers are being analyzed. Approximately 1 μl of the diluted blood sample is injected into the machine by means of a Hamilton syringe. Ethanol has a retention time of about two minutes; propanol, three and one fourth minutes; and the *water* appears in four and one half minutes. There must be no overlap of the compounds. Analysis is achieved by comparison of the digital integrator outputs for the ethanol:propanol ratio with known standards. Peak height measurement can be used provided a single operator standardizes himself; variations between operators are considerable unless the integrator is used. Because the detector behaves similarly to the ethanol and propanol, the calibration curve is constant from month to month and alterations in the injected volumes, column packing, gas flow rates and temperature changes are of no consequence. Isopropanol and chloroform have similar retention times to ethanol, but a second column of 100/120 Porapak Q at 180 degrees C satisfactorily resolves these compounds.

Very low concentrations of alcohol in blood can be measured if the injected volume is increased and the propanol concentration reduced. Propanol solutions of 8 mg/100 ml *lose* propanol even in the dark in a refrigerator at about 1 percent per day, and it is therefore advisable to run standards more frequently than in the routine case.

Because of the high precision of the method, care must also be taken in the preparation of standards. It is advisable to make up direct standards in large quantities, i.e. to weigh 5 g of purified absolute ethanol and dilute to 5 litres with water, and not attempt to weigh 100 mg and dilute to 100 ml. A C o V of 1% can be achieved easily.

When a new column is used large *water* peaks may be found, but these can be diminished by injecting repetitive 50-μl quantities of water to flush out the column. This peak decreases as the column ages. It is most important to get a very stable baseline in this method, and conditioning for forty-eight hours at 120 degrees C with nitrogen passing through the column at 40 ml/min is recommended when a new column is installed. After this, if the apparatus is only used intermittently, purging for two hours at 120 degrees C is usually sufficient.

When the column has been in use for some time, broadening of peaks will occur; instead of repacking the whole column it will be found necessary only to repack the top two to three inches; reconditioning, however, must be done.

An alternative procedure, Machata's head space method, is also in routine use in the Home Office Forensic Science Laboratories. See Machata (1967).

DICHROMATE METHODS. Two methods are recommended, serving slightly different purposes. Both are exactly similar dichromate oxidation methods, but, whereas the former gives a quantitative determination in about half an hour, the latter requires an overnight period for diffusion. The first method is the one used for rapid clinical estimations; the second is suitable if large numbers of determinations from drunken drivers are being routinely analysed.

METHOD 1. Ten ml of a potassium dichromate-sulphuric acid mixture (0.1N $K_2Cr_2O_7$ in 60% v/v H_2SO_4) are placed in tube B (Fig. 7). The tube A is then weighed empty and again after the addition of about 2 g blood; 2 ml of 10% sodium tungstate are then added to the blood followed by about four drops of bench dilute sulphuric acid. The thick protein precipitate can be easily coated over the inner surface of the tube by a flick of the wrist. If urine is used, 2 ml is taken; no protein precipitation is necessary. Alcohol and the aqueous phase are then rapidly and completely volatilised when both tubes are placed in a water bath at 80 degrees C and a stream of air is blown or sucked over the blood into the dichromate mixture in Tube B. Two precautions are necessary—the air must be cleaned by prior passage through a strong chromic acid mixture, and the bubbling orifice into the reaction mixture must be as small as possible to ensure complete oxidation of the alcohol. Physiological quantities of acetone do not interfere under these conditions. When the blood has completely dried, the dichromate is washed into a 1 litre conical flask with about 250 ml of distilled water; 5 ml of 10% potassium iodide are added, and the liberated iodine is titrated with exactly 0.1N sodium thiosulphate using starch solution as the final indicator. A similar titration is then performed on 10 ml of the potassium dichromate-sulphuric acid mixture which has been used in a blank determination.

Let the blank determination be y millilitres and the alcohol determination z millilitres.

Let the weight of blood be w grams.

Then $(y - z)$ millilitres of 0.1N sodium thiosulphate = alcohol from w grams of blood

But 1 ml of 0.1N sodium thiosulphate = 1.15 mg of alcohol

$$\frac{1.15 \times (y - z) \times 100}{w} = \text{milligrams of alcohol per 100 g of blood}$$

or

$$\frac{1.15 \times (y - z) \times 105}{w} = \text{milligrams of alcohol per 100 ml of blood.}$$

METHOD 2 (Nickolls, 1960).

This is a macrodiffusion method using cylindrical jars. About 2 g of blood are accurately weighed into one half of a small petri dish; 1 ml of saturated potassium carbonate solution is then added, and the dish is placed, supported on a small glass tripod, in the jar; 10 ml of the potassium dichromate-sulphuric acid reagent are placed in the base of the jar. A glass plate with ground glass edges makes an airtight seal and is held in place by a metal screw cap. The jar is incubated at 37 degrees C overnight. The titrations and calculations are exactly the same as in Method 1.

The enzymatic method is also most useful and is suitable for routine determinations; it requires a spectrophotometer capable of reading at 340 mμ. The method is based on the oxidation of alcohol to acetaldehyde with diphosphopyridine nucleotide (DPN) as coenzyme. Semicarbazide is used to remove the acetaldehyde; this forces the reaction to completion. Details of the method have been described by Lundquist, (1959) in a review on the determination of ethanol. Reference to the original paper is recommended.

Gas chromatography is now a routine procedure in the Home Office Forensic Science Laboratories for the analysis of blood samples taken in relation to traffic offences and C o V's of better than 1 percent are achieved on 10-μl samples of blood.

It must be stressed that dichromate methods are reliable and accurate for alcohol determinations when the ethanol concentrations are relatively high (over 50 mg/100 ml). Below this figure, and especially if postmortem samples are being analyzed, efforts should be made to use either a gas chromatographic method or ADH.

INTERPRETATION OF RESULTS. It should be noted that, in general, it is extremely difficult to interpret postmortem blood alcohol concentrations when these are below 100 mg/100 ml. Many types of bacteria will produce small amounts of alcohol, and the presence of traces of ethanol in the blood or tissues from a body that has not been autopsied within twenty-four hours of death should be expected and ignored unless circumstances require special investigations such as an intensive bacteriological study. If urine has been obtained the interpretation becomes much easier. If death occurs shortly after the bulk of alcohol ingestion ceased, it is to be expected that the urine concentration will be lower than the blood alcohol concentration; if death occurs over two hours after the ingestion of alcohol then the urine concentration will be higher than the blood alcohol concentration, usually about 33 percent higher. If these generalizations do not fit what the toxicologist is told about the circumstances, the samples should be reinvestigated critically, and, if a dichromate method has been used, the alcohol results double checked by a different method.

To reach a blood alcohol concentration of 200 mg/100 ml a man of eleven stones (154 lb.) would have to drink seven pints of 3% w/v beer (120 g of alcohol) or just over ten ounces of spirits (70 proof spirit, 93.3 g of alcohol). These figures are based on a Widmark factor of 0.90 for beer and 0.70 for spirits. Other figures can be obtained by direct proportion, increasing directly with weight and with blood alcohol concentration.

Normally no difficulty will be experienced in interpreting blood alcohol concentrations in samples from the living patients provided the clinician has not used ethanol to swab down the patient's arm or to sterilize his hypodermic syringe!

It should be remembered that even small amounts of alcohol will be of significance if other depressants of the central nervous system are also present.

In postmortem blood samples two precautions have to be taken. The first is to guard against the postmortem production of alcohol in the blood by yeasts, fungi and bacteria, and the second is to ensure that no diffusion of alcohol has occurred from the gastrointestinal tract into the blood in the period between death and the autopsy. As indicated in Chapter 1, both these precautions are covered by the pathologist taking two separate samples from peripheral parts of the body well away from any injuries and adding a little solid sodium fluoride to one of them. The concentration should be at least 1 percent.

Relation of blood alcohol with clinical effect: (a) 50 mg/100 ml of blood—usually little apparent clinical effect. (b) 80 mg/100 ml of blood—legal limit in the United Kingdom for driving a motor vehicle. Loss of driving license for a twelve-month period is mandatory in addition to a fine or gaol sentence. It is of interest to note that it is the alcohol concentration in the blood sample that is the deciding factor, and not the subsequently back calculated value for the time of the driving offence. This is at variance with the practice of many European countries. (c) 300 mg/100 ml of blood: clinically drunk; increasing tendency to asphyxiate from inhalation of vomit. (d) 460 mg/100 ml: death from respiratory depression.

See Alcohol and Road Traffic, Proceedings Fourth Internation-al Conference (1966); *Alcohol and Traffic Safety, Proceedings Fifth International Conference* (1969); Gormsen (1954); Harger (1961 and 1963); Harger and Forney (1967); Kirk, Gibon and Parker (1958); Kozelka and Hine (1941); Lundquist (1959); Muelberger (1954); Plueckhahn (1967); *The Role of Alcohol to Road Accidents* B.M.A. (1960); Southgate and Carter (1926) and Ward Smith (1965).

ETHCHLORVYNOL

METHOD 1 (Haux, 1972 Courtesy *Clin Chim, Acta*).

REAGENTS

Trichloroacetic acid, 10% (w/v).

Color reagent. Dissolve 0.2 g of diphenylamine (special in-dicator grade) in 50 ml concentrated sulfuric acid (AR). Add this solution slowly to 50 ml of water. Stable for approximately one month at room temperature in the dark.

Stock standard (1 mg/ml). Dissolve 100 mg ethchlorvynol (Placidyl®) in ethanol (USP grade) and make to 100 ml. This will remain stable for approximately one month in the refriger-ator.

Working standard (1 mg/100 ml). Dilute 1 ml of the stock standard to 100 ml with ethanol. Stable for about one month in the refrigerator.

Chloroform. Reagent grade.

PROCEDURE

Unknown. Into 0.5 ml serum or urine blow 3.5 ml cold 10% trichloracetic acid in a strong stream to achieve a fine protein precipitate. Shake vigorously. Centrifuge for five minutes at high speed. Transfer 3 ml of the clear supernatant to a second centri-fuge tube. Add 3 ml of color reagent. Mix and let stand for five minutes. Add 3 ml chloroform and shake well. Centrifuge for one minute to clear the chloroform layer or filter through phase sep-arating paper (Whatman 1 PS). Read the organic layer in a spectrophotometer or colorimeter at 524 nm.

If the color reaction is carried out in a colorimeter cuvette

(Klett tube) the chloroform layer can be read after centrifugation without further manipulation.

Blank. Process 0.5 ml of water as for the unknown.

Standard. Treat 0.5 ml of the working standard as for the unknown.

Calculation.

$$\frac{\text{Absorbance of unknown}}{\text{Absorbance of standard}} \times 1 = \text{mg}/100 \text{ ml ethchlorvynol}$$

If the readings of the unknown are too high, dilute with chloroform and multiply the readings by the dilution factor.

METHOD 2 (Wallace, Hamilton, Riloff, and Blum, 1974 Courtesy *Clin. Chem.*)

Two ml of whole blood, serum or urine, or 2 g of homogenized tissue are mixed vigorously for five minutes with 20 ml of Spectrograde *n*-heptane. The extraction is not pH-dependent, and can be done effectively in a 25-ml stoppered graduated cylinder. After the heptane-specimen mixture has separated (centrifugation is not generally required), an aliquot of 10 to 15 ml of the heptane layer is refluxed with 10 ml of hydrochloric acid (1 mol/liter) for twenty minutes with continuous magnetic stirring. The temperature of the refluxing liquids is 100 ± 3 degrees C. Upon completion of the reflux and cooling (in an ice bath or cool tap water) to near room temperature, the heptane layer (for nontissue specimens) is scanned spectrophotometrically over the range 210 to 360 nm versus a blank of Spectrograde *n*-heptane. For measurements at a single wavelength, the absorbance is measured at 247 nm.

The heptane layer may be extracted (3 min, manual) with an equal volume of semicarbazide (0.5 mol/litre) buffered at pH 3.5 with solid sodium acetate. The molarity of the sodium acetate is not critical, and the semicarbazide solution is stable indefinitely when stored at room temperature in a brown bottle. The aqueous extract containing the semicarbazone of the ethchlorvynol derivative is scanned against a semicarbazide blank, or the absorbance measured at 286 nm. To eliminate interference from ultraviolet-absorbing compounds normally present in tissue and tissue extracts, the semicarbazide reaction is required for the analysis of tissue specimens.

Oxidation of ethchlorvynol results in a product (s) having a well-defined aborption curve (A_{max}, 247 nm) with absorbance/concentration ratio of 0.065. Conversion of the oxidation product (s) to the semicarbazone derivative yields a sharp curve with the maximum at 286 nm and an absorbance/concentration ratio of 0.093. A linear relationship exists between the concentration of the drug, the absorbance of the oxidation product (s) and the formation of the semicarbazone. The linearity exists over the range of ethchlorvynol concentrations usually encountered in biologic specimens. If an exceptionally high absorbance is obtained, it is measured on a dilution of the final solution. Such an application is practical because the oxidation of ethchlorvynol is nearly stoichiometric over a wide concentration range, a marked advantage over available colorimetric procedure that require a new determination with smaller volume of specimen if the initial analysis shows too great an absorbance. Semicarbazone blanks for urine, serum or tissue homogenates should have an absorbance of less than 0.03. Heptane blanks for tissue extracts are often high and variable, necessitating formation of the semicarbazone derivative. The carbonyl and the semicarbazone blanks obtained from oxalated whole blood are equivalent to those obtained with serum.

Heptane extractions recover only unchanged drug and hence results parallel the GC methods.

METHOD 3 (Maes, Hodnett, Landesman, Kananen, Finkle and Sunshine, 1969 Courtesy *J. For. Sci.*

Extraction. Homogenize 3 g of tissue with an equal amount of water. Pipette 5 ml of homogenate (or 5 ml of urine or 5 ml of blood) into a glass-stoppered centrifuge tube or a separatory funnel and add 2 ml of ethyl acetate. Stopper and shake gently for two minutes. Centrifuge at 2,000 rpm (8-in head) for five minutes. For high concentrations transfer 0.5 ml of the supernatant layer into a calibrated centrifuge tube and slowly evaporate the solvent to 0.2 ml using a fine jet of nitrogen. When therapeutic concentrations are to be measured, the respective aliquots should be 0.6 ml evaporated to 0.1 ml. Rinse the walls of the tube twice with 1 to 2 ml of ethyl acetate and evaporate each rinse to 0.2 ml. Inject a 5-μl aliquot into the gas chromatograph. Determine the area of the curve corresponding to ethchlorvynol from the integrator. Analyze a suitable reference solution in an identical manner. The amount of the drug in the sample injected is determined by multiplying the amount in the injected reference solution by the ratio of the integrator readings of the sample and the reference solution. In each series of determinations each reference solution is chromatographed at least two times.

Instrumentation. An F & M Model 402® dual column gas chromatograph equipped with a flame ionization detector and a 1 mV Minneapolis-Honeywell® recorder with a disc-integrator was employed. The column used was a 6 ft. by $\frac{1}{4}$ in. O.D. glass column packed with a 1% Hi-Eff 3–BP (Neopentyl glycol succinate) on 80 to 100 mesh Gas-Chrom Q. The column was conditioned overnight at 140 degrees C. It was periodically reconditioned after each batch of twenty biological samples was analyzed.

The operating conditions were as follows: temperature: column, 110 degrees C; injection port, 150 degrees C; detector block, 130 degrees C; gas flow rates: helium (carrier gas) 35 ml/min., hydrogen, 25 ml/min and air, 500 ml/min. The recorder speed was 15 in/hr. A more recent method has just been published using an internal standard by Evenson and Poquette (1974).

INTERPRETATION OF RESULTS. Therapeutic blood levels even on long-term dosing rarely exceed 1 to 2 mg/100 ml in blood, and Maes and his co-workers (1969) found a maximum of 0.18 mg/100 ml in the blood after ingestion of 200 mg. However, patients rarely take a single dose in isolation, and continued use leads to continued accumulation. A high level reflects a persistent degree of addiction as with a vast number of other drugs, although the current betting would be probably closed at about 4 mg/100 ml of ethchlorvynol in blood. Indeed, Millhouse *et al.* reported a chronic intoxication in a female, aged twenty-nine, with a blood level of 3.7 mg/100 ml. Fatal levels are high in blood, liver and kidney—a level as high as 65 mg/100 g has been reported (Finkle, personal communication). Kimber (personal communication) reports a case where the blood level was only 1.7 mg/100 ml (liver 8.3 mg/100 g), but the patient had died ninety hours after ingestion.

See also Evenson and Poquette (1974) and Millhouse, Davies and Wraith, (1966).

ETHYLENE GLYCOL

METHOD (Harger and Forney, 1959).

Blood. Blood, 1 ml, is diluted with 7 ml water and 1 ml of 10% w/v sodium tungstate solution added. With vigorous shaking add, dropwise, 1 ml of 0.67N H_2SO_4. Shake well, then filter through a small dry filter paper. Place 1 ml filtrate in a small test tube, add 4 ml water and 0.25 ml of a solution of 2.13% w/v $NaIO_4$ in 0.67N H_2SO_4; stand for ten minutes. Quickly introduce 2 ml Schiff's reagent and mix. After twenty-five minutes read at 555 nm. Compare with 10 to 70 μg ethylene glycol determined in the same way. Schiff's reagent is made by adding 0.2 g basic fuchsine to 120 ml almost boiling water. Dissolve and cool in running water. Dissolve 2 g sodium metabisulphite in 20 ml water and add to the cooled fuchsine. Next add 2 ml concentrated HCl and 60 ml water. Keep in a refrigerator and use within two to three weeks.

Tissues. Macerate 50 g tissue with 200 ml water. Take 25 ml, add 15 ml water, 5 ml 10% w/v sodium tungstate and 5 ml 0.67N H_2SO_4; shake and filter. Proceed as for protein-free blood filtrate.

INTERPRETATION OF RESULTS. Even in the refrigerator, loss of ethylene glycol occurs on storage. Harger and Forney note that the blood level in one case dropped from 384 mg/100 ml to 80 mg/100 ml on twelve days' storage.

Fatal blood and tissue levels usually are high if death is rapid —often several hundred milligrams/100 ml. If death is delayed for several days, only traces may be found, and it should be noted that *blank* values up to the equivalent of 35 mg/100 ml in blood have been noted, A method giving blank values as low as 5 mg/100 ml has been published (Russell, *et al.*, 1969).

Oxalic acid determinations (p. 286 are useful confirmatory tests. See also Roscher (1971).

FLUORIDE

METHOD 1

QUANTITATIVE PROCEDURE (Teichmann, Dubois and Monkman, 1963). In this procedure, disposable plastic petri dishes are used. To the inside of the petri dish cover, 0.1 ml of 0.5N sodium hydroxide solution is distributed by successively touching the pipette tip to the plastic. The individual spots dry rapidly; 1 ml of urine or dilute tissue slurry is transferred to the lower section of the dish, and 0.3 g solid silver sulphate added to it; 2 ml of 66% sulphuric acid is placed beside the urine, the vessel tilted to mix the urine and acid and immediately covered with the prepared lid, taking care to maintain the assembly horizontal at all times. After a period of twenty hours at 50 degrees C in an oven, the covers are carefully removed and the sodium hydroxide absorbent is transferred to a 10-ml volumetric flask with successive washings from a 5-ml pipette; 3 ml of Belcher's reagent are added and the volume made up to the mark with water. Readings are taken at 622 nm. Standards of 0 to 4 μg, including the diffusion stage, are similarly prepared.

Belcher's Reagent. 8.2 g sodium acetate in 6 ml glacial acetic acid and sufficient water to effect solution. Transfer quantitatively to a 200-ml volumetric flask. Dissolve 0.0479 g alizarin complexone in 1 ml 20% ammonium acetate with the assistance of 0.1 ml ammonium hydroxide and 5 ml water. Filter this solution through a Whatman No. 1 filter paper into the 200-ml flask. Wash the filter with a few drops of water. Add 100 ml of acetone to the flask slowly with swirling. Dissolve separately 0.0612 g lanthanum chloride in 2.5 ml 2M hydrochloric acid, warming gently, and add this to the contents of the volumetric flask. Dilute to 200 ml with water. Mix well, cool to room temperature and adjust accurately to 200 ml.

Urines should be stored in polyethylene vessels, not glass. The range of the method as described is 0 to 4 μg of fluoride, but increased sensitivity may be obtained by using 281 nm. Urine levels do not normally exceed 50 μg/100 ml.

METHOD 2 (Hall, 1963).

One ml of blood, CSF or urine is mixed with 0.3 ml of N lithium hydroxide and 0.2 ml of 0.2M magnesium succinate in a platinum crucible and dried at 110 degrees C. The crucible is covered with a lid and placed in a small metal cannister having a tightly-fitting lid. This is placed in a cold muffle furnace, and the temperature is slowly raised to 400 degrees C which is maintained for fifteen hours. When cool the ash is transferred to a polythene diffusion bottle together with 0.4 ml of 0.5N perchloric acid and 2 x 0.3-ml portions of water as washings.

Rectangles of 3.0 by 1.2 cm Whatman 541 filter paper, previously washed with hot distilled water and dried, are pushed into the lumen of an adaptor of 5-mm internal diameter polythene tubing inside the well of the bottle cap. The free 2 cm of paper is impregnated with 15 μl of 0.2M magnesium succinate (see below) placed 0.5 cm from the free edge; 2 ml of silver sulphate in perchloric acid (4 g finely powdered silver sulphate with 2 ml water and 23 ml 72% perchloric acid and warmed to 80°C, add 75 ml of 72% perchloric acid and cool) are added immediately from a burette, and the cap is screwed tightly into position. Seal the junction between cap and bottle with a mixture of equal parts of ceresine and carnuba waxes. Diffuse at 60 degrees C for twenty-four hours. Remove the paper with forceps and place in stoppered 5-ml tubes. Add 2 ml lanthanum alizarin complexanate reagent and place in a water bath at 60 degrees C for ten minutes. Cool and extract the blue complex with 1.5, 1.0 and 1.0-ml portions of butanol solvent. Adjust the volume to 4.3 ml with solvent, shake for thirty seconds with 1 ml of water and cool to 0 degrees C. Separate the aqueous phase by centrifuging and adjust the volume to 4 ml. Read at 570 nm. Prepare standards in the same way of 0.1 to 1.0 μg F.

Lanthanum Reagent. Suspend 38.5 mg of reprecipitated alizarin complexone in 2 ml of water in a test tube; add 0.2 ml of M sodium acetate and warm to dissolve. Make up to 200 ml with water. Take 30 ml with constant mixing into 50 ml of succinate buffer (0.4724 g succinic acid in 96 ml water with warming; cool; add 3.2 ml of N sodium hydroxide and make up to 100 ml) and 20 ml of lanthanum nitrate (43.3 mg La

$(NO)_3 \; 6H_2O$ in 100 ml water). Add 25 ml of t-butanol. Prepare fresh each day.

Butanol Solvent. Three ml of hydroxylamine hydrochloride solution (6.95 g recrystallized in 100 ml water) with 97 ml isobutanol, shake until homogeneous.

METHOD 3 (Barnes and Runcie, 1968 Courtesy *J. Clin Path.*).

The fluoride electrode was used in conjunction with a standard calomel reference electrode and an expanded scale *p*H meter (Radiometer 25 SE). Readings were taken on the millivolt scale.

REAGENTS

1. Stock fluoride standard, 1 mg/ml, 2.21 g of sodium fluoride was dissolved in water and diluted to 1 litre

2. M sodium acetate adjusted to *p*H 7.2

3. M sodium acetate adjusted to *p*H 5.4

4. SOLUTION A. Sodium chloride, 5.8 g; potassium chloride, 0.3 g; sodium carbonate, 2.1 g; dissolved in water and diluted to 1 litre

5. SOLUTION B. Sodium chloride, 3.5 g; potassium chloride, 2.5 g; sodium dihydrogen phosphate, anhydrous), 4.8 g; dissolved in water and diluted to 1 litre.

The following solutions were prepared as described by Hall (1963):

6. *Lithium Hydroxide (Fluoride-Free).* About 4 g of metallic lithium, freed from its crust of oxide, was added in small pieces at a time to 500 ml of distilled water. When the metal was dissolved, the normality of the solution was checked by titration against potassium hydrogen phthalate and the concentration adjusted to 1N.

7. *Magnesium Succinate (Fluoride-Free).* About 3 g of magnesium turnings were washed twice with 100 ml of distilled water in an Erlenmeyer flask, and the washings discarded. One hundred ml of distilled water and 50 ml of 5% succinic acid were then added. After about one minute, the acid solution was decanted and the magnesium again washed with 100 ml of water. The turnings were suspended in 100 ml of water and dissolved by the addition of 100 ml of 5% succinic acid. When

the reaction subsided, the solution was filtered through Whatman No. 42 filter paper. The filtrate was evaporated to dryness at 100 degrees C and the white residue ground to a fine powder in a glass mortar. Magnesium succinate solution (0.2 M) was prepared by dissolving 5.13 g of the magnesium succinate in water and diluting to 100 ml. It was stored at 2 degrees C in a polythene container.

METHOD

General Procedure. All glassware was washed in dilute hydrochloric acid and rinsed several times in distilled water.

Standards were prepared in the appropriate solutions to give a similar ionic composition and *p*H to that of the test sample. Approximately 10 ml of the solution were placed in a small polystyrene beaker; the electrodes were just immersed in the liquid which was constantly stirred.

Plasma. To 10 ml of plasma in a glass-stoppered test tube 2.5 ml of 25% trichloracetic acid were added. The tube was shaken vigorously, allowed to stand for twenty minutes and then centrifuged at 4,000 rpm. To 4 ml of the clear supernatant, 3 ml of M sodium acetate (*p*H 7.2) were added. The resultant *p*H was about 4.9.

When 0.5, 0.7, 1.0, 1.5 and 2.0 µg of fluoride were added to 10-ml aliquots of pooled dog plasma the recovery was found to be 90 to 105 percent.

Human plasma, collected from twelve volunteers living in an area where the water contains 0.1 ppm of fluoride, was assayed. A mean value of 0.023 µg/ml ± 0.005 SD was obtained. At these levels, reproducibility is within 2 mV, which represents a variation of about ± 15 percent.

Urine. Twenty-four-hour collections were preserved by the addition of concentrated hydrochloric acid (5 ml/litre). Three-ml aliquots were diluted with two volumes af acetate buffer *p*H 5.4. The mean value of eighteen human samples was found to be 1.16 mg/24 hours ± 0.52 SD. See also Singer *et al.* (1969).

INTERPRETATION OF RESULTS. Normal levels of fluoride in blood, that is the amount to be found in a healthy adult, are of the order 0 to 50 μg/100 ml, and soft tissues may contain up to 80 μg/100 g. In fatal cases of poisoning blood levels rise to about 200 to 300 μg/100 ml. Urinary output in a normal individual is said to be up to 1 mg per day.

Teichman, Dubois and Monkman reporting at the first International Meeting in Forensic Toxicology, London, 1963, surveyed the literature on urinary excretion in persons not exposed to abnormal fluoride and gave mean concentrations of the order of 0.3 to 0.4 ppm (30-40 μg/100 ml). In poisoning cases, high concentrations which can be of the order of several milligrams per 100 ml are found.

Abukurah *et al.* (1972) report the recovery of a man after ingestion of 120 g of sodium fluoride. The initial serum fluoride concentration was 2 μg/ml.

See also Goldstone, (1955); Singer, Armstrong and Vogel, (1969); Stewart and Stolman, (1960) and Linde, (1960).

FLUOROACETATE

Sodium fluoroacetate and fluoroacetamide are widely used as rodenticides, and their detection used to be ensured by the determiniation of organic fluorine, but a gas chromatographic method has been developed which provides a most useful alternative method.

METHOD

Tissue (Ramsey and Clifford, 1949). Grind 10 g of tissue and put in a 100-ml beaker and boil gently with 300 ml water for about half an hour. Transfer and comminute rinsing with 2 × 25 ml water. Add 5 ml of 0.67 N sulphuric acid and 50 to 75 ml 20% w/v phosphotungstic acid to precipitate all the proteins. Add water to make the total weight 600 g. Shake and filter through a Buchner funnel. Add 12 ml 0.67 N sulphuric acid and extract continuously with ether for one hour. Proceed as for ether extract below.

Urine (Sawyer, Cox, Dixon and Thompson, 1967). To an ether extract of urine is added 1 ml of N-methyl-di-N-octylamine and evaporated to approximately 20 ml. The concentrate is poured onto a 2-cm plug of anhydrous sodium sulphate prepared into a 2 cm $\times$ 25-cm column with a tapered tip. Collect the eluate in a Danish-Kuderna flask and evaporate to 1 ml over a boiling water bath. Wash down with 5 to 10 ml, repeat the evaporation and disconnect the 5-ml flask. Remove the remaining ether by blowing air on the surface. Wash down the sides with 0.1 to 0.2 ml ether and evaporate again. Add 10 μl of freshly prepared diazomethane in ether, stopper and stand for one to two minutes. A microlitre aliquot is examined by GLC using a five-foot column of (a) PEG on AW-DCMS Chromosorb W 20/80, and (b) dinonylphthalate on silanised Chromosorb, with an injection block temperature at 100 degrees C and a column temperature at 50 degrees C. Methyl fluoroacetate has retention times of 22.0 minutes and 7.2 minutes on the two columns respectively.

FOOD AND DRINK

The toxicologist is often asked to examine these items in suspected criminal cases or in outbreaks of widespread illness thought to be associated with poisoning. Even sealed pharmaceutical ampoules may come under suspicion. Perhaps the best advice that can be offered is never to taste the offending article. A sample of whisky that turned out to be adulterated with urine is perhaps the example most likely to deter enthusiasts.

The elementary tests of a close visual inspection, coupled with smell, and a pH measurement are the first preliminary tests. The analysis should then follow the procedure outlined for analysis of the alimentary tract (Chap. 7). The variety of potential adulterants is endless and circumstances should not be allowed to stop or distract systematic analysis. Vomiting, diarrhea and convulsions occur from so many adulterants that, as has been said above, guesses only waste valuable material. Biological tests must be considered, especially if sealed ampoules are involved. The substitution of insulin for morphine is a bizarre example in which chemical analysis might only reveal the phenolic preservative, but injection into mice would readily show the presence of the poison.

The toxicologist must be prepared to analyze many of these samples with the assurance of the police that the complaint is from a person of devious psychological personality, and that there is no doubt nothing to be found. The number of times these complaints turn out to be justified must keep the analyst constantly on his guard.

GLUTETHIMIDE

This drug should have been detected if the ultraviolet screen described for "weak acids" page 51 has been followed. It is only a very weak acid and is unstable in alkali, but provided readings have been taken quickly at 235 nm in 0.54N sodium hydroxide, it should have been found and a reasonable estimate of its concentration obtained.

An improved ultraviolet method has been described.

METHOD (Knowlton and Goldbaum, 1969).

To 25 ml of dichloromethane in a 25-ml glass stoppered cylinder, add 2 ml of blood, serum or plasma, and shake approximately one minute. After separation of the phases, remove the aqueous layer by aspiration and filter the solvent layer through fast filter paper (e.g. Whatman No. 41) to remove any remaining aqueous phase. Shake the clear solvent with 5 ml of 0.45N KOH to remove acidic compounds. Separate the aqueous layer and shake the solvent with 5 ml of 0.5N HCl to remove basic compounds. Separate the acid layer and filter the solvent through fast filter paper to obtain a clear aliquot, usually 20 ml. Transfer the measured aliquot to a 50-ml beaker and evaporate to 1 to 2 ml on a steam bath. To prevent loss of glutethimide due to heat, air dry the remaining solvent.

Dissolve the residue in the beaker with 3 ml of ethanol. Transfer 3 ml of the glutethimide reference solution, 10 μg/ml, to a test tube. (Because only an insignificant amount of glutethimide is lost, the reference solution need not be carried through the extraction procedure.) To each solution add 1 ml of 0.2N KOH and mix. The addition to the reference solution and to the unknown should be about fifteen to twenty seconds apart with the same sequence and time interval observed when measuring the absorbance. A few seconds' variation is not significant, and more than one unknown may be read with a single standard.

Turbidity may occur with the addition of alkali, especially

when whole blood or lipemic plasmas are analyzed. If this occurs, dissolve the suspended lipid by addition of 0.5 ml of dichloromethane. Add the same volume of solvent to the reference solution.

Transfer the clear solutions to cuvettes and determine the absorbancies at 235 nm, using as a reference blank 3 ml of ethanol to which has been added 1 ml of 0.2N KOH. If dichloromethane has been added to the test solutions, add an equal volume to the reference blank. The first measurements should be made approximately five minutes after the addition of alkali. Subsequent measurements, in a 1-cm planar cuvette, are made when the decrease in absorbance of the standard is 0.10; then 0.20; and finally, when the absorbance has decreased, 0.30 which is in about twenty minutes. Noting the time for decrease in absorbance in units of 0.10 for the standard is only recommended for ease in making calculations.

When the concentration of glutethimide in the 2-ml sample is 5 μg/ml or more, a significant decrease in absorbance is observed. If the decrease between the first and second measurements is less than 0.05, indicating a concentration of less than 5 μg/ml, it is recommended that a larger sample be analyzed. Extract 3 or 4 ml of the sample in 50 ml of dichloromethane and obtain the residue from 40 ml of the clear solvent for analysis as described.

Positive identification of the presence of glutethimide in the unknown sample is made when the absorption maximum is at 235 nm and the characteristic rate of decrease in absorbance during the several-time intervals is observed just as in the case of the reference glutethimide. The concentration of glutethimide is determined by relating the amount of the decrease in the absorbance of the unknown to that of the standard during the same time interval. If there is no significant change in absorbance of the unknown, glutethimide is considered to be absent. The calculations of the glutethimide concentration in plasma is as follows:

$$\frac{\text{Difference in absorbance of unknown}}{\text{Difference in absorbance of reference standard}} \times \text{Concentration of glutethimide in } \mu\text{g/ml of reference standard} \times$$

$$\text{Volume of alcohol used} \times \frac{\text{Volume of solvent used in extraction}}{\text{Aliquot of solvent evaporated}} \div$$

to dissolve residue

Volume of sample (ml) $= \mu$g of glutethimide/ml of sample

It will be found, however, that if this procedure is applied to urine, the rate of hydrolysis is not the same as that of unchanged glutethimide, but will be considerably slower due to the presence of 2-phenyl glutarimide, a metabolite of glutethimide.

However, recent work (Gold *et al.*, 1974, Ambre and Fischer, 1972) using gas chromatographic procedures have shown that several metabolites are to be expected, and these may contribute to the interpretation of results. Fiereck and Tietz (1971) also describe a GC method for its separation from eleven barbiturates.

INTERPRETATION OF RESULTS. After ingestion of 500 mg of glutethimide in tablet form by six subjects, plasma levels were found to reach as high as 7.9 μg/ml two hours after ingestion, but had fallen to about 2 μg/ml six hours later and 0.4 to 0.9 μg/ml after twenty-four hours (Grierson and Gordon, 1969).

Sunshine and his co-workers, (1968), in reporting serial blood levels of unchanged drug and metabolites in intoxicated patients, again reveal evidence of the "rebound" phenomenon in which blood levels rise again many hours after the original peak. In their cases this occurred as late as fifty hours after the original ingestion. Although they reported that mildly intoxicated patients could usually be aroused at blood levels below 10 μg/ml, severely intoxicated patients had blood levels usually greater than 30 μg/ml in the series of thirty-nine admissions reported by Grierson and Gordon (1969).

No correlation was observed in the moderately and severely intoxicated patients between blood levels and the duration of coma. Moreover, of the twenty comatose patients who survived, six awoke at a time when the blood glutethamide levels were equal to or even greater than the value at admission; only two remained comatose until the blood level had fallen below 50 percent of the admission value. The method used for analysis in these series was the 1960 method of Goldbaum and his co-workers;

it would therefore not fully differentiate between glutethimide and the presence of the metabolites. It is interesting, however, that these workers report levels as high as 60 $\mu g/ml$ with no coma and levels as low as 20 $\mu g/ml$ with severe hypotension and coma. Finkle (1967) reports the results of blood and urine concentrations in a series of sixteen cases, both fatal and nonfatal, and reported that glutethimide was detectable in the urine for almost two days following the ingestion of one 500-mg glutethimide tablet. The maximum concentration in the urine of 70 $\mu g/ml$ was obtained twenty-two hours after ingestion.

Three cases of *drinking drivers* with symptoms of intoxication were found to have blood glutethimide levels of 5, 5 and 8 $\mu g/ml$. In fatal cases very high levels were not found, indeed they were below those noted above in which other patients were conscious.

Gold *et al.* (1974) say that in their series of patients the serum levels at which overdose patients could be aroused was from 0.4 to 1.8 mg/100 ml. (4-18 $\mu g/ml$).

The coma produced by glutethimide may be of long duration, and there can well be a lack of correlation between plasma levels and clinical condition. After 500-mg doses, Curry, S.H. *et al.* (1971) found peak plasma levels of 0..29 to 0.71 mg/100 ml. There is clearly an overlap between sedative and *toxic* levels at about 0.7 to 1.0 mg/100 ml.

See also Ambre and Fischer (1972) and Bohn and Rucker 1968).

IMIPRAMINE (Tofranil®) and DESMETHYLIMIPRAMINE (Pertofran®)

METHOD 1. (Rutter, 1960). Blood, 10 ml, is stirred with 2 ml water and 8 ml concentrated hydrochloric acid and heated in a beaker in a boiling water bath for five minutes. Remove and place in an ice bath. When cool, add 12 ml 60% w/v potassium hydroxide which has been previously washed with ether. Keep cool and check the pH to ensure alkalinity. If acid, add more alkali. Shake with 150 ml ether, breaking any emulsion by centrifuging. Separate and shake the aqueous phase with a further 50-ml portion of ether. Combine the ether fractions and wash in sequence with 10 ml 2.5% sodium hydroxide, 10 ml water and 5 ml water. Extract the ether with 5 ml 0.1N sulphuric acid. To 1.5 ml of this sulphuric acid add 1.5 ml of reagent and transfer immediately to a 1-cm glass cell and into a spectrophotometer already balanced at 580 nm against water. Read continuously until a maximum reading is obtained (about 30 sec). A calibration graph is obtained with standards in the range 0 to 50 μg giving optical density readings in the range 0 to 1.0.

Reagent. This is prepared as follows: mix twenty-five parts 0.2% potassium dichromate, twenty-five parts 30% sulphuric acid, twenty-five parts 20% perchloric acid and twenty-five parts 50% nitric acid.

METHOD 2 (Wallace and Biggs, 1969 Courtesy *J. For. Sci.*). Specimens of oxalated whole blood, urine or homogenized tissues are made alkaline (> pH 9.0) with 1 N NaOH. The specimen is placed in a 500-ml separatory funnel to which 100 to 200 ml of hexane (ACS grade) are added. The mixture is shaken vigorously for three minutes. after which the hexane layer is transferred to a graduated cylinder by filtration through a fast-flowing filter paper. The volume of recovered hexane is recorded, and the loss of hexane is considered in the final calculations. Five ml of 6 N H_2SO_4 are added to the filtered hexane and the mixture is shaken vigorously for three minutes. Two ml of the aqueous layer are added to two ml of the color-developing reagent which consists of a mixture of seventy parts concentrated sulfuric acid (ACS grade) and thirty parts of a 2 mg/ml solution of cerium (IV) sulfate in 1N sulfuric acid. A calibration curve is prepared by mixing the cerium sulfate-sulfuric acid reagent with equal volumes of reference solutions of the drug in 6N sulfuric acid. A Beckman® DK-2A ratio-recording spectrophotometer, employing a tungsten lamp as the light source and a lead sulfide cell as the detector, was utilized for absorbancy measurements. Any stable colorimeter, however, is adequate. ($\lambda_{max} = 620$ nm).

Use 2 to 10 μg/ml of imipramine in the final solution as a reference standard.

INTERPRETATION OF RESULTS. Imipramine is metabolised to desmethylimipramine, and, in patients on long-term therapy of 50 to 300 mg per day, blood levels of total drug and metabolite are in the range of 5 to 60 μg/100 ml. Levels in cases of acute poisoning exceed the upper range figure. There are many metabolites of imipramine and desmethylimipramine; these can be separated on TLC. To the toxicologist requiring to show an overdose had been ingested, the colorimetric method described above will give the answer quickly and simply without recourse to the study of the metabolites. It should be noted that renal failure occurs in imipramine overdose and extremely low, virtually nil levels can be obtained on urinalysis. Liver levels are much higher (see Chap. 6.). See also Bickel; Bickel *et al.* (1967); Consolo *et al.* (1967; Crammer *et al.* (1968); Curry (1964); Douglas and Hume (1967); Evreux *et al* (1969); Fatteh *et al.* (1968); Heitmann and Kunst (1968); Hume and Douglas (1968); Lund-Larsen and Sivertssen (1968); Moody *et al.* (1967); Penny (1968); Ramsey (1967); Sachs *et al* (1968); Steel *et al.* (1967) and Symes (1967). Hammer, *et al.*, (1969).

INSULIN

Proof of insulin poisoning with its clinical picture of hypoglycemic coma, convulsions, sweating and altered size of eye pupils can be obtained either by demonstrating reversal of the condition by oral and intravenous glucose during life and by antemortem blood sugar determinations, or by the demonstration of insulin at the site of the injection in fatal cases.

It is rare that there is any useful purpose served by the measurement of postmortem blood sugar concentrations because glycogenolysis in the liver with consequent diffusion of glucose into the heart raises such levels by many hundreds of milligrams per 100 ml within a few hours of death, and glycolysis lowers the peripheral blood sugar levels at a slower but still significantly rapid rate. The terminal agonal release of adrenaline and, hence, a rise in blood glucose at about the moment of death must also be remembered. However, if analyses are done within an hour or two of death on blood from two or more sites from the body and all show a normal value of glucose, the absence of antemortem sugar abnormalities can probably be excluded.

Tissue taken from injection sites should be kept in the refrigerator up to analysis; once deep frozen it must not be allowed to thaw. Insulin is destroyed in the pancreas very rapidly after death, and there is no fear of artefacts in peripheral injection sites. Insulin is relatively stable in muscle, and a delay of several weeks before analysis is of little consequence. Recovery can be expected to be about 50 percent even after three weeks at 0 degrees C.

The method of processing the tissue for the isolation of the protein is not difficult but requires experience. Anyone wishing to perform the extraction is advised to contact the nearest drug firm processing pancreas for insulin to obtain their guidance. It is most important to test the extraction process by adding insulin to muscle before attempting to isolate any from the case sample. This procedure also provides control extracts for the assay stage. The stability of insulin in muscle and its instability during extraction processes are very pertinent reasons for this advice.

Two methods are available for testing the crude protein extract which usually weighs about 1 g from each 50-g aliquot of tissue; these are to demonstrate its activity on the glucose uptake of the isolated rat diaphragm and to show its hypoglycaemic activity when injected into animals (usually mice). The former is a research technique, and, although very sensitive, its use cannot be recommended for routine use in toxicological analysis. The injection of aliquots of the extract in very weakly acidic saline into mice is a reliable and fairly sensitive procedure; twenty milliunits are usually sufficient to produce convulsions, reversed by an injection of 50 mg of glucose in mice which have not been recently fed. Five mice batches are suitable for rough screening, although several hundred are needed for accurate quantitation. Because 20 mg of extract is a convenient weight for injection, these figures mean that if about one unit of any type of insulin is present in the tissue, its detection should be straightforward.

A a result of the extensive work done in an investigation in a murder case (Birkinshaw *et al.*, 1958) no compound other than insulin was suggested as being capable of reacting in the mouse test exactly in the same way. If, however, further confirmation is required, the following tests were found to be suitable:

1. Abolition of the biological activity in the rat diaphragm test under anaerobic conditions

2. Loss of activity on treatment with cysteine

3. Loss of activity on treatment with proteolytic enzymes such as pepsin and, in particular, insulinase.

4. Comparison of the rate of hypoglycaemic effect in guinea pigs compared with insulin

5. Loss of activity when insulin antisera is added to the extract

6. Chromatographic separation of the insulin from other proteins using paper or columns, and demonstration that the activity parallels that of insulin.

It is obvious that these techniques require experience not usually within that of the average toxicologist. He should, however, be aware of their use and be able to carry out the isolation and the mouse assay.

An immunological method of assaying insulin in plasma using iodine 125 is now available, together with the necessary reagents. A liquid or crystal scintillation counter or windowless gas-flow counter is necessary.

In Los Angeles in 1968, William Dale Archer was convicted on three counts of first degree murder involving insulin, and Professor E.R. Arquilla at UCLA Medical Center gave evidence that the insulin level in the formalin-treated brain which had been preserved for more than a year was higher than in control brain. Biological (alloxan diabetic mice) and radioimmunological assay methods were used. See also Janitzki *et al.* (1960) and Phillips, Webb and Curry (1972).

IODIDE

METHOD. Blood, 10 ml, is mixed with 12 ml of saturated potassium hydroxide in a 300-ml nickel crucible and evaporated on a steam bath. The crucible is then placed in a muffle at 250 degrees C for thirty minutes, and the temperature raised to 360 degrees C where it is kept for ten minutes. On removing and cooling, the potassium iodide is removed from the mass of carbonate and hydroxide by dissolving it first with 25 ml 95% ethanol, then by four further portions of 10 ml ethanol; 0.5 ml saturated potassium hydroxide is added to the combined alcoholic extracts which are evaporated on a steam bath, then in a muffle at 385 degrees C for fifteen minutes. The dried extracts are transferred to a distillation flask and 2 ml 50% sulphuric acid, one drop 10% $Fe_2(SO_4)_3$, and 2 ml 3% hydrogen peroxide are added quickly. A bead is inserted, and the liberated iodine is distilled into water containing 0.2 ml 3% sulphuric acid and 0.2 ml 10% sodium bisulphite. Distillation is carried out almost to dryness with additions of 2 ml 3% hydrogen peroxide at intervals. The distillate is boiled for two minutes, then evaporated to 5 to 6 ml after it has been made alkaline to litmus with 10% potassium hydroxide. Add one drop methanol and enough 3% sulphuric acid to make the solution neutral, then add two drops 3% sulphuric acid and five drops of bromine water. Boil down cautiously to 2 ml which converts the hydriodic acid to iodic acid and removes excess bromine. The solution is cooled, a little boiled starch added together with excess potassium iodide, and the liberated iodine titrated with 0.005N thiosulphate (1 ml of 0.005N thiosulphate is equivalent to 106 μg of iodine).

INTERPRETATION OF RESULTS. Little is known of the toxic concentration of iodide in the blood. Absorption via the bladder when sodium iodide is used as a contrast medium is extremely rapid. It can be detected in the blood within thirty seconds of irrigation. In one fatal case investigated by the author in which the sodium iodide was accidentally left in the bladder for two hours, when a further pint of 10% solution was introduced, the blood level was 100 mg/100 ml.

IRON

Occasionally, when ingestion of ferrous or ferric salts is suspected, a method for iron assay on the acid dialysate from the gastrointestinal tract is of value.

METHOD (Kennedy, 1927).

An aliquot of the dialysate is digested with 5 ml of concentrated sulphuric acid and 2 ml of perchloric acid in a Kjeldahl flask over a flame until white fumes appear.

After cooling, one drop of nitric acid is added and the volume made up to 100 ml. To a 10-ml aliquot is added 0.1 ml of 30% w/v aqueous ammonium persulphate solution and 7 ml of 20% w/v aqueous ammonium thiocyanate solution. The optical density of the solution is measured after two minutes and before thirty minutes at 470 nm.

A 50 mg/100 ml standard gives an optical density of approximately 0.6.

INTERPRETATION OF RESULTS. Whole blood contains about 50 mg/100 ml of iron. Most of this is in the red cells. Because of this very high normal concentration no useful conclusions can be drawn from blood or tissue iron levels after the ingestion of toxic doses of soluble iron salts, but see page 62 for iron in serum. Atomic absorption spectrophotometry is a very easy and rapid method to measure iron concentrations.

ISONICOTINYL HYDRAZIDE

METHOD (Bjornesjo and Jarnulf, 1967).

Mix carefully 2 ml of serum, 4 ml of distilled water and 2 ml of 20% w/v metaphosphoric acid and allow the mixture to stand for ten minutes. The protein precipitate is centrifuged off and 4 ml of supernatant are transferred to another tube and mixed with 2 ml 2N acetic acid and 2 ml of a freshly prepared solution made by mixing aliquots of 2% w/v sodium nitroprusside and 4N sodium hydroxide. The absorbance is measured after exactly two minutes at 440 nm in a 3-cm cell against a reagent blank prepared by mixing 3 ml distilled water, 1 ml 20% metaphosphoric acid, 2 ml 2N acetic acid and 2 ml of the nitritopentacyanoferroate reagent. Standards of 20, 30 and 40 μg isoniazid per millilitre are run in parallel. The drug may also be extracted from tissues by a mixture of n-butanol and ether, and assayed by comparative ultraviolet spectrophotometry.

McBay (personal communication) reported an overdose in a thirteen-year-old girl who was dead on arrival at hospital. Her plasma isoniazid level was 15 mg/100 ml. He used the following procedure.

METHOD. Add 3.2 g ammonium sulphate and 1 ml 0.5N sodium hydroxide to 3 ml plasma. Extract with 40 ml ether-isoamyl alcohol 4:1. Separate, then extract the organic phase with 4 ml of 0.1N hydrochloric acid. Use ultraviolet spectrophotometry against standards for assay. An alternative method is provided by Lever (1972).

METHOD 3 Only the spectrophotometric method is described below.

The blood sample (1.0 ml) is pipetted into a 15 by 100-mm test tube. A solution of 5% (v/v) pentane-2,4-dione (acetylacetone) in aqueous 1 M disodium hydrogen phosphate (1.0 ml) is added and mixed. The tube is heated at 100 degrees for three minutes and cooled. A solution of 5 M potassium carbonate and 1M sodium hydroxide (1.0 ml) is added; the mixture is immediately extracted on a vortex mixer with 1.5 ml hexan-1-ol (or other alcohol of at least 5 carbons). The mixture is centrifuged at 2500 rpm for three minutes and the absorbance of the upper organic phase read with a rapid-sampling spectrophotometer set at 397 nm. A blank (1.0 ml water) is also put through the procedure and its absorbance subtracted.

The intensity of the color can be increased by mixing an aliquot of the organic phase with diethanolamine. The solution obtained is viscous and not readily aspirated into a rapid-sampling system, but can be poured into a standard 1-cm spectrophotometer cuvette.

Serum samples with various isoniazid levels were assayed and compared with results obtained with water and standard solutions of isoniazed in water.

INTERPRETATION OF RESULTS. Pragowski (1963) reported seven cases of lethal suicidal intoxication and noted the clinical signs of convulsions, cyanosis and unconsciousness with autopsy findings of generalized congestion with haemorrhages within the CNS. He noted large quantities of unchanged drug in the alimentary tract and concentrations from 9 mg/100 g in the kidney in one case (with blood and liver levels of 41.0 and 78.5 mg/100 g respective) to 35.18 and 61.64 mg/100 g in liver and kidney in two other cases. Death usually occurred in one to four hours, although one survived two days.

Acute isoniazid overdose was a problem in Alaska (Brown, 1972) where young people took it to *trip out*. A dose of 3 to 5 g is said to produce visual hallucinations. Several cases resulted in fatalities. Treatment with massive infusions of intravenous pyridoxine gave excellent results. Metabolic acidosis sometimes occurs. See also Mitchison (1973).

LEAD

This section has not been enlarged—indeed, it has been reduced in size. The dithizone method is still described, and this is for those toxicologists who do not possess atomic absorption spectrophotometers. For those that do, it is impossible here to describe all the variations such as the flame and flameless techniques, and manufacturers always can supply method sheets with the instrument.

Ingestion of paint by young children often leads to lead poisoning. This clinical entity can undoubtedly be unrecognized, and in any seriously ill child it must be considered. Poisoning of adults is not as common, but the writer has had experience with two cases in which it was used with criminal intent. The adulteration of health salts with powdered metallic lead was one instance. It illustrated that the toxicologist must be on his guard for such bizarre occurrences.

Analyses for metals using dithizone are never simple procedures, and lead is probably the most tedious one. It is advisable to keep a set of lead-free glassware especially for the determination. Every piece of glass should be well washed with hot dilute hydrochloric acid, then stood in concentrated dithizone in chloroform. The glass cells used in the spectrophotometer must not be forgotten. At any filtering stage the filter paper must be precleaned by running hot dilute hydrochloric acid through it, followed by copious amounts of distilled water. It is emphasised that all these procedures are essential.

The dithizone used in the determination should be purified before use by shaking a strong solution in carbon tetrachloride with ammonia. The separated alkaline layer is then shaken with fresh carbon tetrachloride after adding dilute hydrochloric acid to acidity. The purified dithizone is then in the organic solvent. The solution should be shielded from the light and prepared fresh daily.

If reagents are also kept separately after purification by continued washing with dithizone in chloroform, then this too can shorten each subsequent analysis. Potassium cyanide cannot be purified in this way, and special lead-free reagent must be used; this can be purchased. The sulphuric acid used must also be lead-free; this can only be determined by experiment. Hydrochloric acid often contains traces of lead and must be redistilled before use. Care must be taken to use pipettes whose calibrations are not marked in lead paint. This stresses that *every* piece of glassware must be examined and cleaned before use.

METHOD 1 (Tompsett, 1956).

If urine is being analysed a volume of 250 ml is taken and is evaporated directly. It is then treated exactly the same as the phosphate-treated blood. Bone is boiled with N hydrochloric acid until it is dissolved. After dilution it is extracted with three portions of 25 ml ether after addition of 10 ml aqueous 2% sodium diethyl-dithiocarbamate. The ether is evaporated and the analysis continued as for blood. Tissue is homogenised with equal volumes of water and 10% sodium dihydrogen phosphate and the analysis continued as for blood.

If blood is being analysed 20 ml of blood and 100 ml 10% $Na_2HPO_4.12H_2O$ are evaporated on a boiling water bath in a silica dish and are then strongly heated over a bunsen flame to destroy the organic material. A little nitric acid is added and the digest is again heated. The residue is dissolved in 75 ml of water containing 5 ml concentrated hydrochloric acid and filtered into a 250-ml flask. The crucible and filter funnel are washed with 25 ml of water. Add 50 ml 20% sodium citrate and adjust the pH to 7.5 to 8.0 by addition of ammonia. Cool, add 5 ml 10% potassium cyanide and extract with 3 x 50-ml portions of ether, adding 5 ml of 2% sodium diethyl-dithiocarbamate after the first ether portion. Shake each extraction for at least two minutes. Wash the combined ether extracts with water, and, after separating, evaporate the ether. If 20 g of blood are being analysed the residue should be digested by boiling with 0.4 ml of concentrated sulphuric acid and 1 ml of 100 volume hydrogen peroxide. The cooled digest should be dissolved in 0.4 ml glacial acetic acid, 2 ml of 880 ammonia and water to 10 ml. If urine, tissue or bone are being analyzed the expected amount of lead will be higher and the digestion is made with 1 ml of concentrated sulphuric acid and 1 ml of hydrogen peroxide. Dilution to 25 ml is made with 1 ml glacial acetic acid and 5 ml of ammonia and water. To a 10-ml aliquot are added six drops 5% w/v sulphurous acid, 5 ml 1% potassium cyanide and 10 ml carbon tetrachloride. A solution of dithizone in ammonia is then added with vigorous shaking, dropwise, until the brownish color of the dithizone is seen in the aqueous phase. This dithizone reagent is made by shaking 5 ml of 1% dithizone in carbon tetrachloride with 10 ml of 0.1N ammonia solution; the mixture is then centrifuged and the supernatant fluid used. It must be freshly prepared. The optical density readings of the separated carbon tetrachloride layer are then read at 525 nm and at 620 nm. The carbon tetrachloride is then shaken with 5 ml of 0.1N sulphuric acid to decompose the lead dithizonate; the carbon tetrachloride is separated and the readings are taken again at the same wavelengths.

Calculations. The first set of readings give a measure of the lead-dithizone complex at 525 nm and of unreacted dithizone at 620 nm. The second set of readings give the zero reading at 525 nm for lead dithizonate, and also measures the increase in dithizone at 620 nm caused by the decomposition of the lead dithizonate by the sulphuric acid. The optical density difference at 620 nm is therefore directly proportional to the molecular amount of dithizone liberated by the lead in solution, and is independent of the actual amount of dithizone used or of the impurities it contains. The calibration graph using this wavelength (620 nm) difference is therefore a constant, which, if the instrumentation is the same, should be reproducible in every laboratory. The difference in readings at 525 nm is a useful cross-check on the analysis being a normal colorimetric measure of lead dithizonate. In our hands the O.D. difference for 10 μg lead in 10 ml carbon tetrachloride gives an O.D. difference at 620 nm of 0.29.

METHOD 2 ATOMIC ABSORPTION. A suitable method for preparing liver samples for flame atomic absorption is as follows: One g of 1 : 1 macerate of liver is evaporated to dryness in a silica dish on a water bath. The residue is then dampened with 50% w/v magnesium nitrate solution which has been freed of lead by adjusting to pH 9 with ammonia and thymol blue indicator, and extracted repeatedly with a solution of 2 mg/100 ml of dithizone in carbon tetrachloride until successive extracts remain green, and then washed with carbon tetrachloride three times. The dampened residue is again dried and placed in a muffle at 500 degrees C for one hour. The crucible is removed, cooled and the ash dampened with the minimum volume of concentrated nitric acid, dried carefully under an infrared heater, and replaced in the muffle for a further one hour. After cooling, 1 ml lead-free 5N hydrochloric acid is added with agitation, and the solution gently evaporated to dryness with a watch glass three-quarters covering the crucible. The residue is dissolved in 1 ml 0.1N hydrochloric acid and washed with water into a 20-ml vial fitted with a snap-on polythene cap. The pH is adjusted to 2 or 3 using thymol blue and an indicator paper; 0.5 ml of 1% w/v aqueous ammonium pyrrolidine dithiocarbamate is added and the lead chelate extracted in 2.5 ml of water-saturated methyl isobutyl ketone by hand-shaking for two minutes; allow it to stand for five minutes and centrifuge for ten minutes. The top organic layer is aspirated into the atomic absorption flame, and readings are taken at 2833 Å and 2203 Å. The difference reading gives a quantitation. Standards are in the range of 0.2 to 2 μg per 2.5 ml organic solvent.

For urine (5-10 ml) the pH is adjusted to pH 2 or 3 with 5% trichloracetic acid; any precipitate is centrifuged off and the extraction with ammonium pyrrolidine dithiocarbamate and methyl isobutyl ketone is performed direct as described above. Blood is ashed in the same way as diluted macerated tissue. This method is suitable for nontoxic levels; in cases of suspected poisoning an aliquot of the hydrochloric acid extract is taken.

INTERPRETATION OF RESULTS. Levels over 70 μg per 100 ml of lead in the blood of adults are indicative of abnormal exposure.

Koumides (1963) reported that he had not seen a case of lead intoxication in a child at, or within a few days of, the time of onset of the illness in whose blood the concentration of lead was lower than 45 μg/100 g. However, it is clear from this report that levels only slightly above this will be found in children suffering from lead poisoning. Normal blood levels in children not exposed to lead are in the range 0 to 30 μg/100 g.

Urine is extensively used for testing for lead, and it is generally agreed that levels over 8 μg/100 ml are indicative of exposure. Usually a diagnosis is made on a consideration of lead analyses on blood and urine, coupled with a consideration of the clinical symptoms and examination of a blood film for punctate basophilia. In addition, there may be a coproporphyrinuria and an elevated δ-amino laevulinic acid excretion. In fatal cases, which are often unrecognized until they come to the attention of the toxicologist, analyses on the other organs are performed. Tompsett gives the following figures for normal healthy adults. Obviously these should be exceeded for a positive diagnosis. X-ray examination of bone also enables the lead lines to be seen, and if the ingested poison is a lead paint, it too can be seen in the gastrointestinal tract on x-ray.

Normal levels:

Liver: 0.09-0.46 mg/100 g
Kidney: 0.07-0.37 mg/100 g
Brain: 0.02-0.07 mg/100 g
Bone: Rib: 0.05-1.29 mg/100 g
Vertebrae: 0.26-1.47 mg/100 g
Femur: 1.82-10.8 mg/100 g
Tibia: 1.53-9.65 mg/100 g
See also Beattie (1974) and Sayers (1974).

LSD AND OTHER HALLUCINOGENS

Although radioimmunoassay techniques have been reported (Taunton Rigby *et al.*, 1973; Loeffler *et al.*, 1973), the writer knows of no suitable method for screening urine routinely for LSD, but sugar-cubes, blotting paper and other media which might be impregnated with LSD often come to the toxicologists laboratory. LSD is light and heat-sensitive, and precautions to minimise its decomposition must be taken. It is not very soluble in organic solvents, and extraction is achieved at pH 8.5 to 9 from the minimum saturated aqueous sodium chloride solution with at least a three-volume excess of organic solvent which may be chloroform or 2% isoamyl alcohol in n-heptane. LSD can be purified by extraction into 0.01M hydrochloric acid, then re-extracted from alkaline solution into organic solvent. Evaporation should be in the dark under nitrogen and reduced pressure at ambient temperature.

Identification and Assay

The blue fluorescence of LSD in ultraviolet light, which can be seen on sugar cubes, paper, etc., is a most useful screening test; it can be quantitated using a spectrofluorimeter using an excitation wavelength of 335 nm and a fluorescence wavelength of 435 nm. Sensitivities of 10 nanograms/ml can be obtained. A sensitive rapid color test is to evaporate an aliquot on a piece of filter paper and test with 1% p-dimethylaminobenzaldehyde in ethanol containing 10% concentrated hydrochloric acid. On warming, a blue color is obtained. To differentiate LSD from ergot alkaloids and other hallucinogens, paper and thin layer chromatography are used.

METHODS (Clarke, E.G.C. (1967) See Table XXXIV).

Paper Chromatography. System Butanol/citric acid on citrated paper (see Chap 80).

TLC. Silica-Gel G; methanol: 880 NH_3 (100: 1.5).

Tables XXXV and XXXVI give further TLC data and ultraviolet maxima of some hallucinogens.

A full study has been made by Fowler, Gomm and Patterson (1972) of the thin layer chromatography of lysergide and other similar compounds, for example lysergic acid, iso LSD and twenty-

TABLE XXXIV
CHROMATOGRAPHY OF HALLUCINOGENS

Rf on Paper	Compound	Fluorescence 254nm	pDMB Reaction Colour	Rf TLC System
0.05	Psilocybin	dark blue	grey	0.34
0.11	Lysergamide	blue	blue	0.18
0.12	Serotonin	pale yellow	purple	0.25
0.13	6-hydroxy DMT	blue	blue	0.32
0.16	Bufotenin	pale blue	purple	0.32
0.18	7-hydroxy DMT	absorbs	green	0.33
0.18	Lysergic acid	blue	blue	0.33
0.25	Ergometrine	blue	blue	0.23
0.25	5-methoxytryptamine	white	purple	0.25
0.25	Mescalin	nil	faint yellow	0.23
0.26	5-methoxy DMT	white	purple	0.32
0.31	Psilocin	absorbs	grey	0.34
0.35	Tryptamine	blue	purple	0.27
0.38	Dimethytryptamine	blue	purple	0.34
0.40	Methylergometrine	blue	blue	0.30
0.40	N-methyltryptamine	blue	purple	0.16
0.45	Methylsergide	blue	blue	0.49
0.47	LSD	blue	blue	0.63
0.63	Dihydroergotamine	green	blue	0.56
0.65	Ergotamine	blue	blue	0.58
0.65	Ergosine	blue	blue	0.58
0.80	Dihydroergotoxin	green	blue	0.68
0.82	Ergotoxin	blue	blue	0.78

TABLE XXXV
THIN LAYER CHROMATOGRAPHY OF SOME HALLUCINOGENS

Stationary phase	Mobile phase	Psilocybin	Psilocin	Serotin	5-Methoxy DMT	5-Methoxy TRY	5-Methyltryptamine	α-Methyltryptamine	Ibogaine	Bufotenine	D.P.T.	D.M.T.	D.E.T.	Mescaline	3,4,5-TMA	M.D.A.	S.T.P.
Silica Gel	Methanol:0.880 Ammonia 100:1.5	04	34	25	32	25				32		34		23	35		
Eastman® K301 sheet or similar layer	Trichlorethylene:Ethyl Acetate: n-Butanol:Methanol 25:25:35:10								89			34		20		33	26
Silica Gel	Benzene:Ethyl Acetate 5% Diethylamine 7:2:1	00							55			42		16			
Silica Gel	n-Propanol:Ammonia (5%)							31	72		60	70	38	55			28
Silica Gel	Methanol:0,880 Ammonia 100:1.5	18		20			23			32		35		21		33	
Silica Gel 30 g with 0.1N NaOH (60 ml)	Methanol	04		15			18	26		21		27	29	13		24	19

TABLE XXXVI
ULTRAVIOLET MAXIMA OF SOME HALLUCINOGENS

max (nm)	of Other Peaks (nm)	Solvent	$E_{1\,cm}^{1\%}$ max.	Substance
225	290	Methanol	970	Ibogaine
226	298	Ethanol	781	Ibogaine
234	286	Acid	197	MDA
252	258, 264	Chloroform		Methyl Benzilate
257	251, 261	Acid	13.4	LBJ
257	251, 261, 263, 268	Acid	13.8	Benactyzine Hydrochloride
258	251, 261, 263, 272	Acid	14.5	JB 8191
258	252, 261, 263, 267	Acid	13.2	JB 318
267	285, 293	Methanol	282	Psilocin
267	285, 293, (222?)	Methanol	202	Psilocybin
267	290, (220?)	Methanol	222	Psilocybin
268		Acid	39	Mescaline
269		Acid	29	3,4,5-TMA
275		Aqueous		5-Methoxytryptamine
275		Aqueous		5-Methoxy DMT
275		Aqueous		Serotonin
277	296	Acid	269	Bufotenine
277	300	Ethanol	300	Bufotenine
279	287	Acid	162	Methyltryptamine Methane Sulphonate
282	274, 290	Ethanol		DPT
282	290, 276	Methanol	311	DMT
282	291	Methanol		DET
288	220	Acid	150	STP
288	224	Aqueous	224	STP
290		Methanol	319	Ibogaine
298		Ethanol	341	Ibogaine

three ergot alkaloids in thirty-eight combinations of plates and solvent systems. For rapid, routine use they recommend Merck Silica Gel F54 plates (0.255 mm precoated) run in acetone and Merck Aluminium Oxide F_{254} (Type E, 0.25mm precoated) also run in acetone used in combination.

See also Axelrod *et al.*, (1956 and 1957); Aghajanian and Bing, (1964); Dal Cortivo *et al.*, (1966) and Wagner *et al.*, (1968).

MAGNESIUM

This metal is of importance in general medicine but the toxicologist must also bear it in mind in relation to attempts to procure an abortion and in deaths of very young children.

Magnesium values on blood will often be requested in poisonings by phenothiazines and tricyclic antidepressants, and the clinical biochemist will have a routine method available in a hospital laboratory.

MANGANESE

This metal as one of its salts is frequently a component with iron salts in *anaemia tablets.*

METHODS (Copeman, 1955).

In a Kjeldahl flask, 10 to 20 g of tissue are boiled with nitric acid and sulphuric acid to completion of destruction of the organic matter. The volume of sulphuric acid should be 10 to 15 ml; nitric acid is added when charring seen. Cool when complete and make up to 50 ml with water. Take 20 ml and evaporate in a silica basin on a sand bath until no more white fumes are seen, and, finally, over a flame until all traces of sulphuric acid are removed and the residue is clear. Cool and treat with 10 ml of water containing 1 ml of a mixture of equal amounts of sulphuric acid and 80% phosphoric acid. Transfer to a 6 by $1\frac{3}{4}$ Pyrex® testtube and wash with 2×5 ml similar portions. Add 0.2 to 0.3 g potassium periodate and bring to a boil over a flame. Place in a boiling water bath until the permanganate color is fully developed. There should be no covering to the test tube. Match the color against 0.001N potassium permanganate standards; 1 ml is equivalent to 0.011 mg manganese.

Van Ormer and Purdy (1973) have reviewed the atomic absorption literature and published a method for measuring manganese in urine. Normal values were a few parts per billion.

Neutron activation analysis figures largely in the literature for manganese measurements.

INTERPRETATION OF RESULTS. Copeman gives the following figures for normal levels in nontoxic tissue:

	mg/100 g	*Maximum Observed*
Liver	0.13	0.16
Kidney	0.076	0.10
Intestines	0.064	0.083

MEPROBAMATE

One is faced with several alternatives for analysis as far as meprobamate is concerned. Usually a neutral ether extract of a urine sample will give sufficient crystalline product for a mixed melting point, but colorimetry as well as thin layer and gas chromatography are also available.

Meprobamate is a drug in which return to consciousness is followed in a few hours by a return to coma. It is possible that intestinal motality recovers leading to further absorption of the drug. This is known to German workers as *nachslaf*.

METHOD 1 (Madsen 1962: Merli and de Zorzi, 1961).

To 1 ml serum add two drops 25% ammonium hydroxide, 1 ml saturated aqueous potassium chloride and 25 ml of a mixture of equal volumes of carbon tetrachloride and chloroform. Shake and centrifuge, and separate the organic layer. Filter it through glass wool. Wash the glass wool with 10 ml of solvent mixture and evaporate the combined organic fractions. To the extract add 0.2 ml AAA reagent, and 0.2 ml DMB and mix. Add 1 ml ATA and mix. Stopper loosely and heat at 50 degrees C in a water bath for exactly ten minutes. Cool quickly. Add 1 ml benzene and filter through 6-cm-diameter Whatman No. 41H (541) paper into small glass tubes. Read at 550 nm within fifteen minutes.

AAA—Reagent. Three volumes acetone and one volume glacial acetic acid prepared fresh.

ATA—Reagent. A saturated solution of 25% w/v antimony trichloride in chloroform prepared by heating the mixture on a hot plate until complete dissolution. Filter through Whatman No. 41 (H541) paper. Store the bottle in a plastic bag to avoid water absorption.

DMB Reagent. 1% w/v of p-dimethylaminobenzaldehyde in benzene.

METHOD 2. The neutral ether extract can be examined by thin layer chromatography. Thirteen carbamates were found to react with the well-known furfural-hydrochloric acid reagent (McConnell Davies, 1967. See also: Moss and Jackson, 1961); in a TLC system which used three different solvents. Additional spray reagents included furfural-sulphuric acid and vanillin-sulphuric acid. This last reagent consisted of 5 g of vanillin dissolved in 100 ml of concentrated sulphuric acid. The plate was sprayed well but not soaked with reagent, and yellow spots were observed immediately on spraying except for urea, which gave a red spot, and methylpentynol carbamate and emylcamate which gave purple spots. Further discrimination was obtained on heating the plate at 110 degrees until a standard spot of meprobamate turned blue; then, on observing the plate again fifteen minutes after its removal from the oven. The solvent systems used were the lower layer obtained by shaking together acetic acid: carbon tetrachloride:chloroform:water (100:60:90:50), on silica gel G plates. Kieselgel C plates, impregnated with formamide by dipping the plates in a solution of 5% formamide in methanol and allowing them to dry in air for twelve minutes before application of the samples were also used; the solvent was benzene:chloroform (30:120) saturated with formamide, and in the second system carbon tetrachloride saturated with formamide. It was also found useful to look at the plates under 254 nm light before they were sprayed. Two-way TLC systems were described by Haywood, Horner and Rylance (1967) to characterize neutral drugs, including many carbamates, and Kieselgel GF254 plates were activated for one hour at 110 degrees C before use. Their first system used redistilled ethyl acetate, and after drying for not less than twenty minutes in an air stream, the second 90 degree run was in dioxan:methylene chloride:water (1:2:1), allowed to equilibrate and the aqueous phase discarded. Spots which reacted to give a blue color when exposed to chlorine gas for a few seconds were left in the air for about fifteen minutes, then sprayed with 2% starch solution containing 1% potassium iodide, scraped from the plate and eluted in 2 ml methanol by shaking mechanically for ten minutes, followed by spinning in the centrifuge. The supernatant solution was then separated and evaporated in a vacuum oven at 40 degrees C, dissolved in methanol, and run in chloroform:acetone (9:1). It was found that this elution procedure revealed some decomposition that occurred during the chlorine:starch-potassium iodide treatment, but no doubt this phenomenon provided additional criteria of identification.

METHOD 3. Gas chromatography (Maes *et al.*, 1969).

In gas chromatographic systems, as in TLC, meprobamate cannot be considered in isolation, and procedures that have been described involve both drugs and their derivatives. Ethchlorvynol, paraldehyde, meprobamate and carisoprodol were determined in this method, and the operating conditions for meprobamate and carisoprodol involved a column of 3% SE-30 on 80 to 100 mesh Chromosorb WAW-DMDS at 190 degrees. A thin layer chromatographic system on silica gel G using chloroform:acetone (8:2) with the furfural:hydrochloric acid spray was used for identification. The last two drugs have also been investigated (Maes *et al.*, 1970) using OV-101, 3% column on Diataport S at 190 degrees. A similar technique has been used by Douglas and his co-workers (1967) to separate meprobamate, carisoprodol, mebutamate and tybamate on a 3.8% UC-W 98 methyl silicone on Diataport S at 180 degrees; dibutyl phthalate was used as an internal standard. Skinner (1967) and Maddock and Bloomer (1967) have also described the determination of meprobamate by gas chromatography using SE-30 columns.

METHOD 3A. (Martis and Levy, 1974).

Reference to the published method is necessary because of the complexity of the analysis. Hydrolysis with alkali to 2-methyl-2 propyl-1:3-propanediol after ether extraction is followed by reaction with N,O-bis (trimethylsilyl) acetamide, and a gas chromatographic separation with 2-methyl-2 ethyl-1:3 propanediol as an internal standard. After an 800-mg dose a plasma level peaking at about 13 μg/ml was found with a half life of about seven hours.

INTERPRETATION OF RESULTS. Therapeutic levels after the consumption of 1,600 mg are about 1 to 2 mg/100 ml in the blood. At the higher level the patient is difficult to rouse. In a case of poisoning reported by Bedson (1959) consciousness was regained about thirty-five hours after the blood level was 21.5 mg/100 ml.

Maddock and Bloomer (1967) suggest that plasma levels approaching 20 mg/100 ml indicate very profound intoxication. These workers note that urinary excretion is considerable and say that haemodialysis appears to be the most efficient method for removing meprobamate. Marck (personal communication) reported a case in which after a dose of 24 g there was 145 mg of the drug in 30 ml of urine!

There have been other reports of nonfatal poisonings with blood levels as high as 25 mg/100 ml, but patients are usually comatose with levels over 5 mg/100 ml. However, patients taking 0.8 to 4.8 g per day for periods of four months were found to have plasma levels of 2.3 to 6.3 mg/100 ml with virtual disappearance of the drug in ninety-six hours after cessation of intake.

Finkle (1967) reports normal therapeutic blood levels up to 1.5 mg/100 g, but notes that with simultaneous alcohol ingestion, levels of 50 mg/100 ml ethanol and 0.4 mg/100 ml meprobamate, the subject was *very drunk*. His series give results for combinations of meprobamate, glutethimide, barbiturate, benactyzine, dexedrine, etc., found in road accident cases.

The clinical findings in meprobamate poisoning are very well-known and no new factors have been reported recently, except to emphasize the fact that meprobamate is not very soluble in water and consequently further absorption of the drug from the gastrointestinal tract can occur when an unconscious patient is roused or has a change in body position from recumbent to erect. The case reported from the Walter Reed General Hospital (Jenis *et al.,* 1969) emphasizes this in that the patient returned to consciousness ten hours after being found unconscious, but some fifteen hours later she was again found to be unconscious, cyanotic with no pulse or respiration. The original blood level of 14.4 mg/100 ml had risen to 16.5 mg/100 ml at the time of death. At postmorten examination the stomach contents were found to contain 200 g of granular grey-white particulate matter which was found to contain 25 g of meprobamate.

See also: Hoffman and Ledwig (1959); Kanter (1967); Prokes, (1964).

MERCURY

This is an extremely toxic metal when ingested in the form of its soluble salts. The variety of methods whereby absorption of these salts arises is very wide indeed, ranging from homicidal poisoning, the ingestion of calomel by infants, the absorption of mercury vapor from fingerprint powder by police officers, laboratory and industrial workers, skin absorption of mercurial ointments and vaginal pastes to the accidental ingestion by infants of grass treated with mercurial (lawn) sand.

Whenever a method for the estimation of mercury using dithizone is to be used the reader is recommended to read first the paper by Irving, Risdon and Andrew, (1949).

Measurement of urinary excretion is a common method of screening for mercury poisoning but, in sudden deaths from an unknown cause, the kidney should be analyzed. If a high concentration is found in the kidney, the liver should then be examined.

Most mercuric salts are extremely volatile and students should beware of adding, say 5 μg of mercuric chloride in 1 ml of water to a blood sample in beginning a positive control test for mercury, then evaporating the sample on a steam bath; all the mercury will be lost. Even the experienced worker may be misled into underestimating the volatility of mercuric salts, and all stages of the analysis must be included when standard graphs are being prepared.

The use of *reversion technique* of spectrophotometry for mercury, as for lead, means that the calibration is independent of dithizone concentration or impurities.

METHOD 1. Kidney, 2 g, is refluxed with 2 ml of a 50:50 mixture of concentrated nitric and sulphuric acids for thirty minutes to destroy all organic matter. The conditions of refluxing are critical and must be checked by adequate control experiments. The reflux condenser must be especially efficient, being preferably a coil-type; the more usual double surface type is not sufficiently effective to prevent loss of mercury. The temperature of refluxing must be kept low. A microburner is a convenient flame. When heating is finished, cool in ice and pour 40 ml of water down the condenser into the flask. Cool again and add 2 ml of 50% aqueous solution of hydroxylamine hydrochloride and reflux again for one minute. Cool in ice, filter through a previously acid-washed filter paper into a 50-ml flask, and make up to the mark. Transfer to a separating funnel and shake with 2 to 3 ml of chloroform which is discarded. Shake next with 10 ml of an ice-cold solution of dithizone in chloroform which has an optical density at 600 nm of approximately 0.6 to 0.7. Run off 3.5 ml of the chloroform layer into a 1-cm cuvette and read at 600 nm. Next, run off approximately 5 ml of the same solution into a 25-ml separating funnel and shake with 5 ml of a solution of 10.2 g potassium hydrogen phthalate and 30 g potassium iodide made up to 500 ml with water. Read the chloroform layer also at 600 nm. Exact standards are done by adding known quantities of mercuric chloride to tissue that has been shown to be free of the metal. The calibration curve is prepared by plotting the difference in optical density readings at 600 nm between the dithizone solutions before and after shaking with the reversion solution against the known amounts of mercury. In our hands 20 μg of mercury gives a difference reading of 0.695.

Diagnosis of pink disease in children is often confirmed by urinalysis, and tests on laboratory and industrial workers handling mercury are routine. Because of the difficulty in interpreting tissue levels of mercury, the analysis of urine, which does not result in similar difficulties, is attractive.

METHOD (Gray, 1952). Twenty-five ml of urine are refluxed with 50 ml of water, 10 ml of sulphuric acid (1 + 1) and 1 g potassium permanganate for thirty minutes. If the urine was highly colored add a further 0.5 g of potassium permanganate and reflux again; cool. Add 1 ml of 50% hydroxylamine hydrochloride and reflux for one minute. Cool and dilute to 100 ml with water and sufficient dilute sulphuric acid to bring the concentration to 0.25N. From this stage the dithizone assay is exactly as for digested kidney tissue described above. Great care must be taken by the performance of control experiments to show that loss of mercury does not occur during the refluxing.

METHOD 2

Atomic Absorption (Based on Willis, 1962).

Urine: 50 ml are made to pH 2.5-4 with trichloroacetic acid and 1 ml of 1% ammonium pyrrolidine dithiocarbamate added. The mercury complex is extracted by shaking with 2 ml methyl n-amyl ketone for two minutes. The organic phase is separated and centrifuged. This solution is aspirated into a Perkin-Elmer 303 Atomic Absorption Spectrophotometer fitted with a Boling three-slot burner. Standards are made with 1, 2, 5 and 10 μg of mercury in aqueous solution treated in the same way. The 2536 Å line is used.

Tissue. Two g are refluxed with a 1:1 mixture of concentrated nitric and sulphuric acids as described in the dithizone method above. When digestion is complete the solution is cooled, diluted to about 20 ml with water, and adjusted to pH 2 to 3 using ammonia and indicator paper. The extraction then proceeds as for urine above.

INTERPRETATION OF RESULTS. Mercury is a constituent of some livers and kidneys, arising presumably from mercurial amalgams used in dentistry or from the use of ointments. Although normal levels can be as high as 1.72 mg/100 g in liver and 12.7 mg/100 g in kidneys; levels over 1 mg/100 g should be fully investigated. In persons receiving mercurial diuretics, levels of up to 2.5 mg/ 100 g have been found in liver, and 27.5 mg/100 g in kidney. However, normal nontoxic livers should average at less than 0.5 mg/100 g, while in cases of poisoning from mercuric chloride it is likely that the level will be over 2 mg/100 g, and probably will be about 5 mg/100 g.

In two papers, Smith, (Howie and Smith, 1967; Rodger and Smith, 1967), has studied "normal" *dry* tissue mercury levels and concentrations in hair. Their values are as follows:
Their values are as follows:

	mg/100 g
Hair	.003—2.44 median 0.420
Kidney	.008—7.93
Liver	.015—2.0
Blood	.006—.012
Brain	0.12—1.52

These values are difficult to compare accurately with wet tissue levels, but appear to agree with normally accepted values.

Because normal healthy individuals can have such high tissue mercury levels the diagnosis of poisoning can rarely be made solely on the analytical results. Mercury excretion in the urine has been shown to vary considerably from minute to minute, and, in the living patient, eight-hour samples are recommended for analysis. Rodger and Smith found in forty-six people not knowingly exposed to mercury, a median excretion of 1.3 μg/100 ml with a maximum of 13 μg/100 ml. Berman, (1967) is in general agreement; her maximum noted was 3 μg/100 ml. Roger and Smith have found symptoms with levels in the region 30 to 100 μg per day, but in serious poisoning cases, one can expect much higher concentrations—up to many milligrams per day. In one case in the writers experience a transient rise in urinary mercury was observed and the only significant exposure that could be traced was that the patient had swallowed a mercury amalgam tooth filling that had broken off.

Berman reports excretions of 450 μg/litre in a patient addicted to a calomel-containing preparation and 2 and 5 mg/litre in two cases of pink disease.

See also Forney and Harger, (1949) and Curry, A.S., (1972).

METHADONE

Methods

Two basic methods are given below, one based on gas chromatography, the other on spectrophotometry.

METHOD 1 (Robinson and Williams, 1971; Norheim, 1973; Garratt *et al.*, 1973).

All these methods are basically very similar in that the drug and metabolite are extracted with organic solvent (ether or butyl chloride) from alkaline solution, back extracted into N sulphuric acid, and then re-extracted into ether which is evaporated. Robinson and Williams add a known amount of internal standard of benzhexol hydrochloride to the original biological fluid. Five to 20 ml/g samples are usually the size to be processed. Silicone gum columns (SE39, OV17, W98) are used at temperatures of 185 to 230 degrees C.

METHOD 2 (Wallace *et al.*, 1972 Courtesy *J. Pharm. Sci.*).

Preliminary Extraction of Bile and Urine. Five to twenty milliliters of urine (containing 20–150 μg methadone) was placed in a 250-ml separator and adjusted to pH 9 to 12 by the dropwise addition of 5N sodium hydroxide. Fifty milliliters of *n*-hexane was added, the mixture was shaken vigorously for three minutes, and the aqueous layer was discarded.

Preliminary Extraction of Tissues. Tissue specimens were alkaline-digested to release protein-bound methadone. Ten grams of tissue were combined with 10 ml of 30% potassium hydroxide solution. A flask containing the mixture was immersed in a boiling water bath for ten to thirty minutes or until complete disintegration of the tissue was obtained. The solution was cooled, transferred to a separator, adjusted to pH 9 to 12, and extracted into approximately five volumes of *n*-hexane.

General Extraction. Hexane from the preliminary extractions was filtered through filter paper into a 100-ml stoppered graduated cylinder. The hexane was extracted with 10 ml of 4.7 M sulfuric acid. Nine milliliters of the aqueous layer, along with 5 ml of spectrograde *n*-heptane and 325 to 350 mg barium peroxide, were added to a 250-ml round-bottom flask which was subsequently attached to a water-cooled reflux condenser. The mixture was refluxed for forty-five minutes with constant magnetic stirring, utilizing a high reflux rate of approximately 200 drops minute.

After cooling, the heptane was extracted with an equal volume of 1.0 N sodium hydroxide. The heptane was read in the spectrophotometer at 215 to 360 nm against a similarly-prepared *n*-heptane blank. Analysis at a single wavelength was achieved by determining the absorption at 247 nm. For a standard, 9 ml of 4.7M sulfuric acid containing 100 g of methadone was carried through the reflux step. The methadone concentration of an unknown is determined from the following equation:

$$\frac{\text{OD unknown}}{\text{OD standard}} \times$$

Concentration of standard in heptane (2.0 mg %) $\times$

$$\frac{\text{ml hexane used for extraction}}{\text{ml. hexane recovered}} \times$$

$$\frac{\text{ml 4.7 } M \text{ H}_2\text{SO}_4 \text{ used for extraction}}{\text{ml 4.7 } M \text{ H}_2\text{SO}_4 \text{ used in reflux}} \times$$

$$\frac{\text{ml heptane}}{\text{ml (g) specimen}} = \text{mg \%}$$

where OD = optical density. Satisfactory analysis was performed with as little as 5 ml of urine and 2 ml of heptane.

It should be noted that extraction of drug into organic solvent drops rapidly above about pH 10, and solvents such as chloroform and ethylene dichloride will react with methadone.

INTERPRETATION OF RESULTS. Robinson and Williams (1971) give extensive details of methadone and its metabolites' distribution in eleven fatal cases, some of which were associated with other drugs. Blood concentrations varied from 22 to 304 μg/100 ml with liver levels from 25 to 4950 μg/100 g. Urine values were in the range 50 μg to 13.2 mg/100 ml. The metabolite was also quantified in these cases. The proportion of unchanged drug to metabolite varies considerably between individuals and between different workers' results.

Norheim (1973) has reported five cases of death giving blood values from 36 to 100 μg/100 ml; liver, 120 to 310 μg/100 g; and urine 320 to 1800 μg/100 ml.

A high proportion of methadone intake is excreted in the urine, both as unchanged drug and as 2-ethylidene-1,5 dimethyl 3,3,diphenylpyrollidone. The urinary excretion, however, may be affected by change in urinary pH. The plasma levels of patients receiving up to 120 mg a day varied from 20 to 108 μg/100 ml (Inturrisi and Verebely (1972)).

Lung tissue, then liver, kidney and brain are usually at higher levels than the blood.

METHAQUALONE

Considerable apparent differences occur in the concentrations of this drug in biological materials if different methods of analysis are used. Bailey and Jatlow (1973) showed this was due to a metabolite, soluble in chloroform and possibly in ether, having the same ultraviolet spectrum as the unchanged drug. They were able to separate the metabolites from drug by the fact that the former were not soluble in hexane in which methaqualone is soluble. In interpreting results this finding is of great importance; in one of their cases a chloroform/UV method gave a value of 66 mg/100 ml in serum, but gas chromatography gave only a value of 9 mg/100 ml.

It must be remembered that methaqualone is a very weak base and will not be extracted from organic solvents by acid strengths as high as 0.1N. In general, sulphuric acid is preferable to hydrochloric acid although many workers do use hydrochloric.

The drug may be re-extracted after ultraviolet spectrophotometry and can be examined by TLC (See Tables VIII and IX).

METHOD. Blood, 5 ml, is made alkaline by addition of 1 ml 2% sodium hydroxide and extracted with ether (50 ml). Shake slowly or, preferably, use a roller extraction technique. Separate the layers and wash the ether with 5 ml water. Separate and shake the ether with 5 ml of 2N H_2SO_4. Read the aqueous layer from 220 to 290 nm. Methaqualone has a characteristic curve with λ max = 234 nm and $E_{1cm}^{1\%}$ = approximately 1090.

METHOD Berry, (1969 Courtesy of *J. Chromatogr.*).

A sample of 5.0 ml of plasma was made alkaline by the addition of 1.0 ml of 1N sodium hydroxide and extracted with 15 ml of hexane by gentle shaking for ten minutes in a 30-ml centrifuge tube. After centrifugation at 3,000 r.p.m., the organic layer was transferred to a second tube containing approximately 3 g of anhydrous sodium sulphate. On carrying out a second five minutes extraction with 10 ml of hexane, the organic fractions were bulked, thoroughly shaken with the anhydrous sodium sulphate, and left to stand for ten minutes. The extract was then evaporated to dryness under a stream of nitrogen in a 10-ml conical centrifuge-tube to which 1.0 ml of the butobarbitone standard solution had been added, the tube being immersed in a water-bath at 60 degrees. The residue was taken up in 100 μl of absolute ethanol, and 3 to 5 μl of this were injected on to the gas chromatograph.

A Pye® 104 model 24 dual column gas chromatograph, equipped with a flame ionisation detector and a 1m V Honeywell recorder, was used. The column was a 7 foot by $\frac{1}{4}$ inch internal diameter coiled glass tube which had been silanised with a 5% solution of dimethyldichlorosilane in benzene over a period of twenty-four hours. Glass wool was silanised in the same solution. After drying at 100 degrees, the column was packed with 3% cyclohexanedimethanol succinate (CDMS) on 85 to 100 mesh Diatomite CO. This packing was prepared as follows: 0.77 g of CDMS were dissolved in 100 ml of dichloromethane. The support (24 g) was added to the flask and left to stand, with occasional swirling, for two hours. The solvent was removed under vacuum in a rotary evaporator, the final stages of evaporation being completed in a water bath at 100 degrees for thirty minutes. The prepared column was then packed with the coated support by closing one end with silanised glass wool and applying a vacuum. After filling, the other end was closed with silanised glass wool and the packed column conditioned for forty-eight hours at 250 degrees with a nitrogen flow rate of 55 ml/min. At the end of this time the column was tapped down, more coated support added and conditioning for a further twenty-four hours carried out. This column has been in constant use for eighteen months and no significant change in behavior has been observed. The instrument settings were as follows: temperature, column 200 degrees, injection port, 240 degrees; gas flow rates, hydrogen 45 ml/min, nitrogen (carrier gas) 55 ml/min, air 400 ml/min; sensitivity, 2 $\times$ 10^{-10} A.

Butobarbitone was chosen as an internal standard since the column used will separate barbiturates, and this analogue has good resolution from both the solvent peak and the methaqualone peak. Furthermore, the acidic barbiturates will be excluded from the alkaline extract. A range of standard solutions containing 200 μg/ml of butobarbitone and from 20 μg to 200 μg/ml of methaqualone, were made in ethanol. A standard curve was prepared by injecting 3 to 5 μl aliquots of these solutions just prior to measuring unknown samples. The ratio of the peak height of methaqualone to butobarbitone was linear over the range 0.1 μg to 1 μg of methaqualone.

A quicker method using a better internal standard has been described by Evenson and Lensmeyer (1974).

A very sensitive gas chromatographic method for the determination of levels following therapeutic doses has been published by Mitchard and Williams (1972), and use of a *fingerprint* TLC pattern of methaqualone metabolites after various pre-extraction procedures have been described by Goudie and Burnett (1971). Allen *et al.* (1970) have described a similar approach.

METHOD (Allen, Fry and Marks, 1970).

Extract 20 ml of urine with an equal volume of methylene dichloride after making the urine to pH 10 to 11. Separate and dry the organic layer with 1 g of solid sodium sulphate; decant and evaporate. Redissolve in about 60 μl of methanol and apply to a silica gel (Merck F_{254}®) plate and develop in ethyl acetate: methanol:ammonia (170:20:10). After drying view in 254 nm light. The methaqualone metabolite is seen as a dark spot at Rf 0.35, and on spraying with 1 mg/ml of Fast Blue B, salt in 75% methanol/water appears as a blue-mauve spot.

INTERPRETATION OF RESULTS. Therapeutic blood levels are usually well below 0.5 mg/100 ml. In fatal cases noted by Maehly and Bonnichsen (1966) blood levels were in the range 0.5 to 3.2 mg/100 ml with tissue concentrations somewhat higher (3.8-5.8 mg/100 g in liver and 2.2-9.2 mg/100 g in kidney). In the living patient recovery has been noted after haemodialysis with a blood level of 10.5 mg/100 ml.

In Bailey and Jatlow's (1973) series of fifteen cases, unchanged drug levels in serum in overdose cases varied from 0.2 to 2.2 mg/100 ml. Those with levels above 0.8 mg/100 ml were usually unconscious.

The phenomenon of alternating coma-arousal-coma has been well documented in methaqualone cases.

As has been indicated above, therapeutic levels are of the order of 0.1 mg/100 ml. In fatal cases the blood level will usually exceed 0.5 mg/100 ml. It is interesting that in the majority of cases the blood contains about 1.0 mg/100 ml and rarely exceeds 3 mg/100 ml. Tissue concentrations in fatal cases, particularly the liver and kidney, contain somewhat higher concentrations, usually about 7 mg/100 g in the liver and 4 mg/100 g in the kidney. These figures contrast with the series reported by Matthews *et al.*, (1968) who found plasma concentrations of as high as 4 mg/100 ml in conscious patients and, indeed, a value of 8 mg/100 ml gave only a loss of one grade of consciousness. In one patient who was very severely poisoned, the exceedingly high plasma level of 23 mg/100 ml was noted. This situation clearly parallels that in many other areas of toxicology where, in one subject, death has to be ascribed to poisoning, but two or three times the same level in another person can be found associated with little clinical abnormality. It should be noted however that in Matthew's series the ultraviolet of measurement was being used.

See also: Bonnichsen, *et al.*, (1974).

METHANOL

METHOD 1. (Williams *et al.*, 1961).

Deproteinise 0.2 ml of serum with 1.8 ml of a solution made by mixing 10 g of trichloracetic acid with 10 ml of 10% sulphuric acid. To 1 ml of the filtrate or centrifuged supernatant is added 0.1 ml of 5% potassium permanganate. After five minutes a little powdered sodium bisulphite is added until the solution is colorless. Two tenths ml of an 0.5% solution of freshly prepared chromotropic acid is then added with 6 ml of concentrated sulphuric acid. After mixing the solution is heated at 100 degrees C in a boiling bath for five minutes. After cooling the optical density is read at 570 nm. A calibration curve is prepared from exact standards prepared in the same way.

METHOD 2 (Feldstein and Klendshoj, 1954).

Sulphuric acid (2.2 ml of 10%) is pipetted into the center well of a Conway cell. In the outer compartment is placed 1 ml of saturated aqueous potassium carbonate solution. Sealing of the ground glass plate is made with petroleum jelly.

Half millilitre of sample is introduced into the outer compartment; the cell is sealed and tilted several times to thoroughly mix the sample and carbonate. Diffusion is allowed to proceed for two hours at room temperature. At the end of this period 1 ml of the sulphuric acid is pipetted into a 25-ml test tube; one drop of 5% aqueous potassium permanganate is added and the tube shaken. After five minutes at room temperature, drops of a saturated aqueous solution of sodium bisulphite are added until the permanganate is decolorized. After the addition of 0.2 ml of freshly prepared 0.5% aqueous chromotropic acid, the tube is cooled in ice and 4 ml of concentrated sulphuric acid added. The tube is shaken, then immersed in a boiling water bath for fifteen minutes after which it is cooled to room temperature. After making up to exactly 10 ml, readings at 580 nm are taken for the test and controls. Suitable standards are in the range 0 to 80 μg of methanol.

Schiff's reagent can be used to test for methanol by adding it to the permanganate-oxidised distillates made up to 10% with sulphuric acid. Acetaldehyde does not then interfere, and estimates of concentration can be made by comparison with standards.

INTERPRETATION OF RESULTS. Methanol is considerably more toxic than ethanol, and correspondingly lower concentrations are found in cases of poisoning. Levels over 80 mg/100 ml of blood must be considered extremely dangerous to life.

Because ethanol is the most common volatile poison it is probable that analysis will be directed to it first. Methanol however is often a cause of obscure acidotic coma which may not develop for several hours after ingestion of the poison. Although the metabolism of ethanol is relatively rapid, the rate of disappearance of methanol from the blood is so slow that appreciable amounts may be present over forty-eight hours after ingestion. It is therefore important that screening tests for this poison test should be applied routinely.

See also Bamford (1951) and Polson and Tattersall, (1959).

METHYLPENTYNOL

METHOD (Perlman and Johnson, 1952) .

Alkaline Silver Reagent. To a 250-ml volumetric flask add 125 ml of 0.1N silver nitrate and 15 ml 6N sodium hydroxide solution. Dissolve the precipitate in concentrated ammonia and add 10 ml of ammonia in excess; make up to the mark with water. Prepare fresh.

Silver Standard. 177.45 mg of silver nitrate in 500 ml distilled water contains 0.2 mg/ml of silver. For a working standard dilute 1:10.

Rhodanine Solution. A saturated solution of p-dimethylamino-benzal rhodanine in acetone is filtered and diluted 1:5 with acetone.

Ammonium Acetate—Gelatin Solution. To 100 ml of a 1.0% filtered aqueous gelatine solution add 25 g of ammonium acetate. Stir until dissolved.

PROCEDURE. A calibration curve is prepared as follows. To 0 to 80 μg silver from the silver standard solution in 5 ml of solution, 1 ml of gelatin ammonium acetate solution is added followed by 2 ml of diluted rhodanine solution and gently mixed. The optical density is read within five minutes at 550 nm against a blank containing all the reagents with 5 ml of water instead of the silver standard.

Urine. Extract an aliquot of urine with ether after adjusting the pH to 8. Shake the separated ether with 4 ml of alkaline silver reagent for thirty minutes. This volume is sufficient for 8.7 mg of drug. The precipitate is centrifuged and well washed with three portions of distilled water; 2 ml of concentrated nitric acid are added and the precipitate decomposed by immersion of the tube in a steam bath for one hour. The residue is dissolved in water, and after adjusting the pH to 7 is made up to exactly 250 ml. A quantitative silver estimation gives a measure of the amount of the silver acetylide precipitate and, hence, the drug.

Blood. Five to 10 ml oxalated blood samples after dilution with 30 ml of water and adjustment of the pH to 8 are extracted with 3 $\times$ 50-ml portions of ether. The method then is the same as for urine. In the writer's hands it has been found necessary to wash the ether extracts with water before shaking with alkaline silver reagent. This prevents a slight cloudiness and any possible interference with silver chloride. The method is not specific for methylpentynol, but can be used to assay any neutral ether soluble acetylenic compound. One such common drug is ethchlorvynol or 5 chloro-3-ethylpent 1-en-4yn-3ol. If a positive result is obtained in this test, a differentiation must be made. The most probable line of successful attack is undoubtedly gas chromatography, although in fatal cases it is likely that a few milligrams can be isolated and, in this event, infrared examination of the liquid should be attempted.

METHYPRYLON (Noludar®)

METHOD (Xanthaky, Freireich, Matusiak and Lukash, 1966).

Extract 5 ml serum with 70 ml chloroform in a separating funnel. After separation, the chloroform layer is washed first with 30 ml 3% sodium bicarbonate, then with 30 ml 0.5N hydrochloric acid. Filter the washed chloroform layer through Whatman No. 1 paper and evaporate at room temperature in a hood. (Note there is a pronounced loss of drug on prolonged standing at room temperature).

To an aliquot containing 25 to 200 μg of methyprylon, add 3 ml of water, 1 ml of diluted Folin-Ciocalteau reagent (1 part reagent + 2.5 parts distilled water) and 0.45 ml 2N sodium hydroxide. Read at 700 nm after thirty minutes. Standards containing 25, 50 and 100 μg are similarly treated.

INTERPRETATION OF RESULTS. Bailey and Jatlow (1973) say that concentrations above 3 mg/100 ml in the serum are sufficient to account for coma. Methyprylon is said to have a half-life of four hours.

After an overdose of 30 g, a patient was rousable after twelve hours at a serum level of 3 mg/100 ml (Xanthaky *et al.*) ; 98 mg was recovered in 1400 ml of urine over twelve hours.

MONOAMINE OXIDASE INHIBITORS

These drugs are widely used in psychiatric practice, the most common are phenelzine and tranylcypromine. The former is chemically unstable, and so far no results are available on its efficient extraction from blood or tissue and specific assay. However, the substituted derivatives of hydrazine, to which class nearly all these drugs belong, can be salted from stomach contents into ether from ammoniacal-saturated ammonium sulphate solution and detected as blue colors on a butanol-citric acid chromatogram after spraying with a saturated aqueous solution of phosphomolybdic acid and exposing to ammonia fumes. Assay by comparison with standards, and avoid loss of volatile drugs by not allowing the ether extract to evaporate to dryness.

Tranylcypromine is chemically related to amphetamine and it extraction and assay follows the procedure for this compound. (For assay by comparative TLC see Table VI).

An alternative approach is as follows, although the reader is warned that no opportunity has yet been obtained to try the method in actual cases.

METHOD (Curry and Mercier, 1970 Courtesy of *Nature.*).

Rat liver mitochondria provide the MAO; after homogenization of fresh rat livers in 0.3 M sucrose, mitochondria are isolated by the method of Hawkins and stored at −10 degrees C. A suspension of MAO is prepared by diluting 1 ml of the mitochondria preparation with 3 ml of 0.1 M phosphate buffer, pH 7.4. The different MAO inhibitors in the free base form—harmine, iproniazid, isocarboxazid, nialamide, pargyline, phenelzine, pivhydrazine and tranylcypromine as well as isoniazid, a weak MAO inhibitor chemically related to the most potent hydrazine derivatives, are extracted by vigorous shaking with freshly distilled ether from an aqueous solution at pH 10. The organic solvent is dried with solid sodium sulphate, evaporated under nitrogen to near dryness, and transferred to a silica gel G thin layer plate which is then developed in chloroform and ethyl acetate (1 : 1).

After evaporation of the solvent, the plate is sprayed with the enzyme suspension and incubated for fifteen minutes in a moisture tank kept at 37 degrees C. The plate is then developed for MAO activity by spraying with a solution containing 10 mg of nitro blue tetrazolium, 10 mg of tryptamine HCl, and 1 mg of sodium sulphate in 5 ml of 0.1 M phosphate buffer, pH 7.4. The plate is incubated for two hours at 37 degrees C in the moisture tank without being moved. Areas of MAO inhibition appear very distinctively as white spots on a dark blue background at different heights on the plate according to the respective R_F of the drug concerned (Table XXXVII).

TABLE XXXVII
THIN LAYER CHROMATOGRAPHY OF THE DIFFERENT MAO
INHIBITORS ON SILICA GEL G
PLATES IN ETHYL ACETATE: CHLOROFORM (1 : 1)

Drug	Rf
Nialamide	0.00
Harmine	0.04
Iproniazid	0.07
Tranylcypromine	0.11; 0.88
Phenelzine	0.50; 0.68; 0.83
Pivhydrazine	0.58
Isocarboxazide	0.70
Pargyline	0.79

INTERPRETATION OF RESULTS. Monoamine oxidase inhibitors in therapeutic dosage, or even for several days after cessation of therapeutic dosage, can alter the body's biochemistry in such a manner that subsequent therapeutic doses of other drugs, particularly adrenaline type compounds, amphetamine and pethidine, cause serious clinical symptoms and even death. Serious interaction with the amino acid tyramine in such foods as cheese has also been described. The toxicologist is in a difficult position in these cases, as his analyses will only reveal traces of drug and the interpretation as to whether a therapeutic dose or an overdose has been taken will probably depend on the quantity of unchanged drug in the stomach and intestines. Demonstration of about a therapeutic dose several hours after ingestion infers the ingestion of a much larger quantity.

OXALATE

METHOD (Zarembski and Hodgkinson, 1965.)

Whole blood or serum (2 ml) is mixed with 0.5 ml sodium formate (10% w/v), 0.2 ml of 0.1N acetic acid and 4.9 ml water in a 10-ml glass-stoppered tube. The tube is heated in a boiling water bath for five minutes, then 0.4 ml calcium formate (10% w/v) added with mixing and heating continued for a further five minutes. After cooling, the tube is centrifuged and 6 ml of the supernatant is put into a tube and mixed with 98% formic acid (0.8 ml for serum, 0.1 ml for urine) and 10N HCl added to make the final pH 1 (0.7 ml for serum; 0.22 ml for urine). Tri-n-butyl phosphate, 12 ml, is added and the tube rocked gently for five minutes; it is then centrifuged for five minutes and the ester phase transferred to another 25-ml tube with a Pasteur pipette. The extracted oxalic acid is transferred to an aqueous phase by shaking the tri-n-butyl phosphate with 1.9 ml 2N sodium hydroxide for two minutes. After centrifuging, the ester phase is discarded. Any residual ester phase is removed by 3 × 5-ml washes of 40/60 light petroleum, warming gently after the last removal.

One drop bromothymol blue solution is added and the pH adjusted to 7 ± 0.2 with dilute acetic acid and sodium hydroxide (match against standards) ; 2 ml of a saturated solution of calcium sulphate is added followed by 13.5 ml ethanol, mix gently and stand overnight at room temperature. Centrifuge for ten minutes, remove the supernatant and dry the precipitate at 105 to 110 degrees C for thirty minutes. Dissolve in 2 ml 1.25N hydrochloric acid. cool in ice and shake gently for several minutes in a mechanical shaker. A freshly prepared zinc spiral (see below) is introduced and shaking continued at eight to ten strokes per second for a further twenty minutes. The spiral is then raised above the solution by bending the top end of the zinc wire over the lip of the tube and washed with 1 ml of 0.5% resorcinol solution, and the tube centrifuged for three minutes. The dry spiral is now removed, 1.5 ml hydrochloric acid added, and the tube heated in a boiling water bath for five minutes. After cooling, 9.6 ml of 1.8M potassium carbonate is added followed by 1 ml of 10% (w/v) freshly prepared ascorbic acid and 1 ml of EDTA reagent (25 g dipotassium EDTA in 100 ml 1.8M potassium carbonate, prepared fresh). After twenty minutes at room temperature, the solution is diluted to 25 ml with carbonate-bicarbonate buffer (200 ml 0.1 M K_2CO_3 and 800 ml 0.1M $KHCO_3$). After a further ten minutes read the fluorescent intensity at 530 nm with an excitation wavelength of 490 nm (Aminco Bowman) or read the extinction at 490 nm. Calibrate using 0 to 10 μg oxalic acid. (one ml urine and 1 ml water may be used instead of 2 ml serum.)

Zinc Spirals. One-eighth-inch diameter electrolytic zinc wire is flattened with steel rollers to a thickness of about 2 mm. The flattened wire is cleaned with scouring powder, cut into 22-cm lengths and one end of each piece wound into a spiral approximately 1 cm long × 1 cm in diameter. Immediately before use it is placed in silicone MS 550, washed under a running tap, and dipped in 10N nitric acid until brown fumes appear. Wash thoroughly in distilled water and place for about five seconds in a test tube containing 2 ml of 1.25N HCl and one drop 0.5% methylene blue solution. Wash briefly in distilled water and place for five seconds in 1.25N HCl. Repeat before each use; each spiral lasts for about ten analyses.

A simple method for the determination of oxalate in urine has been described by Giterson *et al.* (1970) in which calcium chloride is used to precipitate the oxalic acid, and the calcium surplus is titrated using a routine complexometric method. Twenty-five ml of urine was boiled with 0.5 ml 3% $CaCl_2$ $6H_2O$ cooled. After five hours at room temperature the precipitant was centrifuged and calcium determined in the supernatant. Roscher's histochemical technique (1971) may be applicable.

INTERPRETATION OF RESULTS. Whole blood contains 200 to 320 $\mu g/100$ ml of oxalic acid; serum 135 to 280 $\mu g/ml$. Daily urinary excretion is from 9 to 28.5 mg per twenty-four hours.

In fatal poisoning, blood levels over 1 mg/100 ml can be expected. Recovery has been noted after a blood level of 370 $\mu g/100$ ml. Concentrations in liver tissue can be expected to be higher than in blood. In a fatal ethylene glycol poisoning the concentration of oxalate in the liver was 24.5 mg/100 g.

See also: Zarembski and Hodgkinson (1962); Zarembski and Hodgkinson, (1963); Zarembski and Hodgkinson, (1967).

PARACETAMOL (ACETAMINOPHEN)

A method for paracetamol has been described on page 57. a gas chromatographic method is also available.

METHOD 1 (Prescott, 1971 Courtesy *J. Pharm. Pharmacol*).

Phosphate buffer (1.0 ml, M, pH 7.4) is added to plasma or urine (2.0 ml) containing up to 50 μg of paracetamol in a 15 ml glass-stoppered tube. Redistilled ethyl acetate (5.0 ml) containing N-butyryl-*p*-aminophenol (5 $\mu g/ml$) is then added, and extraction effected by gentle mechanical shaking for ten minutes. After centrifugation, the upper organic phase is transferred with Pasteur pipettes to 10-ml tapered stoppered centrifuge tubes and taken to dryness using a rotary vacuum evaporator. Pyridine (5 μl) and acetic anhydride (15 μl) are then added to the residue, the tubes stoppered and the contents mixed with a vortex mixer. The tubes are incubated on a water bath at 45 degrees for twenty minutes and 1 to 3-μl aliquots are injected directly into the gas chromatograph. Samples containing paracetamol (50-500 μg/ml) are extracted with ethyl acetate containing *N*-butyryl-*p*-aminophenol (50 μg/ml), the residue is dissolved in pyridine (15 μl) and acetic anhydride (30 μl), and one-μl aliquots are injected into the chromatograph. Appropriate dilutions are made of more concentrated samples, and total unchanged and conjugated paracetamol in plasma or urine can be determined by prior hydrolysis with glusulase as described by Prescott (1971).

A Hewlett-Packard Model 402 gas chromatograph with flame ionization detectors and a 2-foot-long, one fourth-inch i.d. U-shaped glass tube column packed with 3% HI-EFF 8BP on 100/120 mesh Gaschrom Q (Applied Science) was used with the column temperature 220 degrees and the nitrogen carrier gas flow rate 80 ml/min. The retention times of phenacetin, paracetamol and *N*-butyryl-*p*-aminophenol were 1.6, 3.4 and 4.5 minute respectively. Satisfactory results were also obtained with four-foot columns of 3% OV17 or 1% Carbowax 20 M on Gaschrom Q. *p*-Aminophenol will yield the same acetylated derivative as paracetamol, but this is of little consequence since, in man, *p*-aminophenol is not detectable in biological fluids following ingestion of paracetamol.

An appropriate aqueous standard of paracetamol is run with the samples, and drug concentrations determined using the peak height ratios of drug to internal standard. The recovery of paracetamol added to plasma, urine or aqueous solutions is identical. A suitable alternative colorimetric method is as follows.

METHOD (Gwilt, Robertson and McChesney, 1963. See also Turner, 1965).

Blood, 2 ml, is mixed thoroughly with anhydous sodium sulphate to form a dry friable mass. This is extracted in a Soxhlet thimble with 150 ml ether and 2.2 ml isopentanol for one hour. The solvent is concentrated to 70 ml and extracted with portions of 0.1N sodium hydroxide (5 ml, 2 ml). The combined aqueous extracts are treated in a covered tube with 1.5 ml concentrated hydrochloric acid for forty-five minutes at 100 degrees C. The solution is cooled to room temperature, five drops of α-naphthol reagent and 2.5 ml 40% sodium hydroxide added, and it is allowed to stand for three minutes. The blue-violet color is then extracted after addition of solid potassium chloride to saturate with 5 ml n-butanol. Read at 635 nm.

α-Naphthol Reagent. 1 ml 5% ethanolic α-naphthol solution is mixed with 10 mg potassium dichromate and 1 ml of 2N hydrochloric acid. After five minutes add 19 ml of 5% α-naphthol in ethanol.

INTERPRETATION OF RESULTS. Forty-five minutes after ingestion of 1 g, blood levels are in the range 0.45 to 2.5 mg/100 ml. No significant difference exists between whole blood and plasma levels. In cases involving large overdoses the rapid excretion of paracetamol results in blood levels in the above range when the blood is not taken for several hours after ingestion. In acute poisoning, however, the blood level would be expected to be several milligrams per 100 ml (see p. 58).

See also Davidson and Eastham, (1966), Heirwegh and Fevery, (1967), Krickler, (1967) and Gwilt, *et al.,* 1963).

PARALDEHYDE

METHOD 1 (Figot, Hine and Way, 1952).

Acetaldehyde is distilled from 0.5 g of blood after adding 10 to 15 ml of distilled water and 3 to 4 ml of concentrated sulphuric acid. The distillate is collected in 30 ml of buffered semicarbazide (0.0067N semicarbazide hydrochloride buffered at pH 7.0: 8.28 g $NaH_2PO_4 \cdot H_2O$ + 19.88 g Na_2HPO_4 anhydrous per litre).

A special apparatus is used to assist the distillation by means of an air stream; seven minutes are required. The distillate is diluted to 100 ml and read against controls and standards at 224 nm.

METHOD 2. Blood (10 ml), or tissue slurry, with 15 ml water and 25 ml dilute (6N) sulphuric acid are distilled; 22.5 ml are collected, the collection tube being cooled in ice. Two and five tenths ml of Schiff's reagent are added, and after exactly twenty-five minutes the violet color is read against exact blood controls containing paraldehyde in the range 0 to 50 mg per 100 ml at 560 nm.

Schiff's Reagent: This is prepared by dissolving 0.2 g basic fuchsin in 120 ml of water, adding 2 g sodium metabisulphite in 20 ml of water, 2 ml concentrated hydrochloric acid and diluting to 200 ml. If necessary the reagent is decolorized with charcoal.

METHOD 3 (Maes *et al.*, 1969). Homogenise 10 g of tissue with 50 ml of water and distill. Collect almost 10 ml of distillate into a chilled flask and make up to 10 ml. Inject 1-μl aliquots into a gas chromatograph using a 7% Halcomid M-18 on 90 to 100 Anakrom AB at 65 degrees C. Compare with aqueous standards similarly processed in the range 5 to 50 mg/100 ml.

INTERPRETATION OF RESULTS. Fifty mg/100 ml of paraldehyde in blood must be considered a serious case of poisoning.

Paraldehyde is frequently used as a sedative in the management of psychotic patients, and even in the treatment of alcoholics. There have been cases in which too enthusiastic therapeutic administration has resulted in profound respiratory depression and death; this can occur with blood levels slightly below 50 mg/100 ml. Often, a history of additional medication with other tranquillizers is noted in such cases. Conversely, in addicts regularly taking large doses over long periods, blood levels over 50 mg/100 ml can be found in a conscious patient. There is no published evidence for paraldehyde accumulation in the body when it is taken in therapeutic amounts. In investigations the author did on the blood of a tetanic patient who was receiving regular repeated doses for several weeks the blood level did not rise over 10 mg/100 ml. (See also Maes *et al.* [1970] who found therapeutic levels did not exceed 15 mg/100 ml in plasma.)

See also: Agranat and Trubshaw, (1955); Copeman, (1956); Stotz, (1943).

PARAQUAT AND DIQUAT

Paraquat (1,1'-dimethyl-4,4'-bipyridilium) dichloride or dimethyl sulphate is a herbicide which has caused death after ingestion of large overdoses. Tadjer (1967) reported the detection of this compound after direct extraction of 100-200 g of tissue with carbon tetrachloride using TLC (six different solvents) and sprays of iodine in chloroform, Dragendorff's reagent and iodoplatinate. The best TLC solvent was methanol:chloroform (19:1). The Rf value is about 0.37. Diquat was found to run best in methanol: chloroform (13:2) with an Rf of 0.84.

METHOD (Daniel, and Gage, 1966).

A 10-mm internal diameter column is prepared from about 1 ml of DOW AG-50W-X8 cation exchange resin. The column is washed with water. Twelve and five tenths ml 25% trichloracetic acid are added to 50 ml of urine and centrifuged. The precipitate is washed with 6 ml 5% trichloracetic acid, centrifuged, and the supernatants combined. The supernatant solution is passed at a rate of 3 to 4 ml a minute down the column which is then washed with 25-ml portions of water.

Paraquat is eluted from the column with 25 ml 5M ammonium chloride at a rate not exceeding 0.5 ml/min. To 5 ml of eluate are added 1 ml 0.2% sodium dithionite in N sodium hydroxide, and readings are taken at 379 nm. in a 1-cm cell. Standards are prepared in the region 10 to 100 μg. Readings must be taken within ten minutes of addition of the dithionate reagent.

Diquat can also be estimated with the following modifications: The column is prepared and washed with 25 ml water, 25 ml 6M sodium chloride and 25 ml water. After passing the TCA-treated urine down the column it is washed with 25 ml water, 25 ml 0.6M sodium chloride and 25 ml water. Diquat is eluted with 25 ml 5M ammonium chloride and estimated at 379 nm by adding 1 ml of 0.2% w/v sodium dithionite in 5% aqueous sodium tetraborate to 5 ml of eluate.

A rapid test for paraquat is to add 0.1 g sodium bicarbonate and 0.1 g sodium dithionite to 5 ml of clear natural gastric contents or urine. A blue color develops almost immediately and 20 μg/ml gives an absorbance of 0.72 at 625 nm in a Unicam® SP600 (Matthew *et al.,* 1968.) .

To analyse tissues, macerate with an equal volume of water and add trichloracetic acid to precipitate protein. After centrifuging, the supernatant is treated as for urine.

The test noted on page 67 only produced blue colors if the paraquat level in the urine exceeded 10 μg/ml.

Berry and Grove (1971) have described a simple test for paraquat in urine with a sensitivity of 0.01 μg/ml in a 250-ml aliquot of urine. This involves ion exchange chromatography and the usual dithionite reduction, but a simple spot test is also described.

METHOD. Ten ml of urine are taken and 2 ml of 1% sodium dithionite in 1N sodium hydroxide are added. Berry and Grove consider that if a blue color is seen, the patient should be hospitalized for the ensuing ten days because the concentration of paraquat in the urine will be greater than 1 ppm.

It is clear that the sensitivity of the dithionite test on urine will depend on the exact conditions employed and on the alkalinity of the final solution. It behoves toxicologists to measure their sensitivities before influencing clinical treatment, especially in an apparently negative case. See also: Heyndrickx, *et al.,* (1967) .

Heyndrickx *et al.* (1969) used methanol:formic acid:water (85:5:10) followed by spraying with potassium iodoplatinate to separate paraquat from diquat.

Fletcher (1974) notes 232 deaths from paraquat in the world in the period from 1964 to 1973. Blood analyses are not recommended, and, in life, urine is the best media for detecting paraquat ingestion.

Carson (1972) gives details of nine fatal poisonings in which seven were detected by chemical analyses. Liver and kidney are the preferred organs for analysis. See also: Bullivant, (1966) .

PARATHION AND OTHER ORGANO-PHOSPHORUS COMPOUNDS

METHOD (Turner, 1965) .
The viscera are made acid to litmus and steam distilled. The

distillate (5-10 ml) is made acid to litmus with dilute hydrochloric acid and extracted several times with ether. The combined ether extracts are dried over anhydrous sodium sulphate, filtered and evaporated. The extract is examined by paper chromatography using 10% aqueous acetonitrile as the stationary phase and light petroleum ether saturated with acetonitrile as the mobile phase. Control spots of parathion, paraoxon, methylparathion and p-nitrophenol are also run. TLC (Machata, 1968) may also be used; a Silica-Gel G plate is run in hexane acetone (4:1 and 9:1).

DETECTION (Thomas and Abbot, 1966).

The most sensitive is by a spray of brilliant green (color index No. 42040) followed by exposing the plate to an atmosphere of ammonia. A spray of 0.5% palladium chloride in 1% hydrochloric acid can also be used. Alternatively, one can demonstrate cholinesterse inhibition by spraying with a solution at 37 degrees C of 10 ml horse or human serum, 30 ml distilled water, 1 ml 0.1N sodium hydroxide and 4 ml 1.2% bromothymol blue in 0.1N sodium hydroxide. The plate is then allowed to incubate for twenty minutes at room temperature without being moved. The plate is then sprayed with 2% acetylcholine bromide in distilled water. Areas of cholinesterase inhibition are seen within two minutes and fully appear as bright blue spots on a yellow background in twenty to thirty minutes. Parathion and other phosphorothionate or phosphorodithioate compounds can be converted on the TLC to corresponding oxons which are highly active inhibitors by spraying with a fresh solution of n-bromosuccinimide in acetone and heating at 60 degrees C for fifteen minutes in a forced air oven. Alternatively, exposure to bromine vapor may be used. The cholinesterase spray reagent is then used on top.

Hladka and Hladky (1966), separated the p-nitrophenol and p-nitrometacresol in urine in persons exposed to parathion by hydrolysing the urine with HCl (5:1) for one hour on a boiling water bath. Extraction is with four parts petrol ether and one part ether. The concentrated extract is run in 20% acetone and 80% hexane on TLC plates of Silica-Gel containing 15% plaster; it is then inspected under ultraviolet light to give black spots at Rf 0.33. Yellow colors are seen after exposure to ammonia vapor.

Heyndrickx, Maes and de Leenheer (1964) present the alternative method to steam distillation for the isolation of the OP compounds; they extract blood four times with petroleum:ether (40:70) and examine the evaporated extracts by TLC (hexane:acetone, 4:2.5) followed by the bromine vapour/plasma-acetylcholine bromide technique described above. They were able to detect and estimate parathion in approximately 3-ml samples of blood and milk from a poisoned cow.

Parathion is relatively stable in buried bodies and exhumation is well worth trying if parathion poisoning is suspected. Van Hecke, Derveaux and Hans-Berteau, (1958) give an account of criminal poisoning by parathion that illustrates the high degree of awareness that forensic pathologists and toxicologists must possess if homicide is to be detected. These workers also showed the Stas-Otto process followed by benzene and ether extraction stages also isolated parathion.

Vercruysse and Deslypere, (1964), in a comprehensive paper, suggest after elution in hexane:acetone (4:2), an alternative spraying procedure that will detect 0.1 μg of parathion. After exposure to bromine vapor for five minutes and aeration, the plate is sprayed with fresh horse serum. After thirty minutes the thin layer plate is further treated with an alcohol solution of phenyl acetate (0.25%), then with 25 mg of Fast Blue RR salt in 10 ml water and 10 ml pH 7 buffer (0.2M $Na_2 HPO_4$ 35 ml + 0.1M citric acid 7.5 ml). White spots are seen on a red background.

See also: El-Rejal and Hopkins, (1965).

Malathion:

Method (Lewin, *et al.*, 1973).

A distillate of acidified stomach contents and tissues is extracted with hexane which is separated and evaporated. The residue in methanol gives a characteristic ultraviolet spectrum with λ max = 326 nm. TLC on Merck Kieselgel F_{254} plates developed in hexane:acetone (80:20) gives a yellow spot at Rf 0.52 on spraying with acidic palladium chloride solution. Gas chromatography on 5% DC200 on 60 to 80 Chromosorb W at 200 degrees C shows malathion with a retention time of two minutes on a 1.4-metre column.

See also: Farago, (1967).

PROPOXYPHENE (Darvon®)

METHOD (McBay, Turk, Corbett and Hudson, 1974 Courtesy *J. For. Sci.*)

Ten ml of blood and 15 ml concentrated hydrochloric acid are placed in a 60-ml test tube. The mixture is heated in a boiling water bath for twenty minutes with occasional stirring. Ten-g amounts of homogenized tissue, 10 ml of water and 15 ml of concentrated hydrochloric acid are treated in the same way. Cool and add 15 ml of 50% sodium hydroxide solution in a 500-ml Erlenmeyer flask. Cool; add 150 ml ether and shake vigorously. Separate the ether layer and filter through a dry Whatman No. 1 filter paper. Wash the filtrate with 10 ml water and separate. Record the volume of ether for subsequent correction factor. Shake with 5 ml of 0.25N hydrochloric acid. A peak at 255 nm in this acid extract indicates propoxyphene. Dilute with 0.25N hydrochloric acid to give an absorbance of about 0.3. Irradiate in a quartz cuvette for five minutes a few millimeters from a 257.3 nm ultraviolet light. Ten μg/ml equivalent of hydrolysed irradiated propoxyphene then has an absorption peak at 255 nm of about 0.62. A TLC separation on Silica Gel G using an iodoplatinate spray in ammonia: methanol (1.5:100) gives an Rf of 0.65 for hydrolysed, UV-irradiated tissue extracts.

Evenson and Koellner (1973) have described a rapid GC method using only 1 ml of serum. After a dose of nearly 200 mg, a volunteer's blood level reached only 27 μg/100 ml.

INTERPRETATION OF RESULTS. In overdose cases, liver levels are much higher than blood levels. In liver, values range from 1.5 to 30 mg/100 g where the corresponding blood values are 0.2 to 1.5 mg/100 ml. Cravey, *et al.* (1974) have reported 238 cases, and, in general, agree with these figures although their liver values reached 55 mg/100 g and blood values were as high as 6.0 mg/100 g. Both sets of authors note that multiple drug intake was often involved.

Worm (1971) described nine cases of fatal poisoning which were analyzed using gas chromatography. He also noted the fact that liver levels were higher than blood values, but his highest concentration in liver was only 2.2 mg/100 g. Bile concentrations appeared to be even higher.

See also Thompson *et al.,* (1970) and Valentour *et al.,* (1974).

QUATERNARY AMMONIUM COMPOUNDS
*Including pancuronium, succinylcholine, tubocurarine
and hexamethonium*

METHOD (Stevens and Moffat: Personal communication).

A reasonably rapid and simple method of extracting quaternary amines from urine or tissue is to utilize the formation of solvent-soluble ion-pair compounds in either the urine directly or in the filtrate obtained after deproteinizing a tissue slurry.

For large molecular weight compounds, such as d-tubocurarine and pancuronium, iodide was used to form the ion-pair, while for small molecule quaternaries bromothymol blue had to be used as no pairing with the iodide ion appeared to take place with these compounds. Pancuronium was not extractable as an ion-pair with bromothymol blue.

Pancuronium (bromide) was decomposed in N HCl solution (100 μg drug per 0.1 ml) in about ten minutes at 80 degrees C so hot acid conditions must be avoided. The compound was stable when allowed to stand in aqueous ammonia overnight.

For the isolation of pancuronium from tissue, cold acid conditions had to be employed for protein precipitation as follows: Liver (200 g) was macerated with water (300 ml) and 200 ml of aluminium chloride reagent (10% w/v $AlCl_3$ + 10% w/v citric acid in 2N HCl) was added with stirring. After standing for five minutes to allow coagulation of protein to take place, the mixture was filtered through two thicknesses of fluted Whatman No. 114 paper. The filtrate was made alkaline by the addition of strong ammonia and saturated with sodium or potassium chloride. To this solution potassum iodide (100 g) in water (100 ml) was added and the mixture shaken with 200 ml of dichloromethane.

To break the emulsion formed it was drawn through a cotton-wool plug (approximately 5 cm x 5 cm diameter), and this had to be replaced by a fresh plug several times before all the emulsion had passed through. The lower layer of dichloromethane was then separated and filtered and evaporated to dryness. If the dichloromethane did not sink in the broken emulsion, then the density of the aqueous portion was reduced by the addition of water.

After evaporating off the dichloromethane, the residue was dissolved in a minimum volume of dichloromethane and spotted onto a *Camlab*® cellulose TLC plate. This was run against a 1-μg spot of pancuronium bromide in the tetrahydrofuran solvent used for the other quaternary amines, and the pancuronium detected colorimetrically on the plate (see below).

The recovery of the drug added to blood samples (100 μg to 50 ml blood) did not exceed 20 percent, and the difficulties due to this low recovery are enhanced by the small amount that needs to be administered owing to its potency and rapid action as a muscle relaxant. In a fatal poisoning case no more than 8 mg was injected into the arm, and the amount found in a 200-g sample of liver was of the order of 5 μg. None of the drug could be found in a 40-ml sample of blood or in the urine.

Extracts of Tissue Containing Added Tubocurarine

One mg of d-tubocurarine chloride in aqueous solution was added to 50 g of liver made into a slurry with water. Water (200 ml) and 25% w/v sodium tungstate solution (50 ml) was added to the slurry, followed, after stirring, by the addition of a 50% w/v solution of sodium bisulphate (50 ml) and placing the mixture in a boiling water bath for fifteen minutes, during which time it was stirred rapidly with an electric stirrer.

The hot mixture was filtered through Whatman No. 114 paper, and the cooled filtrate, after shaking with dichloromethane (200 ml) to remove acidic and neutral compounds, was made alkaline with ammonia (Sp. Gr. 0.91) and saturated with ammonium sulphate. The mixture was shaken with an equal volume of dichloromethane to remove interfering basic material, and the upper aqueous layer retained. This was then saturated with potassium iodide by adding the powdered salt, and the resulting mixture shaken with a fresh portion of dichloromethane to extract tubocurarine. The organic layer was separated and washed with a mixed saturated solution of ammonium sulphate and potassium iodide. Finally, tubocurarine was removed from the dichloromethane extract by shaking the latter with 5 ml of 0.5N sulphuric acid. The optical density of the final acid extract was read at 280 nm and again at 292 nm after the addition of one or two drops of strong caustic alkali (60% KOH or 40% NaOH). Recoveries of tubocurarine varied from 50 to 75% of the added drug.

Interference from Other Bases

The presence of certain putrefactive bases, arising from the liver sample, in the final acid extract could cause serious interference. It is interesting to note that tyramine, a base which appears very early in the process of putrefaction, possesses very similar maxima to tubocurarine in the acid (275 nm) and alkaline (294 nm) media. The shape of the tyramine curve is also somewhat similar to that of tubocurarine.

Fortunately, however, the method of deproteination prevents most of the tyramine in the sample from reaching the aqueous filtrate, and the first alkaline clean up removes any of this base which gets through into the filtrate. It was found that 1 mg of tyramine base was virtually completely removed by shaking with two successive portions of dichloromethane.

Thymine (λ max = 265 nm, rounded peak), which sometimes occurs in livers with mould growing on them, was much more difficult to remove by the alkaline dichloromethane clean-up procedure due to its limited solubility in organic solvents.

To cater for the contingency of both tyramine and thymine being present in the extracted tubocurarine fraction, a thin-layer chromatography system using Merck® precoated aluminia plates was employed. The mobile phase was prepared by shaking 100 ml methyl acetate with 50 ml of dilute aqueous ammonia (strong ammonia, Sp. Gr. 0.91, : water, $2\frac{1}{2}$: $97\frac{1}{2}$ by volume).

A 7-cm run took approximately ten to fifteen minutes, and the plate was developed by examining it in ultraviolet light (254 nm) followed by lightly spraying with Folin-Ciocalteau reagent, and then with 2N sodium hydroxide. Rf values in this system were tubocurarine 0.05, thymine 0.2 and tyramine 0.4, and the best resolution was obtained if the surrounding temperature did not exceed 70 degrees F (21°C). Prior equilibration of the chromatographic tank with the solvent vapour was also necessary for satisfactory separation.

By this means a portion of the dichloromethane extract could be set aside for thin layer chromatography to supplement the ultraviolet data previously obtained.

In a case of poisoning by tubocurarine, 80 μg was isolated from 100 g of liver.

For small molecular weight compounds the analytical procedure used for the screening of urine samples for suxamethonium (succinylcholine) is typical. Suxamethonium presents special problems in that analysis of blood or tissue cannot be accomplished because cholinesterase activity in blood and plasma causes rapid breakdown of the drug into succinic acid and choline, both of which are present in normal body tissues.

The method used to screen urines to which suxamethonium chloride had been added (500 μg to 100 ml), and also case samples of urine obtained from patients who had been injected with the drug (100-200 mg) as a muscle relaxant prior to surgery, was a modification of the method described by Ballard *et al.* (1954).

Twenty ml urine (or whatever volume was available) were adjusted to pH 7.5 by dropwise addition of a saturated solution of Na_3PO_4, and 10 ml of 0.15% w/v bromothymol blue solution (0.3 g bromothymol blue dissolved in 10 ml warm methanol and diluted with water to 200 ml) added. Dichloromethane (30 ml) was added and the mixture shaken vigorously for a few seconds. After standing for one to two minutes, the (emulsified) lower layer of dichloromethane was drawn through a cotton-wool plug (3-4 cm long packed fairly tightly into a glass tube 25 cm x 1 cm in diameter) to break the emulsion. The liquid layers resulting from the broken emulsion were then shaken together to re-extract any ion-pair complex which had been dissociated by the cotton-wool back into the dichloromethane. The large dichloromethane:water ratio prevented the emulsion from reforming.

The dichloromethane extract was filtered and evaporated to dryness on a boiling water bath. Centrifuging the emulsion was not advised as inferior recoveries of suxamethonium were obtained. The orange residue (of ion-pair complexes from all the urinary amines) was dissolved in 1 ml of dichloromethane, and aliquots of this solution, starting with 0.2 ml and increasing if negative results are obtained, were repeatedly streaked over a 1.5-cm length of the starting line on (1) a Camlab silica plate (7 cm x 7 cm) and (2) a Camlab cellulose plate (7 cm x 7 cm). Reference spots containing 1 μg of suxamethonium chloride (0.001 ml of an aqueous standard solution containing 1 mg per ml; spot diameter = 2 nm) were placed alongside the colored band on each plate and dried in a current of warm air.

The *cellulose plate* was run in a tetrahydrofuran solvent mixture (1% w/v ammonium formate in 5% v/v formic acid : 30 vols, tetrahydrofuran : 70 vols) in a well-equilibrated tank (7 cm x 7 cm) for ten to fifteen minutes, then removed and dried in warm air. It was sprayed with potassium iodoplatinate solution, followed by a light spray of 25% w/v ammonium formate solution, and placed in an oven at 100 degrees C for two to three minutes. This procedure faded the background color of the iodoplatinate and left suxamethonium as a pale reddish-violet band of Rf value 0.35 to 0.40 on a white background. Because of the faded background amounts of the drug, 1 to 2 μg could be detected after extraction from urine.

The *silica plate* was run in a solvent mixture containing methanol, 80:0.2 N HCl, 20 for about twenty to twenty-five minutes. As the silica was more retentive than cellulose to the ion-pair compounds, the orange band had frequently scarcely cleared the starting line by the time the solvent front had reached the end of the plate. If this occurred, the plate was withdrawn and dried, and a fresh 1-μg reference spot of suxamethonium placed on the starting line. The plate was rerun in the same solvent mixture, and when dried was sprayed with iodoplatinate, but *not* given any ammonium formate treatment as all iodoplatinate-produced spots were slowly faded on silica by this treatment. Suxamethonium gave a purple spot or band in this system at Rf 0.1.

Estimation of amounts extracted was performed by simple visual comparison of the width and depth of color of the band on the cellulose plate after iodoplatinate-formate treatment, with the 1-μg standard spot which was run on the same plate. Recovery of suxamethonium after addition to urine samples was approximately 40 to 50 percent.

In large samples of urine which were weak in suxamethonium (3-20 μg per 100 mls), the drug could be concentrated by precipitation with sodium tungstate and sodium bisulphate. The mixture was centrifuged (3600 r.p.m. for 5 min, and the supernatant liquid discarded. The precipitate was suspended in 10 to 20 mls of water, and the pH of the mixture was adjusted to 7.5. Analysis then proceeded as described using bromothymol blue. This procedure increased sensitivity of detection and reduced the solution to be extracted to a conveniently small bulk.

Suxamethonium levels in the case urines. Results indicated that excretion of the drug was very rapid, but that urinary levels depended upon the dilution incurred due to the time urine was held in the bladder. These levels ranged from approximately 20 μg per 100 ml, where urine had been retained for up to twenty-two hours after injection of 100 mg of the drug, to 1600 μg per 100 ml, where urine had been voided ten to fifteen minutes after injection.

In one case of incontinence after injection the subsequent sample of urine did not contain a detectable quantity of suxamethonium.

When the urine samples were analysed for the drug some four months after receiving them, positive results were obtained on some of them, the levels varying from 1 to 25 μg per 100 ml. Four samples furnished negative results. The pH values of the samples varied between 5.5 and 9.0, and various types of fungal growth were present in some samples. There was, however, no clear relationship between the pH value, the presence or absence of fungal growth, and the presence or absence of the drug.

Other methods of detecting suxamethonium. Owing to its small size, instability and chemical inertness, the suxamethonium molecule possesses no distinct color reactions (other than with iodoplatinate) or diagnostic U.V., I.R. or mass spectra, and cannot be detected *per se* by gas chromatography.

If *at least 10 to 20 μg* of the drug is available in a band on the cellulose plate, then the following gas-chromatographic method was found to be suitable. This depended on the conversion of aliquots of the drug to the methyl, propyl and 2-chloroethyl esters of succinic acid as follows: After spraying a cellulose plate with iodoplatinate reagent, the band due to the suspected succinylcholine was scraped into a small glass tube. A few drops of 2N sodium hydroxide solution were added to hydrolyse the drug, and after a few minutes the solution was removed and taken to dryness on a water bath with a stream of nitrogen. A few drops of a solution of hydrogen chloride in ether were added to liberate succinic acid which dissolved in the ether. Esterification was achieved by the addition of a few drops of (a) an ethereal solution of diazomethane, (b) boron trifluoride/propanol or (c) boron trichloride/2-chloroethanol to the separated ether solution. The ether solutions were then chromatographed using a Perkin Elmer F11 gas chromatograph with oven temperatures of respectively (a) 120 degrees, (b) 180 degrees or (c) 220 degrees. Reagent a was prepared by distilling N-methyl N-nitrosotoluene-4-sulphonamide, B.D.H., 5 g in 50 ml ether, by dropwise addition to 1.5 g KOH in 15 ml warm 50% ethanol.

The esters of succinic acid produced by this procedure were identified by their retention times, which had previously been determined using standard solutions. These retention times were (a) methyl ester, 2.7 minutes at 120 degrees C; (b) propyl ester, 4.0 minutes at 180 degrees C; and (c) 2-chloroethyl ester, 4.7 minutes at 220 degrees C.

Control samples, using areas of the same cellulose plate containing no suxamethonium, were taken through the same procedure and showed no peaks at these retention times.

Attack by cholinesterase was used as an additional recognition test for suxamethonium on a cellulose plate as follows: After running a band of ion-pair residue on the cellulose plate together with a number of 1-μg spots of standard suxamethonium solution placed at either side of the band, one half of this plate was sprayed with cholinesterase solution in phosphate buffer pH 8, and the other half with phosphate buffer (pH 8) as a control. The damp plate was then placed in a moisture chamber at 37 degrees C for seventy-five to ninety minutes. It was then removed and dried, and sprayed with potassium iodoplatinate and 25% w/v ammonioum formate and placed in an oven at 100 degrees C for two to three minutes. The half of the plate which had been sprayed with enzyme showed no suxamethonium, while the buffer-sprayed half gave the usual reddish-purple band and control spots of the drug. In addition to suxamethonium, suxethonium was attacked by cholinesterase, but drugs like hexamethonium and decamethonium which are not choline esters were unaffected. The cholinesterase used was Type IV from horse serum; 2 mg in 2 ml phosphate buffer was used.

Stability of Suxamethonium and Conditions of Storage of Urine

Suxamethonium is very labile at pH values exceeding 8.5. One hundred μg of the drug in 50 ml of aqueous solution of pH 9 had disappeared on standing at room temperature for twenty minutes. In contrast, no significant loss occurred when it was subjected to N HCl at 78 degrees C for ten minutes or boiled under reflux for one hour in 0.1N HCl. Urine samples, which contained 5 μg suxamethonium per ml, were made 0.1N in HCl and stored at 4 degrees C. Approximately a 30 percent loss of drug resulted in some urines after ten days, and total loss after twenty-eight days storage.

If the concentration of the acid in urine was reduced to 0.01N (0.1 ml of 10N HCl added to 100 ml urine), no appreciable loss of drug occurred if the urine was stored for six to eight weeks at 4 degrees C. The pH of the acidified urine was about 5 initially and did not change more than 0.1 to 0.2 units during the period of storage.

In view of the tendency of untreated stored urine to rise in pH by as much as one pH unit per month at 4 degrees C due to bacterial action, these precautions are advised to maintain the sample at pH 5 at which suxamethonium has been reported to be most stable.

A phenonmenon was encountered in samples of urine obtained from one person in that after addition of suxamethonium to the urine to give a calculated level of 5 μg per ml, analysis directly after addition always furnished negative results unless the urine had been boiled before addition of the drug.

It was concluded that the urine contained cholinesterase, and this occurrence has been encountered previously by other workers.

Extraction of Other Quaternary Amines from Urine

The method of extraction using bromothymol blue as the ion-pair forming agent was successfully applied to extract other quaternary amines after addition to urine samples. Estimation of amounts extracted was performed by simple visual comparison of the width and depth of color of the bands on the cellulose plate with iodoplatinate, with 1-μg standard spots which were run on the same TLC plate.

Recoveries of decamethonium and hexamethonium after addition to urine approximated to 50 percent.

In Table XXXVIII the Rf values and colour responses to iodo-platinateformate and cobalt thiocyanate (3 g Co $(NO_3)_2$ + 9 g KCNS in 50 ml water) are given for the fifteen quaternaries examined.

Twelve tertiary amine drugs were added, in turn, to different samples of urine to give a level of 5μg of each drug per ml. The drugs were then extracted by the described ion-pair method, and the extracts obtained were run in the cellulose-tetrahydrofuran and silica-methanol TLC systems.

It was found that all twelve travelled well ahead of suxamethonium in both systems. They would, therefore, not interfere in the detection of suxamethonium on the plates. The drugs tested were chlordiazepoxide, chlorpromazine, codeine, methadone, methaqualone, morphine, nicotine, pethidine, phenazone, phenelzine, quinine and strychnine.

If other quaternary amines were present which were stable to alkali, removal of the tertiary amine drugs by solvent extraction from alkaline solution could be carried out prior to extraction by the ion-pair method.

Extraction of Quaternary Amines from Blood and Tissue

The extraction of pancuronium and d-tubocurarine as iodides has already been mentioned. For tubocurarine tungstic acid was used to precipitate protein, but its use is not advised with certain other quaternary amines, especially guanethidine, hexamethonium paraquat, suxamethonium and suxethonium, as these compounds form precipitates with tungstic acid.

After addition of hexamethonium to blood (200 μg to 20 mls), satisfactory recovery (30-50%) was obtained using a hot acid protein precipitant such as Nickoll's hydrochloric acid-ammonium sulphate at 60 degrees C, keeping the acid concentration N in the mixture or $AlCl_3$-HCl precipitation at 50 degrees to 60 degrees C. The filtrate in each method was adjusted to pH 7.5 using 40% w/v

TABLE XXXVIII

RF VALUES AND COLOUR RESPONSES OF QUATERNARY AMINE COMPOUNDS IN CELLULOSE AND SILICA TLC SYSTEMS. THOSE MARKED * WERE SUCCESSFULLY EXTRACTED AFTER ADDITION TO URINE SAMPLES.

Quaternary Compound	Approx. Rf value		UV light (254 nm)	Colour responses on cellulose to:			Colour response on silica to iodoplatinate
	Cellulose	Silica		iodoplatinate	after H.COONH$_4$ (100°C)	Co (CNS)$_2$	
*Atropine methonitrate	0.95	0.35	—	bluish purple	reddish purple	blue	bluish purple
*Azamethonium	0.40	0.10	—	greyish blue	greyish blue	blue (weak)	greyish blue
*Bretylium	0.94	0.40	—	greyish blue	greyish purple	blue	bluish purple
Cetrimide	1.0	0.50	—	grey (weak)	pale brown	blue	reddish purple
*Decamethonium	0.56	0.16	—	violet blue	violet blue	blue (weak)	bluish purple
Gallamine	0.34	0.05	—	purplish grey	grey	blue	grey - purple grey
*Guanethidine	0.56	0.50	—	greenish blue	bluish grey	—	greyish blue
*Hexamethonium	0.36	0.10	—	violet blue	reddish purple	blue	greyish blue
*Paraquat	0.22	0.10	absorbs	greenish blue	bluish grey	blue	greyish blue
Suxamethonium	0.35	0.10	—	reddish purple	reddish purple	blue	bluish purple
*Suxethonium	0.40	0.23	—	bluish purple	reddish purple	blue	greyish blue
*Tubocurarine	0.85	0.40	absorbs (weak)	purplish brown	orange brown	blue	purple
Acetylcholine	0.70	0.60	—	purple	greyish purple	blue	purple
*Choline	0.60	0.60	—	bluish grey	grey	blue	grey
Pancuronium[1]	0.80	not tried	—	purplish brown	purplish brown	not tried	not tried

[1]does not form ion-pair with bromothymol blue. Iodide in the presence of ammonia is required for extraction of pancuronium into dichloromethane.

sodium hydroxide with cooling, then analysed in the manner described for suxamethonium in urine.

The same protein precipitation techniques were successfully applied to samples of blood and drinking chocolate to which atropine methonitrate had been added.

Vidic *et al.*, (1972) have described a gas chromatographic method for the determination of such quaternary ammonium compounds as scopolamine-butyl bromide, d-tubocurarine, methylcurarine, neostigmine and choline esters. See also Stevens and Fox (1971): Stevens and Moffat, (1974).

THIORIDAZINE (Mellaril®)

METHOD (Zehnder and Tanner, 1961).

Blood, 10 ml, is stirred with 2 ml water and 8 ml concentrated hydrochloric acid and heated in a beaker in a boiling water bath for five minutes. Remove and place in an ice bath. When cool, add 12 ml 60% w/v potassium hydroxide which has been previously washed with ether. Keep cool and check the pH to ensure alkalinity. If acid, add more alkali. Shake with 150 ml ether, breaking any emulsion by centrifuging. Separate and shake the aqueous phase with a further 50-ml portion of ether. Combine the ether fractions and wash in sequence with 10 ml 2.5% sodium hydroxide, 10 ml water and 5 ml water. Shake with 4 ml 0.1N sulphuric acid which is separated; to it add 2 ml of 50% sulphuric acid and 0.1 ml of 0.375% ferric nitrate hydrate. Read immediately at 635 nm. Standards should be made in the range of 0 to 100 μg giving optical density readings in the range 0 to 0.3 with a 1-cm cell. Gas chromatography can also be used (Curry, S.H. and Mould, 1969).

INTERPRETATION OF RESULTS. In general, blood levels over 0.1 mg/100 ml will be found in cases of sudden death following an acute overdose (see also Chap. 6), although Tompsett (1968) found a mean plasma level of 0.18 mg/100 ml after a single oral dose of 200 mg.

Curry and Mould, (1969) also showed high therapeutic doses (300 mg twice daily) could give plasma levels up to 0.18 mg/100 ml.

WARFARIN

This rodenticide interferes with the clotting mechanism of the blood and extensive internal haemorrhages are found at autopsy. Pribilla (1963) reported a case of murder involving this poison and extremely low levels in the tissues were found (liver, 180 μg; kidneys, 30 μg; total musculature, 1200 μg, stomach contents, 3.9 μg). These levels show the care that must be exercised in a search for this poison, Fishwick and Taylor, (1967) extract exhaustively dilute acidified macerated tissue with ether and purify by passage down a Silica-Gel column. After re-extraction into chloroform and evaporation, TLC separation is done using Kieselguhr GF254 plates using ether:hexane:acetic acid (7:25:1) as a solvent. Inspection under 254 nm light reveals the spot at Rf 0.46 which can be eluted with ethyl acetate. Ultraviolet spectrophotometry in 5 ml isopropyl alcohol with 1% acetic acid shows the characteristic curve with max = 305 nm and $E_{1cm}^{1\%}$ of 361.

A gas chromatographic method has also been described.

METHOD (Funnell *et al.,* 1970 Courtesy *J. For. Sci.*)

Fifty grams of homogenized liver was vigorously shaken for forty-five minutes with 10 ml of 15% trichloracetic acid and 100 ml of chloroform. The mixture was filtered through a Buchner funnel containing a one-half-inch layer of sand and washed with chloroform.

The filtrate was transferred to a 250-ml separatory funnel (equipped with a Teflon stopcock), and 50 ml of water were added. Following brief shaking the phases were allowed to separate and the aqueous phase was discarded.

The chloroform phase was passed at a rate of 2 ml per minute through a basic alumina column (aluminium oxide, basic, Brockman activity Grade 1) (6 in high by $\frac{3}{4}''$ in diameter). The column was subsequently washed with 50 ml of chloroform followed by the same quantity of ether, then dried with compressed air.

The warfarin was eluted from the column at a rate of 0.5 ml per minute with 50 ml of ethyl alcohol: acetic acid, 99:1, and the eluate retained in the column was blown through with compressed air. The total eluate was transferred to a 250-ml separatory funnel and 150 ml of water and 3 ml of 2N sulfuric acid were added. The mixture was shaken vigorously for ten minutes with three successive 15-ml portions of chloroform after which the aqueous phase was discarded.

The combined chloroform extracts were transferred to a 250-ml separatory funnel, then extracted with three successive portions of 40 ml of 5% sodium bicarbonate buffered to pH 9.5 by the addition of saturated sodium carbonate. The pH was readjusted to 9.5 following the shaking to prevent formation of an emulsion. The presence of an emulsion is an indication of a pH lower than 9.5 which should be corrected appropriately. The chloroform phase was discarded. The combined alkaline extract was acidified to pH 1 by the careful addition of 50% sulfuric acid, cooled to room temperature and extracted three times with 15-ml portions of chloroform.

The combined chloroform extracts were dried with anhydrous sodium sulfate, filtered through a Whatman-IPS phase-separating silicone-treated paper and reduced in volume to about 2 to 3 ml by means of gentle heat and a stream of dry nitrogen.

To the final chloroform extract in a glass-stoppered flask 0.1 ml of silylating agent bis(trimethylsilyl) trifluoroacetamide (Regisil®) was added and the flask stoppered, and heated to 60 degrees C for fifteen minutes. The solution was then allowed to cool to room temperature, made up to 5 ml with water-free chloroform and 1 to 2 microliters were injected into the chromatograph.

The Beckman Model GC-5 gas chromatograph was used, equipped with a flame ionization detector and a ten-inch linear recorder (Model 1005) with integrator. The column was stainless steel tubing, 0.115 in o.d., 0.093 in i.d., and 6 ft long, packed with 10% SE-30 on acid-washed 60 to 80 mesh Chromosorb W support. The operating conditions were: injector, detector line and detector temperature, 270 degrees C; column temperature, 240 degrees C; nitrogen flow ml/minute.

A method involving extraction, TLC and fluorimetry has also been described (Lewis *et al.*, 1970).

Steady state plasma warfarin levels, when used as anticoagulants vary from about 40 to 320 μg/100 ml (Breckenbridge and Orme, 1973). See also Corn and Berberich (1967).

ZINC

Nowadays, only atomic absorption spectrometry can be considered in the context of zinc analyses (e.g. Hauck, 1973) and method sheets are generally available. McBean *et al.*, (1972) have published *normal* zinc concentrations in bone, muscle, liver, pancreas and kidney in seventeen patients. Zinc concentrations vary—up and down—in disease states.

REFERENCES

Abukurah, A.R., Moser, A.M., Baird, C.L., Randall, R.E., Setter, J.G., and Blanke, R.V.: Acute sodium fluoride poisoning. *JAMA, 222*:816, 1972.

Abul-Haj, S.K., Ewald, R.A., and Kazyak, L.: Fatal mushroom poisoning. Report of a case confirmed by toxicological analysis of tissue. *N Engl J Med, 269*:223, 1963.

Adamovic, V.M.: Aromatic amines as spray reagents in the thin layer chromatography of chlorinated organic pesticides. *J Chromatogr, 23*:274, 1966.

Aghajanian, G.K., and Bing, O.H.L.: Persistence of LSD in the plasma of human subjects. *Clin Pharm Ther, 5*:611, 1964.

Agranat, A.L., and Trubshaw, W.H.D.: Two cases of poisoning from deteriorated paraldehyde. *S Afr Med J, 29*:1021, 1955.

Agurell, S., Gustaffson, B., Holmstedt, B., Leander, K., Lindgren, J.E., Nillson, I., Sandberg, F., and Asberg, M.: Quantitation of Δ' tetrahydrocannabinol in plasma from cannabis smokers, *J Pharm Pharmacol, 25*:554, 1973.

Ainsworth, C.A., Schoegel, E.L., Domanski, T.J., and Goldbaum, L.R.: A gas chromatographic procedure for the determination of carboxyhaemoglobin in post-mortem samples. *J Forensic Sci, 12*:529, 1967.

Alcohol and Traffic Safety, Proceedings Fourth International Conference. Bloomington, Indiana University, 1966.

Alcohol and Road Traffic, Proceedings Fifth International Conference. Frieburg, 1969.

Allen, J.T., Fry, D., and Marks, V.: Urine spot test for methaqualone. *Lancet, 1*:951, 1970.

Ambre, J.J., and Fischer, L.J.: Glutethimide intoxication: plasma levels and a metabolite in humans, dogs and rats. *Res Commun Chem Pathol Pharmacol, 4*:307, 1972.

Amundson, M.E., and Mathey, J.A.: Excretion of nortriptyline hydrochloride in man. *J Pharm Sci, 55*:277, 1966.

Asberg, M., Cronholm, B., Sjöqvist, F., and Tuck, D.: Correlation of subjective side effects with plasma concentrations of nortriptyline, *Br Med J, 4*: 18, 1970.

Axelrod, J., Brady, R.O., Witkop, and Evarts, E.V.: The metabolism of LSD. *Nature, 178*:143, 1956.

idem: The distribution and metabolism of LSD. *Ann NY Acad Sci, 66*:435, 1957.

Bailey, D.N., and Jatlow, P.I.: Methaqualone overdose: Analytical methodology and the significance of serum drug concentrations. *Clin Chem, 19*:615, 1973a.

Bailey, D.N., and Jatlow, P.I.: Methyprylon overdose: Interpretation of serum drug concentrations. *Clin Toxicol, 6*:563, 1973b.

Balazar, A., Åsberg, M., and Tuck, D.: Relationship between the steady state plasma concentration of nortriptyline and some of its pharmacological effects in "Biological effects of drugs in relation to their plasma concentrations." In Davies, D.S., and Prichard, B.N.C.: London, MacMillan Press, 1973.

Ballantyne, B.: The forensic diagnosis of acute cyanide poisoning. In Ballantyne, B. (Ed.): *Forensic Toxicology*. Bristol, John Wright and Sons Ltd., 1974, p. 99.

Ballard, C.W., Isaacs, J., and Scott, P.G.W.: The photometric determination of quaternary ammonium salts and of certain amines by compound formation with indicators. *J Pharm Pharmacol, 6*:971, 1954.

Bamford, F.: *Poisons, their isolation and detection,* 3rd ed. London, Churchill, 1951, p. 40.

Barnes, F.W., and Runcie, J.: Potentiometric method for the determination of inorganic fluoride in biological material. *J Clin Path, 21*:668, 1968.

Barnes, R.J., Kong, S.M., and Wu, R.W.Y.: Electrocardiographic changes in amitriptyline poisoning. *Br Med J, 3*:222, 1968.

Barrowcliffe, D.: The Stoneleigh Abbey Poisoning Case. *Med Leg J, 39*:79, 1971.

Beattie, A.D.: Clinical and biochemical effects of lead. In Ballantyne, B. (Ed.): *Forensic Toxicology*. Bristol, John Wright and Sons, 1974.

Beckett, A.H., Tucker, G.T., and Moffat, A.C.: Routine detection and identification in urine of stimulants and other drugs some of which may be used to modify performance in sport. *J Pharm Pharmacol, 19*:273, 1967.

Bedson, H.S.: Coma due to meprobamate intoxication, report of a case confirmed by chemical analysis. *Lancet, i*:288, 1959.

Beharrell, G.P., Hailey, D.M., and McLaurin, M.K.: Determination of nitrazepam (Mogadon) in plasma by electron capture gas chromatography: *J Chromatogr, 70*:45, 1972.

Benyon, K.I., and Elgar, K.E.: The analysis for residues of chlorinated insecticides and acaricides. A Review. *Analyst, 91*:143, 1966.

Berlin, A., Agurell, S., Borga, O., Lund, L., and Sjoqvist, F.: Micromethod for the determination of diphenylhydantoin in plasma and CSF. A comparison between gas chromatographic and spectrophotometric method. *Scand J Clin Lab Invest, 29*:281-287, 1972.

Berlin, A., Siwers, B., Agurell, S., Hiort, A., Sjoqvist, F., and Ström, S.: Determination of bioavailability of diazepam in various formulations from steady state plasma concentration data. *Clin Pharmacol Ther, 13:*733, 1972.

Berman, E.: Determination of cadmium, thallium and mercury in biological material. *Perkin Elmer Atomic Absorption Newsletter, 6:*57, 1967.

Berry, D.J.: Gas chromatographic analysis of commonly prescribed barbiturates at therapeutic and overdose levels in plasma and urine. *J Chromatogr, 86:*89, 1973.

Berry, D.J., Gas chromatographic determination of methaqualone at therapeutic levels in human plasma. *J Chromatogr, 42:*39, 1969.

Berry, D.J., and Grove, J.: The determination of paraquat in urine. *Clin Chem Acta, 34:*5, 1971.

Betke, K., and Kleihauer, E.: Cytological demonstration of carboxyhaemoglobin in human erythrocytes. *Nature, 214:*188, 1967.

Betts, T.A., Kalra, P.L., Cooper, R., and Jeavons, P.M.: Epileptic fits as a probable side-effect of amitriptyline. *Lancet, 1:*390, 1968.

Beyer, K.H. and Sadee, W.: Chemistry and analysis of benzodiazepine derivatives. V. Spectrophotometric determination of 5-phenyl-1, 4-benzodiazepine derivatives and metabolic studies of nitrazepam. *Arzneimittelforschung, 19:*1929, 1969.

Bickel, M.H.: Metabolism and structure-activity relationships of thymoleptic drugs. *Proc First Int Symp Antidepressant Drugs,* Milan, 3.

Bickel, M.H., Brochon, R., Friolet, B., Herrman, B., and Stofer, A.R.: Clinical and biochemical results of a fatal case of desipramine intoxication. *Psychopharmacologia (Berlin), 10:*431, 1967.

Birkinshaw, V.J., Gurd, M.R., Randall, S.S., Curry, A.S., Price, D.E., and Wright, P.H.: Investigations in a Case of Murder by Insulin Poisoning. *Br Med J, ii:*463, 1958.

Bjornesjo, K.B., and Jarnulf, B.: Determination of isonicotinic acid hydrazide in blood serum. *Scand J Clin Lab Invest, 20:*39, 1967.

Blackmore, D.J., and Jenkins, R.: Exclusion of urinary barbiturates by gas chromatography. *J For Sci Soc, 8:*34, 1968.

Blackmore, D.J.: The determination of carbon monoxide in blood and tissue. *Analyst, 95:*439, 1970.

Blackmore, D.J.: Distribution of HbCO in human erythrocytes following inhalation of CO. *Nature, 227:*386, 1970.

Blackmore, D.J.: Interpretation of carboxyhaemoglobin found at post mortem in victims of aircraft accidents. *Clin Aviation Aerosp Med, 41:*757, 1970.

Blackwell, B.: Another amitriptyline side effect? *Lancet, 1:*426, 1968.

Blazek, J., and Hroníková, M.: Thin layer chromatographic separation of amitriptyline from nortriptyline. *Cesk Farm, 16:*41, 1967.

Block, S.S., Stephens, R.L., Barreto, A., and Murrill, W.A.: Chemical identification of the amanita toxin in mushrooms. *Science, 121:*505, 1955.

Bohn, G., and Rucker, G.: Use of a combination of thin layer chromatography and mass spectrometry in the determination of glutethimide in organ material. *Arch Toxikol, 23:*221, 1968.

Bolt, A.G., Forrest, I.S., and Serra, M.T.: Quantitative studies of urinary excretion of chlorpromazine metabolites in chronically-dosed psychiatric patients. *J Pharm Sci, 55:*1205, 1966.

Bonnichsen, R., and Maehly, A.C.: Poisoning by volatile compounds: hydrocyanic acid. *J Forensic Sci, 11(4):*516-528, 1966.

Bonnichsen, R., Maehly, A.C., and Skold, G.: A report on autopsy cases involving amitriptyline and nortriptyline. *J Leg Med, 67:*190, 1970.

Bonnichsen, R., Mårde, Y., and Ryhage, R.: Identification of free and conjugated metabolites of methaqualone by gas chromatography-mass spectrometry. *Clin Chem, 20:*230, 1974.

Bowden, C.H., and Woodhall, W.R.: The determination and significance of low blood carboxyhaemoglobin levels. *Med Sci Law, 4:*98, 1964.

Bowen, D.A.L., Lewis, T.L.T., and Edwards, W.R.: Acute arsenical poisoning due to acetarsol pessaries. *Brit Med J, 1:*1282, 1961

Braithwaite, R.A., and Widdop, B.: A specific gas chromatographic method for the measurement of "steady state" plasma levels of amitriptyline and nortriptyline in patients. *Clin Chem Acta, 35:*461, 1971.

Breckenbridge, A., and Orme, M. L'E.: Measurement of plasma warfarin concentrations in clinical practice. Davies, D.S., and Prichard, B.N.C. (Eds.): *Biological Effects of Drugs in Relation to Their Plasma Concentrations.* New York, MacMillan Press, 1973.

Brown, C.V.: Abuse of isoniazid. *Lancet, 1:*743, 1972.

Brown, V.K.H., Hunter, C.G., and Richardson, A.: A blood test diagnostic of exposure to Aldrin and Dieldrin. *Br J Ind Med, 21:*283, 1964.

Bruno, B., and Lambliase, M.: Acute poisoning by an antidepressant (amitriptyline hydrochloride) in an infant. *Rass Int Clin Ter, 49:*836, 1969.

Bullivant, C.M.: Accidental poisoning by paraquat: Report of two cases in man. *Br Med J, i:*1273, 1966.

Burston, G.R.: ECG changes in amitriptyline poisoning. *Br Med J, 3:*500, 1968.

Carson, E.D.: Fatal paraquat poisoning in Northern Ireland. *J Forensic Sci Soc, 12:*437, 1972.

Cate, J.C., and Jatlow, P.I.: Chlordiazepoxide overdose; interpretation of serum drug concentrations. *Clin Toxicol, 6:*553, 1973.

Cernik, A.A.: A preliminary procedure for the determination of cadmium in blood. *Perkin Elmer Atomic Absorption Newsletter, 12:*163, 1973.

Charalampons, K.D., and Johnson, P.C.: Studies of C14 protriptyline in man: plasma levels and excretion. *J Clin Pharmacol, 7:*93, 1967.

Chin, D., Fastlich, E., and Davidow, B.: The determination of dilantin in serum by gas chromatography. *J. Chromatogr, 71:*545, 1972.

Christoph, G.W., Schmidt, D.E., Davis, J.M., and Janowsky, D.S.: A method for determination of chlorpromazine in human blood serum. *Clin Chem Acta, 38:*265, 1972.

Chu, R.C., Barron, G.P., and Baumgarner, P.A.W.: Arsenic determination at sub-nanogram levels by arsine evolution and flameless atomic absorption spectrophotometric technique. *Anal Chem, 44:*1476, 1972.

Clarke, E.G.C.: The identification of some proscribed psychedelic drugs. *J Forensic Sci Soc, 7:*46, 1967.

Coble, Y., Hildebrandt, P., Davis, J., Raasch, F., and Curley, A.: Acute Endrin poisoning. *JAMA, 202:*489, 1967.

Collison, H.A., Rodkey, F.L., and O'Neal, D.J.: Determination of carbon monoxide in blood by gas chromatography. *Clin Chem, 14:*162, 1968.

Consolo, S., Dolfini, E., Garattini, S., and Valzelli, L.: Desipramine and amphetamine metabolism. *J Pharm Pharmacol, 19:*253, 1967.

Conway, E.J.: *Microdiffusion Analysis and Volumetric Error,* 3rd Ed. London, Crosby Lockwood, 1950, p. 257.

Cooper, A.G.: *Carbon Monoxide, A Bibliography with Abstracts.* US Department of Health, Education and Welfare, Public Health Service, Washington, 1966.

Cooper, R.G., Greaves, M.S., and Owen, G.: Gas liquid chromatographic isolation, identification and quantitation of some barbiturates, glutethimide and diphenylhydantoin in whole blood. *Clin Chem, 18:*1343, 1972.

Copeman, P.R. v. d. R.: The significance of manganese in human tissue: 1. the determination of manganese in biological material. *J For Med, 2:*55, 1955.

Copeman, P.R. v.d. R.: Review of analytical findings in cases of poisoning by paraldehyde. *J Forensic Med, 3:*80, 1956.

Corn, M., and Berberich, R.: Rapid fluorometric assay for plasma warfarin. *Clin Chem, 13:*126, 1967.

Crammer, J.L., Scott, B., Woods, H., and Rolfe, B.: Metabolism of ^{14}C-imipramine. 1. Excretion in the rat and in man. *Psychopharmacologia (Berlin), 12:*263, 1968.

Cravey, R.H., Shaw, R.F., and Nakamura, G.R.: Incidence of propoxyphene poisoning. A report of fatal cases. *J Forensic Sci, 19:*72, 1974.

Cueto, C., and Biros, F.J.: Chlorinated insecticides and related materials in human urine. *Toxic Appl Pharmacol, 10:*261, 1967.

Curry, A.S.: *Advances in Forensic and Clinical Toxicology.* Cleveland, CRC Press, 1972.

Curry, A.S.: Cyanide poisoning. *Acta Pharmacol Toxicol, 20:*291-294, 1963.

Curry, A.S.: The isolation and detection of ergometrine in toxicological analysis. *J Pharm Pharmacol, 11:*411, 1959.

Curry, A.S.: Seven fatal cases involving imipramine in man. *J Pharm Pharmacol, 16:*265, 1964.

Curry, A.S., and Fox, R.A.: Thin layer chromatography of common barbiturates. *Analyst, 93:*834, 1968.

Curry, A.S., and Knott, A.R.: Normal levels of cadmium in human liver and kidney in England. *Clin Chim Acta, 30:*115, 1970.

Curry, A.S., and Mercier, M.: Detection and identification of monoamine oxidase inhibitors in biological samples. *Nature, 228*:281, 1970.

Curry, A.S., Price, D.E., and Rutter, E.R.: The production of cyanide in post-mortem material. *Acta Pharmacol Toxicol, 25*:339, 1967.

Curry, A.S., Walker, G.W., and Simpson, G.S.: Determination of ethanol in blood by gas chromatography. *Analyst, 91*:742, 1966.

Curry, S.H.: Plasma protein binding of chlorpromazine. *J Pharm Pharmacol, 22*:193, 1970.

Curry, S.H., and Marshall, J.H.L.: Plasma levels of chlorpromazine and some of its relatively non-polar metabolites in psychiatric patients, *Life Sci, 7*: 9, 1968.

Curry, S.H., and Mould, G.P.: Gas chromatographic identification of thioridazine in plasma and a method for routine assay of the drug. *J Pharm Pharmacol, 21*:674, 1969.

Curry, S.H., Riddall, D., Gordon, J.S., Simpson, P., Binns, T.B., Rondel, R., and McMartin, B.: Disposition of glutethimide in man. *Clin Pharmacol Ther, 12*:849, 1971.

Dal Cortivo, L.A., Broich, J.R., Dihrberg, A., and Newman, B.: Identification and estimation of LSD by TLC and fluorimetry. *Anal Chem, 38*:1959, 1966.

Dalziel, K., and O'Brien, J.R.P.: Kinetics of reduction of oxyhaemoglobin by sodium dithionite. *Biochem J, 67*:122, 1957.

Daniel, J.W., and Gage, J.C.: Absorption and excretion of Diquat and Paraquat in rats. *Brit J Ind Med, 23*:133, 1966.

Davidson, D.G.D., and Eastham, W.N.: Acute liver necrosis following overdose of paracetamol. *Br Med J, ii*:497, 1966.

de Bruin, A.: Carboxyhaemoglobin levels due to traffic exhaust. *Arch Environ Health, 384*:15, 1967.

de Faubert Maunder, M.J., Egan, H., Godly, H., Hammond, E.W. Roburn, J., and Thomas, J.: Clean-up of animal fats and dairy products for the analysis of chlorinated pesticide residues. *Analyst, 89*:168, 1964.

de Silva, J.A.F., Koechlin, B.A., and Bader, G.: Blood-level distribution patterns of diazepam and its major metabolite in man. *J Pharm Sci, 55*:692, 1966.

de Silva, J.A.F., and Puglisi, C.V.: Determination medazepam (Nobrium®) diazepam (Valium®) and their major biotransformation products in blood and urine by electron capture gas-liquid chromatography. *Anal Chem, 42*: 1725, 1970.

Dill, W.A., Chucot, L., Chang, T., and Glazko, A.J.: Simplified benzophenone procedure for determination of diphenylhydantoin in plasma. *Clin Chem, 17*:1201, 1971.

Divatia, K.G., Hine, C.H., and Burbridge, T.N.: A simple method for the determination of tetraethyldithiuram disulphide (ANTABUSE) and blood levels obtained exeprimentally in animals and clinically in man. *J Lab*

*Clin Med, 39:*974, 1952.

Doherty, J.E., Perkins, W.H., and Flanigan, W.J.: The distribution and concentration of tritiated digoxin in human tissues. *Ann Int Med, 66:*116, 1967.

Dominguez, A.M., Halsted, J.R., and Domanski, T.J.: The effect of postmortem changes on carboxyhaemoglobin results. *J Forensic Soc, 9:*330, 1964.

Dominguez, A.M., Christensen, H.E., Goldbaum, L.R., and Stembridge, V.A.: A sensitive procedure for determining carbon monoxide in blood and tissue utilising gas-solid chromatography. *Toxic Appl Pharmacol, 1:*135, 1959.

Douglas, B.H., and Hume, A.S.: Placental transfer of imipramine, a basic lipid-soluble drug. *Am J Obstet Gynecol, 99:*573, 1967.

Douglas, J.F., Kelley, T.F., Smith, N.B., and Stockage, J.A.: Gas chromatographic determination of meprobamate in plasma and urine. *Anal Chem, 39:*956, 1967.

Drabner, J., Bauer, H., and Schwerd, W.: Detection of opipramol (Insidom) and Nortriptyline (Nortrilen) in urine. *Arch Toxikol, 21:*367, 1966.

Driscoll, J.L., Martin, H.F., and Gulzinowicz, B.J.: A gas chromatographic method for quantitative analyses of some urinary metabolites of chlorpromazine. *J Gas Chrom, 2:*109, 1964.

Dubowski, K.M., and Luke, J.L.: The determination of carboxyhaemoglobin and carbon monoxide in blood. Colloquium on Aviation Toxicology, Joint Committee on Aviation Pathology, Oklahoma City, October 12 to 19, 1970. In *Aerosp Med, 41*(7):743-808, 1970.

Edson, E.F.: Agricultural pesticides. *Br Med J, i:*841, 1955.

El-Rejal, A., and Hopkins, T.L.: Thin layer chromatography and cholinesterase detection of several phosphorothiono insecticides and their oxygen analogues. *J Agric Food Chem, 13:*477, 1965.

Eschenhof, E., and Rieder, J.: Studies of the fate of the antidepressant amitriptyline in the organisms of rat and man. *Arzneimittelforschung, 19:*957, 1969.

Evenson, M.A., and Koellner, S.: Rapid method for quantitation of propoxyphene in serum by gas liquid chromatography. *Clin Chem, 19:*492, 1973.

Evenson, M.A., and Lensmeyer, G.L.: Qualitative and quantitative determination of methaqualone in serum by gas chromatography. *Clin Chem, 20:*249, 1974.

Evenson, M.A., and Poquette, M.A.: Rapid gas chromatographic method for quantitation of Ethchlorvynol ("Placidyl") in serum. *Clin Chem, 20:*212, 1974.

Evreux, J.C., Armand, J., and Motin, J.: Evolution clinique et biologique d'une intoxication aigue par la chlorprimipramine (Anafranil®). *Bull Med Leg Tox Med, 1:*37, 1969.

Farago, A.: Fatal suicidal Malathion poisoning. *Arch Toxicol, 23:*11, 1967.

Farago, A.: Thin layer chromatographic detection and quantitative determination of Malathion in biological materials. *J Forensic Sci, 12*:547, 1967.

Fatteh, A., Blanke, R., and Mann, G.T.: Death from imipramine poisoning. *J Forensic Sci, 13*:124, 1968.

Feldstein, M.: Methods for determination of carbon monoxide. In Stolman, A. (Ed): *Progress in Chemical Toxicology*. New York, Academic, vol. 3, 1967.

Feldstein, M., and Klendshoj, N.C.: Determination of methanol of biological fluids by microdiffusion analysis. *Anal Chem, 26*:932, 1954.

Feldstein, M., and Klendshoj, N.C.: The determination of carbon monoxide by micro-diffusion. *Can J Med Technol, 16*:81, 1954.

Feldstein, M., and Klendshoj, N.C.: The determination of volatile substances by microdiffusion analysis. *J Forensic Sci, 2*:39, 1957.

Fenimore, D.C., Freeman, R.R., and Loy, P.R.: Determination of Δ^9 tetrahydrocannabinol in blood by electron capture gas chromatography. *Anal Chem, 45*:2331, 1973.

Fenwick, M.L., and Parker, V.H.: The determination of 3:5—dinitro-cresol in the presence of β-carotene in biological tissues. *Analyst, 80*:774, 1955.

Fiereck, E.A., and Tietz, N.W.: A gas chromatographic method for separating and measuring barbiturates and glutethimide in blood. *Clin Chem, 17*: 1024, 1971.

Figot, P.P., Hine, C.H. and Way, E.L.: Estimation and significance of paraldehyde levels in blood and brain. *Acta Pharmacol Toxicol, 3*:290, 1952.

Finkle, B.S.: The identification, quantitation, determination and distribution of meprobamate and gluthethimide in biological material. *J Forensic Sci, 12*:509, 1967.

Fishbein, L.: Chromatographic and biological aspects of polychlorinated biphenyls. *J Chromatogr* (Chromatographic Reviews), *68*:345, 1972.

Fishwick, F.B., and Taylor, A.: The determination of warfarin in animal relicta. *Analyst, 92*:192, 1967.

Flanagen, R.J., and Withers, G.: A rapid micro-method for the screening and measurement of barbiturates and related compounds in plasma by gas liquid chromatography. *J Clin Pathol, 25*:899, 1972.

Fletcher, K.: Paraquat poisoning. In Ballantyne, B.: *Forensic Toxicology*. Bristol, John Wright and Sons, 1974, p. 86.

Forbes, G., Weir, W.P., Smith, H., and Bogan, J.: Amitriptyline poisoning. *J Forensic Sci Soc, 5*:183, 1965.

Foreman, J.K., Gough, T.A., and Walker, E.A.: The determination of beryllium in human and rat urine samples by gas chromatography. *Analyst, 95*:797, 1970.

Forney, R.B., and Harger, R.N.: Mercury content of human tissues from routine autopsy material. *Fed Proc, 8*:292, 1949.

Foster, L.B., and Frings, C.S.: Determination of diazepam (Valium®) concentrations in serum by gas-liquid chromatography. *Clin Chem, 16:*177, 1970.

Fowler, R., Gomm, P.J., and Patterson, D.A.: TLC of lysergide and other ergot alkaloids. *J Chromatogr, 72:*351, 1972.

Freireich, A.W., and Landau, D.: Carbon monoxide determination in postmortem clotted blood. *J Forensic Sci, 16:*112, 1971.

Funnell, H.S., and Platanow, N.: Determination of Warfarin in liver tissue by gas chromatography. *J Forensic Sci, 15:*601, 1970.

Gard, H., Knapp, D., Walle, T., and Gaffney, T.: Qualitative and quantitative studies on the disposition of amitriptyline and other tricyclic antidepressants in man as it relates to the management of the overdosed patient. *Clin Toxicol, 6:*571, 1973.

Garattini, S., Marcucci, F., and Mussinin, E.: Gas chromatographic analysis of benzodiazepines. In Porter, R. (Ed.): *Gas Chromatography in Biology and Medicine.* London, J. and A. Churchill, 1969, p. 161.

Garratt, J.C., Sturner, W.Q., and Mason, M.F.: Toxicologic findings in six fatalities involving methadone. *Clin Toxicol, 6:*163, 1973.

Garrett, E.R., and Hunt, C.A.: Picogram analysis of tetrahydrocannabinol and application to biological fluids. *J Pharm Sci, 62:*1211, 1973.

Gee, D.J.: in "The Poisoned Patient"; Ciba Foundation Symposium. *Elsevier,* 1974.

Gee, D.J., Dalley, R.A., Green, M.A., and Perkin, L.A.: Post mortem diagnosis of barbiturate poisoning in Forensic Toxicology, editor, Ballantyne, B. John Wright and Sons, Bristol, 1974.

Gerade, H.W., and Skiba, P.: Toxicological studies on hydrocarbons: VI. A colorimetric method for the determination of kerosine in blood. *Clin Chem, 6:*327, 1960.

Gettler, A.O., and Baine, J.O.: The toxicology of cyanide. *Am J Med Sci, 195:*182, 1938.

Gettler, A.O., and Goldbaum, L.: Detection and estimation of microquantities of cyanide. *Anal Chem, 19:*270, 1947.

Giterson, A.L., Slooff, P.A.M., and Schouten, H.: Oxalate in urine. *Clin Chem Acta, 29:*342, 1970.

Gjerris, F.: Poisoning with chlordiazepoxide. *Danish Med Bull, 13:*170, 1966.

Gold, M., Tassoni, E., Etzl, M., and Matthew, G.: Concentration of glutethimide and associated compounds in human serum and CSF after drug overdose. *Clin Chem, 20:*195, 1974.

Goldstone, N.I.: The microchemical detection of fluorides by the sodium fluorosilicate crystal test. *Anal Chem, 27:*464, 1955.

Goodwin, J.: Colorimetric measurement of serum bromide with a bromate-rosaniline method. *Clin Chem, 17:*544, 1971.

Goralski, H., and Januszko, L.: Psychiatric and neurological aspects of poisoning with carbon monoxide. *Neurol Neurochir Pol, 18:*633, 1968.

Gormsen, H.: Alcohol production in the dead body. *J Forensic Med, 1:*170, 1954.

idem: Alcohol production in the dead body. *J Forensic Med, 1:*314, 1954.

Goudie, J.H., and Burnett, D.: A rapid method for the detection of methaqualone metabolites. *Clin Chem Acta, 35:*133, 1971.

Grade, R., Forter, W., and Schulzeck, S.: An improved method for the isolation of heart glycosides from tissues using Sephadex G200. *Biochem Pharmacol, 16:*1299, 1967.

Gramer, L., and Ruof, H.: Serum enzyme and protein changes in severe acute carbon monoxide poisoning. *Deut Med Wochenschr, 93:*2275, 1968.

Gray, D.J.S.: The determination of mercury in urine by the reversion technique. *Analyst, 77:*436, 1952.

Greaves, M.S.: Quantitative determination of Medezepam, Diazepam and Nitrazepam in whole blood by flame ionisation gas-liquid chromatography. *Clin Chem, 20:*141, 1974.

Grierson, P., and Gordon, J.S.: The assay of glutethimide in plasma. *J Chromatogr, 44:*279, 1969.

Gutsche, B., and Herrmann, R.: Flame photometric determination of bromine in urine. *Analyst, 95:*805, 1970.

Gwilt, J.R., Robertson, A., Goldman, L., and Blanchard, A.W.: The absorption characteristics of paracetamol tablets in man. *J Pharm Pharmacol, 15:*445, 1963.

Gwilt, J.R., Robertson, A., and McChesney, E.W.: Determination of blood and other tissue concentrations of paracetamol in dog and man. *J Pharm Pharmacol, 15:*440, 1963.

Hall, R.J.: The spectrophotometric determination of sub-microgram amounts of fluorine in biological specimens. *Analyst, 88:*76, 1963.

Hall, T.C.: Rapid test for bromide in blood and urine. *Lancet, ii:*355, 1943.

Halstrom, F., and Moller, K.: The content of cyanide in human organs from cases of poisoning with cyanide taken by mouth. *Acta Pharmacol Toxicol, 1:*18-28, 1945.

Hammar, C-G., and Holmstedt, B.: Mass fragmentography. Identification of chlorpromazine and its metabolites in human blood by a new method. *Anal Biochem, 25:*532, 1968.

Hammar, C.G., and Holmstedt, B.: The identification of chlorpromazine metabolites in human blood by gas-liquid chromatography. *Experientia, 24:*98, 1968.

Hammer, W., Martens, S., and Sjöqvist, F.: A comparative study of the metabolism of desmethylimipramine, nortriptyline and oxyphenbutazone in man. *Clin Pharmacol Ther, 10:*44, 1969.

Hannsson, E., and Cassano, G.B.: Distribution and metabolism of antidepressant drugs. *Proc 1st Int Symp Antidepressant Drugs*, Milan, 1966, p. 10.

Hansen, A.R., and Fischerm, L.J.: Gas chromatographic simultaneous analysis for glutethimide and an active hydroxylated metabolite in tissues, plasma and urine. *Clin Chem, 20:*236, 1974.

Hansen, E., and Moller, K.O.: Arsenic content of organs after fatal poisoning with arsenic trioxide and other arsenical compounds. *Acta Pharmacol Toxicol, 5:*135, (1949).

Haqqani, M.T., and Gutteridge, D.R.: Two cases of clomipramine hydrochloric (Anafranil) poisoning. *Forensic Sci, 3:*83, 1974.

Harger, R.N.: In Stewart, C.P. and Stolman A. (Eds.): *Toxicology Mechanisms and Analytical Methods.* New York, Academic, 1961, vol. II, pp. 86-147.

Harger, R.N.: In Stolman, A. (Ed.): *Progress in Chemical Toxicology.* New York, Academic, 1963, vol. 1, p. 54.

Harger, R.N., and Forney, R.B.: A simple method for detecting and estimating ethylene glycol in body materials: analytical results in six cases. *J For Sci, 4:*136, 1959.

Harger, R.N., and Forney, R.B.: In Stolman, A. (Ed.): *Progress in Chemical Toxicology.* New York and London, Academic, 1967, vol. III, p. 1.

Hauck, G.: Erfahrungen mit der flammenlosen Atomabsorption dei der Untersuchung biologischen Materials auf Spuren von Schwermettalen. *Z Anal Chem, 269:*337, 1973.

Haun, E.C.: Fatal Toxaphene poisoning in a 9 month infant. *Am J Dis Child, 113:*616, 1967.

Hauser, T.R., Hinners, T.A., and Kent, J.L.: Atomic absorption determination of cadmium and lead in whole blood by a reagent free method. *Anal Chem, 44:*1819, 1972.

Haux, P.: Ethchlorvynol (Placidyl) determination in urine and serum. *Clin Chim Acta, 43:*139, 1972.

Haywood, P.E., Horner, M.W., and Rylance, H.J.: Thin layer chromatography of neutral drugs. *Analyst, 92:*711, 1967.

Heirwegh, K.P.M., and Fevery, J.: Determination of unconjugated and total NAPA in urine and serum. *Clin Chem, 13:*215, 1967.

Heitmann, R., and Kunst, H.: Fatal poisoning with desipramine. *Deutsch Med Wschr, 93:*117, 1968.

Henwood, C.S.: Instability of amitriptyline base. *Nature, 216:*1039, 1967.

Hessel, D.W., and Modglin, F.R.: The determination of carbon monoxide in blood by gas-solid chromatography. *J Forensic Sci, 12:*123, 1967.

Heyndrickx, A., Maes, R., and de Leenheer, A.: Intoxication of a child due to parathion by drinking poisoned milk. *J Pharm Belge, 34:*161, 1964.

Heyndrickx, A., Schepens, P., and Scheiris, C.: Toxicological analysis of a fatal poisoning by paraquat in man. *J Eur Toxol, 4:*178, 1969.

Heyndrickx, A., Vercruysse, A., and Noe, M.: A review of forty-one cases of parathion poisoning in man. *J Pharm Belge, 3-4:*127, 1967.

Hodge, H.C., Boyce, A.M., Deichmann, W.B., and Kraybill, H.F.: Toxicology and no-effect levels of Aldrin and Dieldrin. *Toxic Appl Pharmacol, 10:*613, 1967.

Hoffman, A.J., and Ludwig, B.J.: An improved colorimetric method for the determination of meprobamate in biological fluids. *J Am Pharm Assoc, 48:*740, 1959.

Hladka, A., and Hladky, Z.: Separation of p-nitro phenol and p-nitro-m-cresol from urine pigments by TLC. *J Chromatogr, 22:*457, 1966.

Holt, D.W., and Benstead, J.G.: Postmortem assay of digoxin by radioimmunoassay. *J Clin Path. 28:*483, 1975.

Hoover, W.L., Melton, J.R., Howard, P.A., and Bassett, J.W.: Atomic absorption spectrometric determination of arsenic. *J A O A C, 57:*18, 1974.

Howie, R.A., and Smith, H.: Mercury in human tissue. *J Forensic Sci Soc, 7:* 90, 1967.

Huang, C.L.: Isolation and identification of urinary chlorpromazine metabolites in man. *Int J Neuropharmacol, 6:*1, 1967.

Hucker, H.B., and Miller, J.K.: A technique for the improvement of gas chromatographic properties of tertiary amines such as amitriptyline. *J Chromatogr, 32:*408, 1968.

Hume, A.S., and Douglas, B.H.: Placental transfer of desmethylimipramine. *Am J Obstet Gynecol, 101:*915, 1968.

Hunter, C.G., Robinson, J., and Richardson, A.: Chlorinated insecticide content of human body fat in Southern England. *Br Med J, i:*231, 1963.

Iisalo, E., and Nuutila, M.: Myocardial digoxin concentrations in fatal intoxications. *Lancet, 1:*257, 1973.

Inturrisi, C.E., and Verebeley, K.: The levels of methadone in plasma in methadone maintenance. *Clin Pharmacol Ther, 13:*633, 1972.

Irving, H., Risdon, J., and Andrew, J.: The absorptiometric determination of traces of metals: Reversion: A new procedure. *J Chem Soc, 537* and *541,* 1949.

Janitzki, von U., Proch, W., Schleyer, F., Ditschuneit, H., and Pfeiffer, E.: Detection of insulin in cadavers after insulin poisoning: 1. Forensic Medicine: Clinical Picture, Cadaver findings and pretreatment of materials (p. 17-24). II. Experimental detection procedures (p. 24-32). *Med Exptl,* 3, 1960.

Jatlow, P.: Ultra-violet spectrophotometric measurement of chlordiazepoxide in plasma. *Clin Chem, 18:*516, 1972.

Jelliffe, R.W.: A chemical determination of urinary digitoxin and digoxin in man. *J Lab Clin Med, 67:*694, 1966.

Jenis, E.H., Payne, R.J., and Goldbaum, L.R.: Acute meprobamate poisoning. A fatal case following a lucid interval. *JAMA, 207:*361, 1969.

Kanter, S.L.: Acetone as a source of error in the colorimetric determination of meprobamate. *Clin Chim Acta, 17:*147, 1967.

Karjalainen, J., Ojala, K., and Reissell, P.: Tissue concentrations of digoxin in an autopsy material. *Acta Pharmacol Toxicol, 34:*385, 1974.

Kaul, P.N., Conway, M.W., and Clark, M.L., Sensitive quantitative determination of chlorpromazine metabolites. *Nature, 226:*372, 1970.

Kennedy, R.P.: The quantitative determination of iron in tissues. *J Biol Chem, 74:*385, 1927 (modified).

Kingsley, G.R., and Schaffert, R.R.: Microdetermination of arsenic and its application to biological material. *Anal Chem, 23:*914, 1951.

Kirk, P.L., Gibon, A., and Parker, K.P.: Determination of blood alcohol;

improvements in chemical and enzymatic procedures. *Anal Chem, 30:*1418, 1958.

Klinge, D., and Beyer, K.H.: Eine einfache Nachweis-und Bestimmungs-methode fur Imipramin (Tofranil) und seine Derivate bei chemisch-toxikologischen Untersuchungen. *Dtsch Apoth Zig, 108(22):*780, 1968.

Knowles, J.A., and Ruelius, H.W.: Absorption and excretion of oxazepam in humans. *Arz Forsch* (Drug Res), *22:*687, 1972.

Knowlton, M., and Goldbaum, L.R.: An improved rapid method for the determination of glutethimide. *J Forensic Sci, 14:*129, 1969.

Koechlin, B.A., and D'Arconte, L.: Determination of chlordiazepoxide (Librium®) and of a metabolite of lactam character in plasma of humans, dogs and rats by a specific spectrofluorimetric micro method. *Anal Biochem, 5:* 195, 1963.

Korczak-Fabierkiewicz, C., Robinson, D.W., and Lucas, G.H.W.: Conversion of chlorpromazine sulphoxide to chlorpromazine by use of metals in acid solution. *J Chromatogr, 31:*538, 1967.

Koumides, O.,: *Proc First International Meeting in Forensic Toxicology.* London, 1963.

Kovacs, M.F.: Rapid detection of chlorinated pesticide residues by an improved TLC technique: $3\frac{1}{4} \times 4''$ micro slides. *JAOAC, 49:*365, 1966.

Kozelka, F.L., and Hine, C.H.: A method for the determination of ethyl alcohol for medico-legal purposes. *Ind Eng Chem, Anal Ed, 13:*905, 1941.

Kragh-Sorensen, P., Asberg, A., and Eggert-Hansen: Plasma nortriptyline levels in endogenous depression. *Lancet, 1:*113, 1973.

Krickler, D.M.: Paracetamol and the kidney. *Br Med J, ii:*615, 1967.

Larsen, N-E., Naestoft, J., and Hvidberg, E.: Rapid routine determination of some anti-epileptic drugs in serum by gas chromatography. *Clin Chim Acta, 40:*171, 1972.

Leach, H., and Toseland, P.: The determination of barbiturates and some related drugs by gas chromatography. *Clin Chim Acta, 20:*195, 1968.

Lever, M.: Rapid fluorometric or spectrophotometric determination of Isoniazid. *Biochem Med, 6:*65, 1972.

Lewin, J.F., Norris, R.J., and Hughes, J.T.: Three cases of Maldison (Malathion) poisoning. *Forensic Sci, 2:*101, 1973.

Lewis, G.P., Jusko, W.J., and Coughlin, L.L.: Cadmium accumulation in man: influence of smoking, occupation, alcoholic habit and disease. *J Chrom Dis, 25:*717, 1972.

Lewis, R.J., Ilnicki, L.P., and Carlstrom, M.: The assay of Warfarin in plasma or stool. *Biochem Med, 4:*376, 1970.

Linde, H.W.: The estimation of fluoride in body fluids (an enzymatic method). *Anal Chem, 31:*2092, 1960.

Loeffler, L.J., and Pierce, J.V.: Radioimmunoassay for Lysergide (LSD) in illicit drugs and biological fluids. *J Pharm Sci, 62:*1817, 1973.

Lukkari, I., and Alha, A.: Forensic chemical detection of digitalis glycosides in autopsy material. *Anal Abstr, 1556, 1967.*

Lund-Larsen, G., and Sivertssen, E.: Imipramine cardiopathy. *Nord Med, 80:* 986, 1968.

Lundquist, F.: Ethyl alcohol in blood and tissues. In Glick, D. (Ed.), Methods of Biochemical Analysis. New York, Interscience, 1959, Vol. 7, p. 217.

Maas, A.H.J., Hamelink, M.L., and de Leeuw, R.J.M.: An evaluation of spectrophotometric determination of HbO, HbCO and Hb in blood with the Co-oximeter IL 182. *Clin Chim Acta, 29:*303, 1970.

Machata, G.: Die differenzierung der Kohlenoxidvergiftung. *Arch Toxikol, 23:*136, 1968.

Machata, G.: Uber die gaschromatographische Blutalkoholbestimmung. *Blutalkhol, 4:*252, 1967.

Maddock, R.J., and Bloomer, H.A.: Meprobamate overdosage; evaluation of its severity and method of treatment. *JAMA, 201:*123, 1967.

Madsen, O.D.: Colorimetric determination of meprobamate in blood. *Clin Chim Acta, 7:*481, 1962.

Maehly, A.C.: Methods of forensic science. In Lundquist, F. (Ed.): New York, Interscience, 1962, vol. 1.

Maehly, A.C., and Bonnichsen, R.: Fuenf löedliche Vergiftungen mit Methaqualone. *Deut Z Ges Gericht Med, 57:*446, 1966.

Maes, R., Bouche, R., and Laruelle, L.: Détermination quantitative de méprobamate et de Carisoprodol par chromatographie in phase gazause dans différents cas d'intoxications. *Eur J Toxicol, 2:*140, 1970.

Maes, R., Hodnett, N., Landesman, H., Kananen, G., Finkle, B., and Sunshine, I.: The gas chromatographic determination of sedatives (ethchlorvynol, paraldehyde, meprobamate and Carisprodol) in biological material. *J Forensic Sci, 14:*235, 1969.

Malik, M.O.A., and Martin, J.: Chlorpromazine levels in the blood following Largactil® (chlorpromazine hydrochloride) therapy and poisoning. *J Forensic Med, 17:*58, 1970.

Manley, C.H., and Dalley, R.A.: Analytical findings in a death following inhalation of cadmium fumes. *Analyst, 82:*287, 1957.

Mant, A.K.: A review of 100 cases of carbon monoxide poisoning. *Medicolegal J, 28:*31, 1960.

Markiewicz, J.: Investigations on endogenous carboxyhaemoglobin. *J Forensic Med, 14:*16, 1967.

Martis, L., and Levy, R.H.: GLC Determination of Meprobamate in Water, Plasma and Urine. *J Pharm Sci, 63:*834, 1974.

Matthew, H., Logan, A., Woodruff, M.F.A., and Heard, H.: Paraquat poisoning—lung transplantation. *Br Med J, ii:*759, 1968.

Matthew, H., Proudfoot, A.T., Brown, S.S., and Smith, A.C.A.: Mandrax poisoning: conservative management of 116 patients. *Br Med J 2:*101, 1968.

Maybury, R.B., and Cochrane, W.P.: Evaluation of chemical confirmatory tests for analysis of dieldrin residues. *JAOAC, 56:*36, 1973.

McBay, A.J., Turk, R.F., Corbett, B.W., and Hudson, P.: *J Forensic Sci, 19:* 81, 1974.

McBean, L.D., Dove, J.T., Halsted, J.A., and Smith, J.C.: Zinc concentration in human tissue. *Am J Clin Nutr, 25*:672, 1972.

McCallum, R.I., Rannie, I., and Verity, C.: Chronic pulmonary berylliosis in a female chemist. *Br J Indust Med, 18*:133, 1961.

McConnell Davis, T.W.: Thin layer chromatography of thirteen medicinally important carbamates. *J Chromatogr, 29*:283, 1967.

McCredie, R.M., and Jose, A.D.: Analysis of blood carbon monoxide and oxygen by gas chromatography. *J Appl Physiol, 22*:863, 1967.

Meijer, J.W.A.: Simultaneous quantitative determination of antiepileptic drugs including carbamazepine in body fluids. *Epilepsia, 12*:341, 1971.

Merli, S., and de Zorzi, D.: Clinical and experimental studies of Meprobamate poisoning. *Zacchia, 24*:274, 1961.

Michel, H.O.: Electrometric method for the determination of red blood cell and plasma cholinesterase activity. *J Lab Clin Med, 34*:1565, 1949.

Millhouse, J., Davies, D.M., and Wraith, S.K.: Chronic ethchlorvynol intoxication. *Lancet, ii*:1251, 1966.

Milner, G.: Amitriptyline potentiation of alcohol. *Lancet, 1*:222, 1967.

Milner, G.: Cumulative lethal dose of alcohol in mice given amitriptyline. *J Pharm Sci, 57*:2005, 1968.

Mitchard, M., and Williams, M.E.: An improved quantitative GLC assay for the estimation of methaqualone in biological fluids. *J Chromatogr, 72*:29, 1972.

Mitchison, D.A.: Plasma concentrations of isoniazid in the treatment of tuberculosis. In Davies, D.S., and Pritchard, B.N.C. (Eds.): *Biological Effects of Drugs in Relation to Their Plasma Concentrations.* New York, MacMillan Press, 1973.

Moody, J.P., Tait, A.C., and Todrick, A.: Plasma levels of imipramine and desmethylimipramine during therapy. *Br J Psy, 113*:183, 1967.

Moss, M.S., and Jackson, J.V.: A furfural reagent of high specificity for the detection of carbamates on paper chromatograms. *J Pharm Pharmacol, 13*:361, 1961.

Muehlberger, C.W.: Medico-legal aspects of alcohol intoxication. In Gradwohl, R.H.B. (Ed.): *Legal Medicine.* St. Louis, Mosby, 1954, pp. 754-796.

Munksgaard, E.C.: Concentrations of amitriptyline and its metabolites in urine, blood and tissue in fatal amitriptyline poisoning. *Acta Pharmacol, 27*:129, 1969.

Naestoft, J., and Larsen, N.E.: Quantitative determination of clonazepam and its metabolites in human plasma by gas chromatography. *J Chromatogr, 93*:113, 1974.

Nickolls, L.C.: A modified Cavett method for the determination of alcohol in body fluids. *Analyst, 85*:840, 1960.

Noble, J., and Matthew, H.: Acute poisoning by tricyclic antidepressants: clinical features and management of 100 patients. *Clin Toxicol, 2*:403, 1969.

Norheim, G.: Methadone in autopsy cases. *Z Rechsmedizin, 73*:219, 1973.

Norheim, G.: The simultaneous determination of amitriptyline and nortriptyline in post-mortem blood and urine using gas chromatography. *J Chromatogr, 88*:403, 1974.

Obersteg, J., Im, and Delay, F.: Six years' experience with detoxicated coal gas. *Deutch Z Ges Gerichtl Med, 58*:122, 1966.

Olsen, O.V.: A simplified method for extracting phenytoin from serum and a more sensitive staining reaction for quantitative determination by TLC. *Acta Pharmacol Toxicol, 25*:123, 1967.

Orepoulos, D.G., and Lal, S.: Recovery from massive amitriptyline overdosage. *Lancet, 2*:221, 1968.

Palmer, L., and Kolmodin-Hedman, B.: Improved quantitative gas chromatographic method for the analysis of small amounts of chlorinated pesticides in human plasma. *J Chromatogr, 74*:21, 1972.

Palyza, V.: Chromatographie der amanita toxins. II Neue methode zur identifizeirung von amanita-toxinen durch dunnschichtchromatographie. *J Chromatogr, 64*:317, 1972.

Palyza, V., and Kulhanek, C.: Uber die chromatographische analyse von toxinen aus amanita phalloides. *J Chromatogr, 53*:545, 1970.

Papadopoulous, A.S., Baylis, E.M., Fry, D.E., and Marks, V.: A rapid micromethod for determining four anti-convulsant drugs by gas-liquid chromatography. *Clin Chim Acta, 48*:135, 1973.

Paton, W.D.M., and Crown, J. (Eds.) *Cannabis and its Derivatives.* Oxford University Press, 1972.

Patterson, D.A., and Stevens, H.M.: Identification of cannabias. *J Pharm Phrmcol, 22*:391, 1970.

Patty, F.A.: The production of hydrocyanic acid by bacillus pyocyaneus. *J Infect Dis, 29*:73-77, 1921.

Paulet, G., and Chevrier, R.: Rapid estimation of carboxyhaemoglobin by reflectometry. *Ann Biol Clin, 26*:651, 1968.

Pearson, E.F., and Pounds, C.A.: A case involving the administration of known amounts of arsenic and its analysis in hair. *J Forensic Sci Soc, 11*: 229, 1971.

Penny, R.: Imipramine hydrochloride poisoning in children. *Am J Dis Child, 116*:181, 1968.

Perlman, P.L., and Johnson, C.: The metabolism of Dormison and methods for its estimation in biological materials. *J Amer Pharm Assoc, 14*:13, 1952.

Peterson, G.C., Welford, G.A., and Harley, J.H.: Spectrographic microdetermination of beryllium in air dust samples. *Anal Chem, 22*:1197, 1950.

Pettigrew, A.R., and Fell, G.S.: Microdiffusion method for estimation of cyanide in whole blood and its application to the study of conversion of cyanide to thiocyanate. *Clin Chem, 19*:466, 1973.

Phillips, A.R., Webb, B. and Curry, A.S.: The detection of insulin in post mortem tissues. *J Forensic Sci, 17:*460, 1972.

Pickering, R.G., and Martin, J.G.: Modification of the Michel pH Method for the estimation of plasma, erythrocyte and brain cholinesterase activities of various species of laboratory animals. *Archiv für Toxikol, 26:*179, 1970.

Plueckhahn, V.D.: The significance of blood alcohol levels at autopsy. *Med J Aust, 2:*118, 1967.

Polson, C.J., and Tattersall, R.N.: *Clinical Toxicology.* London, English Univ. Press, 1959, pp. 383-387.

Porter, K., and Volman, D.H.: Flame ionisation detection of carbon monoxide for gas chromatographic analysis. *Anal Chem, 34:*748, 1962.

Pragowski, T.: *Proc Third Int Meeting in Forensic Medicine, Pathology and Toxicology,* London, 1963.

Prescott, L.F.: Gas-liquid estimation of paracetamol. *J Pharm Pharmacol, 23:* 807, 1971.

Prescott, L.F.: The gas-liquid chromatographic estimation of phenacetin and paracetamol in plasma and urine. *J Pharm Pharmacol, 23:*111, 1971.

Pribilla, O.,: *Proceedings of the First International Meeting in Forensic Toxicology,* London, 1963.

Prokes, L.H.J.: The oscillopolarographic determination of meprobamate in biological material. *Chemicke Zvesti, 18:*425, 1964.

Ramsey, I.D.: Survival after imipramine poisoning. *Lancet, 2:*1308, 1967.

Ramsey, L.L., and Clifford, P.A.: The determination of monofluoroacetic acid in foods and biological material. *JAOAC, 32:*788, 1949.

Randolph, W.C., Walkenstein, S.S., Joseph, G.L., and Intoccia, A.P.: Rapid ultra-violet procedure for measuring doxepin metabolites in human urine. *Clin Chem, 20:*692, 1974.

Report of a special Committee of the British Medical Association. *The Relation of Alcohol to Road Accidents.* London, British Medical Association, 1960.

Richardson, A., Hunter, C.G., Crabtree, A.N., and Rees, H.J.: Organochloro insecticide content of human adipose tissue in South East England. *Br J Industr Med, 22:*200, 1965.

Richardson, A., Robinson, J., Bush, B., and Davies, J.M.: Determination of Dieldrin (HOED) in blood. *Arch Environ Health, 14:*703, 1967.

Richardson, S.J.: Thin layer chromatography of the common barbiturates. *Proc Assoc Clin Biochem, 3:*140, 1964.

Rieder, J.: A fluorimetric method for determining nitrazepam and the sum of its main metabolites in plasma and urine. *Arz Fasch* (Drug Res), *23:*207, 1973.

Rieder, J.: Plasma levels and derived pharmokinetic characteristics of unchanged diazepam in man. *Arz Forsch* (Drug Res), *23:*212, 1973.

Roberts, P.A., Blossom, C., and Lacefield, D.J.: The stability of carboxyhaemoglobin in the presence of bacteria at three storage temperatures. CAA, Oklahoma City, in press.

Robinson, A., and Williams, F.M.: The distribution of methadone in man. *J Pharm Pharmacol 23:*353, 1971.

Robinson, J., and Hunter, C.G.: Organochlorine insecticides: concentrations in human blood and adipose tissue. *Arch Environ Health, 13:*558, 1966.

Roche, L., Lejeune, E., Bachelor, M., and Versinin, C.: Evolution de l'oxycarbonemic dans les intoxications aigues par l'oxyde de carbone. *Ann Med Leg* (Paris), *40:*132, 1960.

Rodger, W.J., and Smith, H.: Mercury absorption by fingerprint officers using grey powder. *J Forensic Sci Soc, 7:*86, 1967.

Roscher, A.A.: A new histochemical method for the demonstration of calcium oxalate in tissues following fatal ethylene glycol poisoning. *Am J Clin Pathol, 55:*99, 1971.

Russell, J.C., Chesney, E.W., and Golberg, L.: Reappraisal of the toxicology of ethylene glycol. 1. Determination of ethylene glycol in biological material by a chemical method. *Fd Cosmet Toxicol, 7:*107, 1969.

Rutter, E.R.: based on Forrest, I.S., Forrest, F.M., and Mason, A.S.: A rapid colour test for imipramine (Tofranil). *Amer J Psy, 116:*928, 1960.

Sachs, H.W., and Calker, J. van: Zur oralen cadmium vergiftung. *Deut z fur Gericht Med, 49:*157, 1959.

Sachs, M.H., Bonforte, R.J., Lasser, R.P., and Dimich, I.: Cardiovascular complications of imipramine intoxication. *JAMA, 205:*588, 1968.

Saltzman, B.E.: Colorimetric determination of cadmium with dithizone. *Anal Chem, 25:*493, 1953.

Sawyer, R., Cox, B.G., Dixon, E.J., and Thompson, J.: Separation, identification and determination of fluoroacetamide residues in water, biological materials and soils. II. Identification and determination by gas-liquid chromatography. *J Sci Fd Agric, 18:*287, 1967.

Sayers, H.P.: Screening for lead absorption. In Ballantyne, B.: *Forensic Toxicology.* Bristol, John Wright and Sons, Ltd., 1974.

Schafer, M.L., and Campbell, J.E.: The distribution of pesticide residues in human body tissues from Montgomery County, Ohio. In *Organic Pesticides in the Environment.* Advances in Chemistry Series 60, A.C.S. publication 1966, p. 89.

Simon, G.E., Jatlow, P.I., Seligson, H.T., and Seligson, D.: Measurement of 5:5 diphenylhydantoin using thin layer chromatography. *Am J Clin Pathol, 55:*145, 1971.

Simpson, K.: Carbon monoxide poisoning. Medico-legal problems. *J Forensic Med, 2:*5, 1955.

Singer, L., Armstrong, W.D., and Vogel, J.J.: Determination of fluoride content of urine by electrode potential measurements. *J Lab Clin Med, 74:*354, 1969.

Sisenwine, S.F., Knowles, J.S., and Ruelius, H.W.: A specific and highly sensitive method for the determination of protriptyline in body fluids and tissues. *Anal Lett, 2:*315, 1969.

Sjöqvist, F.: Mekanismer bakom desberoende biverkningar. *Svensk Tandiak T,* 65, Suppl. IV, 34, 1968.

Skinner, R.F.: The determination of meprobamate in blood, urine and liver by gas chromatography. *J Forensic Sci, 12:*230, 1967.

Smith, H.: The distribution of antimony, arsenic, copper and zinc in human tissue. *J Forensic Sci Soc, 7:*97, 1967.

Smith, H.: The estimation of arsenic in biological material by activation analysis. *Anal Chem, 31:*1361, 1959.

Smith, H.: The interpretation of the arsenic content of human hair. *J Forensic Sci Soc, 4:*192, 1967.

Smith, J.C., Kench, J.E., and Lane, R.E.: Observations on urinary excretion of cadmium. *Biochem J, 61:*698, 1955.

Smith, W.C., Goudie, A.J., and Sivertson, J.N.M.: Colorimetric determination of trace quantities of boric acid in biological materials. *Anal Chem, 27:*295, 1955.

Smyth, D., and Pennington, G.W.: Identification reactions of chlordiazepoxide (Librium) and the products of hydrolysis 2-amino-4-chloro-benzophenone. *Arch int Pharmacodyn,* 145, 1963.

Smythe, L.E., and Whittem, R.N.: A review of the analytical chemistry of beryllium with 159 references. *Analyst, 86:*83, 1961.

Somogyi, G., Kaldor, A., and Jankovics, A.: Plasma concentrations of cardiac glycosides in digitalis intoxication. *Eur J Clin Pharmacol, 4:*158, 1972.

Southgate, H.W., and Carter, B.: Alcohol in urine as a guide to alcoholic intoxication. *Br Med J, 1:*463, 1926.

Srch, M.: Significance of carbon monoxide from cigarette smoking inside a car. *Deutsch Z Ges Gerichtl Med, 60:*80, 1967.

Steel, C.M., O'Duffy, J., and Brown, S.S.: Clinical effects and treatment of imipramine and amitriptyline poisoning in children. *Br Med J, 3:*663, 1967.

idem, ibid. The detection and excretion of chlordiazepoxide in human plasma and urine. 154, 1963.

Stevens, H.M.: Faster extraction of phenylbutazone of phenylbutazone from blood and plasma. *Clin Chem, 16:*437, 1970.

Stevens, H.M.: A spectrophotometric method for screening urine samples for amines including amphetamine and methylamphetamine. *J For Sci Soc, 13:*119, 1973.

Stevens, H.M., and Fox, R.H.: A method for detecting tubocurarine in tissue. *J Forensic Sci Soc, 11:*177, 1971.

Stevens, H.M., and Jenkins, R.W.: The chromatographic separation of mixtures of benzidiazepine drugs. *J For Sci Soc, 11:*183, 1971.

Stevens, H.M., and Moffat, A.C.: A rapid screening procedure for quaternary ammonium compounds in fluids and tissues with special reference to suxamethonium (succinylcholine). *J Forensic Sci Soc, 14:*141, 1974.

Stewart, C.P., and Stolman, A.: *Toxicology, Mechanisms and Analytical*

Methods. New York, Academic, 1960, vol. I.

Stinnelt, J.L., Valentine, J., and Abrutyn, E.: Nortriptyline hydrochloride overdosage. *JAMA, 204:*69, 1968.

Stitch, S.R.: Trace elements in human tissue. 1. A semi-quantitative spectrographic survey. *Biochem J, 67:*97, 1957.

Stone, H.M., and Stevens, H.M.: The detection of cannabis constituents in the mouth and on the fingers of smokers. *J For Sci Soc, 9:*31, 1969.

Stotz, E.: The determination of acetaldehyde in blood. *J Biol Chem, 148:* 585, 1943.

Street, H.V.: Determination of bromide in blood. *Clin Chim Acta, 5:*938, 1960.

Struempler, A.W.: Adsorption characteristics of silver, lead, cadmium, zinc and nickel on borosilicate glass, polyethylene and polypropylene container surfaces. *Anal Chem, 45:*2251, 1973.

Sunshine, I., and Baumler, J.: A fatal case of poisoning with amitriptyline. *Nature, 199:*1103, 1965.

Sunshine, I., and Finkle, B.: The necessity for tissue studies in fatal cyanide poisonings. *Int Arch Gewerbepath, 20:*558-561, 1964.

Sunshine, I., Maes, R., and Faracci, R.: Determination of glutethimide (Doriden®) and its metabolites in biological specimens. *Clin Chem, 14:*595, 1968.

Sunshine, I., Yaffe, S.J.: Amitriptyline Poisoning. *Amer J Dis Child, 106:*501, 1963.

Symes, M.H.: Monochloroimipramine: A controlled trial of new antidepressant. *Int J Neuropsychiatry, 3:*60, 1967.

Szadkowski, D., Schröter, U., Essing, H.G., Schaller, K.H., and Lehnert, G.: Ein gaschromatographisches Nachweisverfahren für benzol and toluol in kleinsten Blutproben. *Int Arch Arbeitsmed,* 27:300, 1971.

Tadjer, G.S.: The identification of paraquat in biological material using TLC. *J Forensic Sci, 12:*549, 1967.

Taunton Rigby, A., Sher, S.E., and Kelley, P.R.: Lysergic acid diethylamide: Radioimmunoassay, *Science, 181:*165, 1973.

Taylor, M.L., and Arnold, E.L.: Ultra-trace determinations of metals in biological specimens. *Anal Chem, 43:*1328, 1971.

Taylors Principles and Practice of Medical Jurisprudence, 11th ed. London, J. & A. Churchill, 1956-57, vol. II, p. 359.

Teichmann, T., Dubois, L., and Monkman, J.L.: The determination of fluoride by microdiffusion. *Proc First Intern Meeting on Forensic Toxicol,* London, 1963.

Thomas, J., and Abbot, D.C.: *Pesticide Residues.* Lecture series 1966, No. 3, Royal Institute of Chemistry.

Thompson, E., Villandy, J., Plutchak, L.B., and Gupta, R.D.: Spectrophotometric determination of d-propoxyphene (Darvon) in liver tissue. *J Forensic Sci, 15:*605, 1970.

Thürkow, I., Wesseling, H., and Meijer, D.K.F.: Estimation of phenytoin in body fluids in the presence of sulphonyl urea compounds. *Clin Chim Acta, 37:*509, 1972.

Tompsett, S.L.: The determination and distribution of lead in human tissues and excreta. *Analyst, 81:33,* 1956.

Tompsett, S.L.: Determination and identification of cyanide in biological material. *Clin Chem, 5:*587, 1959 (modified).

Tompsett, S.L.: The detection and determination of phenothiazine drugs blood serum. *Acta Pharmacol Toxicol, 26:*298, 1968.

Tompsett, S.L.: The detection and determination of phenothiazine drugs in urine. *Acta Pharmacol, 26:*303, 1968.

Tompsett, S.L.: Mogadon® in blood serum and urine and Librium® in urine. *J Clin Pathol, 21:*366, 1968.

Tompsett, S.L.: The spectrofluorimetric determination of phenothiazine drugs in blood serum. *Acta Pharmacol, 26:*298, 1968.

Turner, L.K.: In Curry, A.S. (Ed.): *Methods of Forensic Science.* New York, Interscience, 1965, vol. 4.

Valentour, J.C., Aggarwal, V., and Sunshine, I.: Sensitive gas chromatographic determination of cyanide. *Anal Chem, 46:*924, 1974.

Valentour, J.C., Monforte, J.R., and Sunshine, I.: Fluorometric determination of propoxyphene. *Clin Chem, 20:*275, 1974.

Van Hecke, W., Derveaux, A., and Hans-Berteau, M.J.: A case of criminal poisoning by parathion. *J Forensic Med, 5:*68, 1958.

Van Kampen, E. J., and Klouwen, H.M.: Spectrophotometric determination of carbon monoxide-hemoglobin using the Beckman DU spectrophotometer. *Chem Abs, 48:*4616, 1954.

Van Ormer, D.G., and Purdy, W.C.: The determination of manganese in urine by atomic absorption spectrometry. *Anal Chem Acta, 64:*93, 1973.

Vercruysse, A., and Deslypere, P.: Acute parathion poisoning. *J Forensic Med, 11:*107, 1964.

Vidic, J.H.V., Dross, H., and Kewitz, H.: Eine gaschromatische Bestimmung quaternärer Ammoniumvergingen. *Z Klin Chem Klin Biochem, 10:*156, 1972.

Wagner, J.G., Aghajanian, G.K., and Bing, O.H.L.: Correlation of performance test scores with "tissue concentration" of LSD in human subjects. *Clin Pharm Ther, 9:*1985, 1968.

Wallace, J.E., and Biggs, J.D.: Colorimetric determination of imipramine in biologic specimens. *J Forensic Sci, 14:*528, 1969.

Wallace, J.E., and Dahl, E.V.: The determination of amitriptyline by ultraviolet spectrophotometry. *J Forensic Sci, 12:*484, 1967.

Wallace, J.E., Hamilton, H.E., Payte, J.T., and Blum, K.: Sensitive spectrophotometric method for determining methadone in biological specimens. *J Pharm Sci, 61:*1397, 1972.

Wallace, J.E., Hamilton, H.E., Riloff, J.A., and Blum, K.: Spectrophotometric determination of ethchlorvynol in biological specimens: *Clin Chem, 20:*

159, 1974.

Ward Smtih, H.: Methods for determining alcohol. In Curry, A.S. (Ed.): *Methods of Forensic Science.* London and New York, Interscience, 1965, vol. IV, p. 1.

Warren, R.J., Thompson, W.E., Zarembo, J.E., and Eisdorfer, I.B.: Ultraviolet and attenuated total reflectance spectra of chlorpromazine metabolites, *J Pharm Sci, 56:*1496, 1967.

Wechsler, M.B., Wharton, R.N., Tanaka, E., and Malitz, S.: Chlorpromazine metabolite pattern in psychotic patients. *J Psychiatr Res, 5:*327, 1967.

Weist, F.R.: Detection of oxazepam in biological fluids by thin layer chromatography. *Arzneimittelforschung, 18:*87, 1968.

Whittaker, J.H., and Price Evans, D.A.: Genetics control of phenylbutazone in man. *Br Med J, 4:*323, 1970.

Wieland, T., and Schmidt, G.: Amanita toxins VIII. *Annalen, 577:*215, 1952.

Williams, L.A., Linn, R.A., and Zak, B.: Rapid microscreen test for methanol in serum and cerebrospinal fluid. *J For Sci, 6:*119, 1961.

Willis, J.B.: Determination of lead and other heavy metals in urine by atomic absorption spectroscopy. *Anal Chem, 34:*614, 1962.

Wilson, W.E., Johnson, S.A., Perkins, W.H., and Ripley, J.E.: Gas chromatographic analysis of cardiac glycosides and related compounds. *Anal Chem, 39:*40, 1967.

Winek, C.L., Fochtman, F.W., and Collom, W.D.: Suicide with amitriptyline-perphenazine combination. *Pa Med, 71:*71, 1968.

Worm, K.: Determination of dextropropoxyphene in organs from fatal poisoning. *Acta Pharmacol Toxicol, 30:*330, 1971.

Worm, K.: Fatal amitriptyline poisoning. Determination of the drug in forensic chemical material. *Acta Pharmacol Toxicol, 27:*439, 1969.

Xanthaky, G., Freireich, A.W., Matusiak, W., and Lukash, L. Hemodialysis in methyprylon poisoning. *JAMA, 198:*1212, 1966.

Zarembski, P.M., and Hodgkinson, A.: Fluorimetric determination of oxalic acid in blood and other biological materials. *Biochem J, 96:*717, 1965.

Zarembski, P.M., and Hodgkinson, A.: The oxalic acid content of English diets. *Br J Nutr, 16:*627, 1962.

Zarembski, P.M., and Hodgkinson, A.: The fluorometric determination of oxalic acid in blood and other biological materials. *Biochem J, 96:*717, 1967.

Zarembski, P.M., and Hodgkinson, A.: The renal clearance of oxalic acid in normal subjects and in patients with primary hyperoxaluria. *Invest Urol, 1:*87, 1963.

Zeegers, J.J.W., Maas, A.H.J., Willebrands, A.F., Kruyswyk, H.H., and Jambroes, G.: The radioimmunoassay of plasma digoxin. *Clin Chim Acta, 44:*109, 1973.

Zehnder, K., and Tanner, P.: Quoted by Neve, H.K.: *Acta Pharmacol Toxicol, 17:*404, 1961.

Zingales, I.A.: Determination of chlordiazepoxide plasma concentrations by electron capture gas chromatography. *J Chromatogr, 61:*237, 1971.

NAME INDEX

333

SUBJECT INDEX